PREGNANT BY MISTAKE

THE STORIES OF SEVENTEEN WOMEN

Katrina Maxtone-Graham

PREGNANT BY MISTAKE

THE STORIES OF SEVENTEEN WOMEN

Rémi Books

NEW YORK

Copyright © 1973, 1990 by Katrina Maxtone-Graham
All Rights Reserved

Library of Congress Cataloging in Publication Data

Maxtone-Graham, Katrina.
  Pregnant by mistake : the stories of seventeen women / Katrina
  Maxtone-Graham
      p.   cm.
  "A new edition with index and new preface"–T.p. verso.
  ISBN 0-943362-01-6 :   ISBN 0-943362-02-4 (pbk.):
  1. Abortion—United States.   2. Adoption—United States.
  3. Unmarried mothers—United States.   I. Title.
  HQ767.5.U5M37   1987
  363.4'6—dc19   87-28353
                                                                 CIP

ISBN 0-943362-01-6 (hardcover)
ISBN 0-943362-02-4 (paperback)

A new edition with index and new preface
Originally published by Liveright Publishing Corporation

First printing: February 1990

Rémi Books, Inc.
205 East 78th Street
New York, NY 10021
(212) 570-6265

Manufactured in the United States of America

For my sisters and brothers
literally and figuratively

CONTENTS

PREFACE

There are no statistics in this book, and no commentaries. There are simply seventeen women who, having faced an unwanted pregnancy, tell what they did and how they felt. All I knew about each of these women before I met her was whether she was planning to talk about abortion, adoption, or single parenthood. Our meeting—which lasted about an hour—began with my describing the project. I explained that I would have to edit the interview and that all names would be changed. Then we started to record. I had not realized—until the first few minutes of the first interview—how incredibly easy, how thoroughly comfortable it would be. Each interview was a fascinating and moving experience, and all are included in the book. These seventeen women have provided me with a vivid reaffirmation of the individuality and significance of every human being.

Editing was agony: to cut when needed, to clarify without distorting, to communicate exactly what each person was communicating meant pondering over every comma and every "you know." Of course it was necessary to remove some seemingly repetitious passages, but even for this I am sorry.

There is no need to be "pro" or "con" any of the issues raised. Obviously, we each have our personal frame of reference; but it does not necessarily fit anyone else's reality. These stories are unlikely to change people's convictions about themselves in their own situations, but I sincerely hope they will make for greater understanding of *other* people in *other* situations, and that this greater understanding will pave the way for greater tolerance.

Although my own point of view has no bearing on what other people do or did, it is, nonetheless, relevant to why I was compelled to make this book: I feel that every child should be a wanted child. I have felt this, intensely, for as long as I can remember. It follows, of course, that I believe in contraception: pregnancy by choice, not pregnancy by mistake. Abortion—necessarily much discussed in the book—is not the book's subject. Abortion is simply one of the options available after *unwanted pregnancy* has occurred.

*   *   *

With those four paragraphs, I opened the preface to the 1973 edition of this book. Little—and much—has happened in the nearly fourteen years since.

Contraception is ever imperfect. Far better than nothing, it still has far to go. The pill, now given in smaller doses, is probably safer; IUD's have fallen into disfavor; diaphragms, condoms, foam, and the like seem about the same as before: often they work, but not always.

The decision to give up a child for adoption derives as it always has, not from the "unwantedness" of the child, but from the poverty of the parent—poverty not only of financial resources, but also of family supportiveness and of humane public policy.

Outsiders—social services, church, parents, in-laws, neighbors—continue to make a critical difference. Some still do it by asserting their own will upon individuals. While such manipulation may be human nature, it serves to weaken the spirit of the already vulnerable and to promote self-destroying decisions. Others—compassionate friends and strangers, whether individuals or organizations—continue to provide the emotional support that nurtures self-confidence and increases personal options.

The availability of safe, legal abortion, which became assured in January 1973 with the Supreme Court decision in *Roe* v. *Wade*, also has continued to the present—and it is still a subject of heated, angry dispute.

As for the greater understanding and tolerance that I dreamed of: no, they don't seem to have happened.

I had decided to write the book that became *Pregnant by Mistake* in October of 1970. Abortion had been illegal in the United States throughout most of our lifetimes and was performed legally only rarely, on rigidly defined grounds. During the late 1960's, however, legal abortions had become more available, as some states began either to tolerate more liberal interpretations or actually to lessen the restrictions of their abortion laws. The legal event of greatest importance to the writing of this book was the passage in 1970 of the Abortion Reform Bill of New York State. On July 1, 1970, abortions until the twenty-fourth week of pregnancy—with no restrictions—became legally available in the State of New York.

By October of 1970, three months later, it was apparent that the free availability of abortions in New York was in jeopardy. In violation of the state legislature's intent, there were systematic attempts to limit facilities, to "establish guidelines," and to impose controls that would deny abortions to some of the women who wanted them. And I wondered if the people fighting for such restrictions were fully informed. They professed compassion for women caught in extreme situations. But what of "ordinary" situations? I suspected that it was lack of knowledge which made those people see one case as "justified," and another as "merely a whim." I was confident that, whatever the situation leading to an abortion, *there must have been reasons*, and I wanted to present those reasons in a human, real way. I decided to find women—any women who had been through the experience of unwanted pregnancy—and to record their stories.

Originally, I had imagined a book about the underlying reasons for the choice to terminate pregnancy. But as soon as I began interviewing, I discovered that the scope was going to be much larger: contraception, unwanted pregnancy in general, adoption (as it was generally understood at the time), parental relationships, marital and lover relationships, poverty, the women's movement, human decency and helpfulness, and all the issues of people's lives. I did not choose to exclude men. The one man who agreed to be interviewed—his wife had died of an illegal abortion many years earlier—later changed his mind.

The interviews came to me solely through the grapevine. Once the project was begun, I talked about it to friends and acquaintances. They spoke to other friends and acquaintances, and out of the blue another interview would come my way. I welcomed every person who offered to talk to me, and I included every interview. Finally I had to stop mentioning the project altogether, for fear of stumbling upon another interview—which I knew I neither had space for, nor could bear to refuse.

The interviews were conducted between February 1971 and October 1972. I worked on the editing simultaneously, beginning in February of 1971 and continuing into the spring of 1973, when my manuscript was accepted for publication.

The first edition of *Pregnant by Mistake* appeared the year that *Roe* v. *Wade* gave women the right to have legal abortions. The long era of punitive, restricting laws had ended, but full understanding was yet to be achieved. These interviews could help to increase that understanding, I thought; my book would serve its niche in time, and then, within a few years, even the dark days of misunderstanding and intolerance would be in the past.

Alas.

These are the areas in which so little has happened.

What is vastly different now—both for this country and for myself—is the development of the adoption reform movement. Although its seeds had been planted in the 1950's, the movement did not take hold until the early 1970's. For me, the possibility of adoption change burst upon my consciousness between the time of the acceptance of the manuscript to this book in April 1973 and the completion, several weeks later, of my preface to that first edition.

Abruptly I had discovered the stunning fact that my longing, as an adopted person, to know who I was, was not a perverse failing of one isolated individual with a particularly inadequate character. My life-long craving for knowledge of the people and circumstances of my birth and my first three years was, I learned, a normal human urge that was shared by other adopted people.

Mind-blowing—to learn that finding my birth parents and foster families was not an insane, unthinkable dream; that seeking my identity was not a shameful pursuit which could cause some mysterious, yet certainly awful, devastation upon people who had once cared for me; that adoptees, like "real" people, had origins; that we, too, were connected to the history of humankind. Soon came evidence in instance after instance that women who have given up children for adoption do not, as society had managed to convince most of us, cease caring for them. And finally I would personally discover the obvious human truth that reunion between long-separated blood relations can be an experience of ecstatic beauty.

These discoveries began, extraordinarily, on the very day I signed my contract with Liveright, the publisher of the original edition of *Pregnant by Mistake*. On that day, April 26, 1973, I returned to the agency from which I had been adopted. There and then, I had my first insights into the myths and deceptions of this country's adoption practices.

The essential precursor to that event had come during the fourth interview in this book. From Allison, I had heard for the first time that adoption agencies keep secret files on adopted people.

Ultimately, I wrote a book about the experiences which evolved from my visit to the adoption agency; and I refer to Allison's gift to me in the first chapter of that book, *An Adopted Woman*. Similarly, what I learned from Gail about maternity homes became relevant to the later events. There are a number of ways in which my two books, and these life experiences, keep spiraling around each other. To me such loops are stirring confirmation of the connections, continuing connections, of the positive forces in life. Nor have they stopped: when I finally found a long-lost foster brother, he shared his news with a neighbor—who then lent him a copy of *Pregnant by Mistake* and confided that she was one of the seventeen women. And portions of this present preface are closely paraphrased from the Postscript of that other book.

An Adopted Woman carries the subtitle, "Her Search. Her Discoveries. A True Story." The fact that this first book is subtitled "The Stories of Seventeen Women" tells something quite personal about me, directly related: in 1973 I could make a book about others, but not about myself. As I observed in the conclusion of that 1973 preface, "Surely the eighteenth person, and the nineteenth, and the twentieth . . . thousand" would all be equally worthy; however, though I did not say it, there was still one person unworthy: me. Now that, too, has changed. Now I feel equal. For me, personally, this is a most tremendous change.

The truth, of course, is that all of us are equal; we are all equally worthy to be heard, and all equally worthy to have choices. The choice to have a child or not. The choice to have relationships with blood family, with non-biological family, with non-family. The choice to be kind, considerate, and loving, to the best of our abilities. Freedom to choose is a theme of both books.

Other developments, less striking but still evolutionary, also mark important differences between the present and those first interviews sixteen years ago. Some of the issues raised here, both by me and by the women I spoke with, noticeably pertain to that earlier point in time. ("Point in time," itself, is a phrase that bolted into our lives the summer that this book was being set in galleys.) Among the anachronisms is, of course, the assumption that adoption reunions are impossible and—because of this assumed impossibility—that they are somehow undesirable.

Further, many subjects are publicly discussed today that were rarely mentioned even in private then. Surrendering children for adoption, abuse of children, incest, all of which seemed not to exist in the early 1970's, have now been addressed on national television by victims and perpetrators alike. In the same vein, though conversely, the topics of women's groups and consciousness raising might be less directly spoken of today, even though the influence of the women's liberation movement is significantly greater these sixteen years later.

Unfortunately, not all the news is good news. Even the adoption reform movement, which has had an enormous national impact, has achieved but a small portion of its potential. Although more and more families are being reunited, and although the general population has become considerably more aware of the complexities of adoption, this same growth has not taken place in adoption agency policy nor in adoption law. Except in Alabama, Alaska, and Kansas, adults who were adopted still do not have the simple right that other citizens have to see their own birth certificates. Adopted people remain without legal recourse, bound by contracts they never signed. Adoption is ever rife with secrecy—"in the best interests" of, as always, the secret-makers.

And now we have the new atrocities of step-parenthood by means of "donors" and "surrogates," and, frequently, cover-ups of these realities. Both the practices and their cover-ups are abuses of children. I guess I should amend my 1973 declaration that "every child should be a wanted child" to include, "but not so wanted that the desire is carried out no-matter-how unnaturally and with no-matter-what inhumanity inflicted on someone else."

In sum, although certain of the subjects and attitudes are distinctly of the period of these interviews, February 1971–October 1972, the underlying issues of human relations, and the hopes to procreate with love and wisdom and to give to our children a life worth living, are still completely current. Forgive the narrators, and me, those exchanges that reflect the confines of our box in time, and read these stories for their continuing present humanity. The need for understanding—and the yearning of these seventeen women, and myself, to contribute to that understanding—belongs to 1987, as it belonged to 1973.

Something else happened that is relevant to the history of this book. In the late summer of 1981, I learned from Liveright that a James Burtchaell was requesting permission to quote "about 5,000 words" from *Pregnant by Mistake*. Burtchaell was hoping to use my material in the lead essay of his forthcoming book of five essays. Liveright asked for a copy of the manuscript, and Burtchaell sent the essay, "Rachel Weeping," subtitled "The Veterans of Abortion."

I could not believe what I was reading: condescension, disdain, and disrespect for the women I had interviewed; innuendos and insults; distortions of the contexts of my quotations; inaccurate identifications and attributions; petty sloppinesses and gigantic misrepresentations. Excerpts from adoption stories were passed off as quotations about abortions. And Burtchaell's omissions—sometimes withholding a key fact from the description of the person quoted, other times withholding crucial phrases from the quoted material itself—furtively changed the meaning of the words being quoted.

I was appalled. How could someone so abuse people and their personal experiences, so abuse another author's work, and—my God!—so abuse the truth of what had been spoken and written?

The permissions editor at Liveright, aware that I might refuse permission, had already recommended to Burtchaell that he "rely on paraphrasing" or that he "have a stand-by chapter ready." But Burtchaell had refused. His book was about to go to press, he told her; besides, he "had based his book" on mine. I discussed the problem with her, and together we struggled to come up with a solution. Burtchaell's book was to contain five essays, couldn't he skip this one and use just four? Could he revise the essay to delete my material? As he had received permission to quote extensively from another author's interviews, he had ample quotations about abortion experiences already. I wanted to refuse permission, but at the same time I was trying to find a way that could be a happy outcome for everyone. Despite all, I felt sorry for a poor struggling author.

Then one day I remembered that, at the very beginning of my first interview, Antonia had said she wanted it clearly understood that she did not wish her words "to be given to the other side and twisted." I had been startled; I couldn't imagine such an ugly possibility. But she was older (and wiser) than I; and I had been content to accept her terms. I had gone out of my way after that to assure each new interviewee, whether she had asked or not, that I would not allow her material to be distorted by anyone.

This memory of Antonia and the others was so vivid. I was surprised it had not returned sooner; I rejoiced that it had returned at all. I couldn't give permission; I had given my word: the interviewees had consented to discuss their experiences in order to further understanding. Considering Burtchaell's misrepresentations and distortions, he certainly was not furthering understanding. On the contrary, he was *obstructing* it.

I telephoned Liveright and they accepted my decision without argument.

(I have since learned that many of my "facts" were mistaken. I had not, as I had thought, needed to have "a reason"; one's reasons for refusal are irrelevant. It had not, technically, been up to me to say yes or no; the decision had been Liveright's contractual prerogative, they had been granting me a courtesy. And the helpless little author of my imagination was in fact the University of Notre Dame's Provost from 1970 to 1977, James Tunstead Burtchaell, C.S.C., a Roman Catholic priest who was at that time, and still is in 1987, a professor of theology at Notre Dame.)

Liveright telephoned Burtchaell to inform him of my decision. A month later I received a letter from Burtchaell, asking again. I refused permission again, this time in writing. Surely this was the end of the matter, I thought, and I wrote as politely as possible. I expressed my sympathy to him as an author facing a disappointment, but explained that my obligation was to the women I had interviewed and to their intention of contributing to understanding.

Neither I nor Liveright heard anything further.

Two years later I discovered, by coincidence, that Burtchaell had used my material anyway.

Rachel Weeping was published in hardcover by Andrews and McMeel in April 1982—without removal of the unauthorized quotations, and misquotations, from *Pregnant by Mistake*. I later learned that a paperback reprint, carrying the subtitle "The Case Against Abortion," was published by Harper and Row in 1984.

Having a copyright, like much else in life, does not seem so important until someone takes it away. I was indescribably distraught.

And I felt the obligation again to say "No." In February 1985 I filed suit against Burtchaell and his two publishers for willful copyright infringement.

To be sure, I had no idea what I was in for. There were depositions—being grilled under oath for nine hours about what seemed like everything I had done since graduating from high school. There were arguments about the tapes of the interviews, which I refused to turn over. There were arguments about the stacks of manuscript drafts which I carried to the depositions in an assortment of shopping bags to demonstrate their bulk—but also refused to turn over. There was a lot of counting of words (7,176 were taken from *Pregnant by Mistake*) and computing of percentages (the quotations from *Pregnant by Mistake* comprise 19 percent of Burtchaell's essay). As my lawyer said to me at some point in the midst of all this, "You know the expression, 'Don't make a federal case of it?' Well, *this* is what they mean."

In April 1986, the U.S. District Court ruled that Burtchaell's use of my quotations was a "fair use." I appealed from that decision to the Court of Appeals for the Second Circuit. In October 1986, the Court of Appeals, in a decision written by Judge Irving Kaufman, also ruled against me.

The Court of Appeals did, however, acknowledge Burtchaell's distortions and inaccuracies, observing that "Burtchaell did portray some of the excerpts in a misleading light" and declaring, "[A]fter comparing the two books, we conclude that many of [Maxtone-Graham's] charges are well-founded— especially those relating to the muddling of adoption and abortion experiences. Burtchaell's scholarship clearly leaves something to be desired, and it is equally unfortunate that the numerous inaccuracies in *Rachel Weeping* escaped the editors' attention."

Now I am appealing once again to a higher court, the Supreme Court of the United States. To be reviewed by the Supreme Court one must ask to be heard. (Of the 4,000 to 5,000 cases every year that request review, fewer than 200 are accepted.) My petition was filed last February. An *amicus curiae* brief in support of my position has recently been filed by the American Society of Journalists and Authors. The Supreme Court will make its decision on whether to hear my appeal probably sometime in May 1987, so at this writing I do not know the outcome. But by the time these words are in print and available to readers, the question of review will be resolved.

What Burtchaell did with the material he quoted is now, and could be forever, completely legal. But if you are in school in the seventh grade and you try the same thing—writing a paper in which you copy out quotations inaccurately and misrepresent their original contexts—you'll get an F, and maybe worse.

And I'd be leery, as well, of taking things from other people after they've asked you not to, even when you figure you can get away with it.

The Supreme Court judges will decide again, or leave as it

stands, the question of the legality of Burtchaell's taking of this copyrighted work. But in the meantime—and afterwards—you, reader, can decide not the legal issue but the human one: would you say, as did Burtchaell, that these women are "incoherent," with "some kind of ego deficiency sapping the[ir] pursuits," "persons in disorder," and that they "do not present themselves attractively?" Or, do you, like me, feel "grateful for the experience of knowing such people"?

In the 1973 edition of *Pregnant by Mistake*, I gave special thanks to Joanna Caplan, then a Referral Consultant at Pregnancy Counseling Service in Boston; it was she who had been willing to "ask around" and introduced me to the first woman I interviewed. I am ever grateful to Joanna and to all the people at Pregnancy Counseling Service. For me they were the beginning of an interstate grapevine. My affection for the friends I made at PCS extended to the institution itself, which, staffed by volunteer counselors, was a non-profit agency offering assistance to pregnant women and counseling in family planning. Also I would like to reiterate my appreciation for the help and advice, over the nearly three years of creating that first edition, of friends Susan Hartung and Bev Placzek.

For this second edition my thanks go both to those who have participated in its preparation and to those who have supported me in my copyright battle against Burtchaell. Inasmuch as there is a long list of people who have assisted in one or another meaningful way, I'll mention them in chronological order of appearance on one or another of the scenes: Ian Maxtone-Graham, Martus Granirer, David Barus, Kim Kowalke, Roger Zissu, Fred Kleeberg, Larry Lader, Lucinda Cissler, Alice Acheson, Mary Ryan, Victor Schmalzer, the American Society of Journalists and Authors, Evelyn Kaye, Sally Olds, Bill Patry, Ken Geller, Lonnie Danchik, Nancy Brooks—and especially Dodi Schultz and Steve Abel.

To conclude, I repeat exactly what I wrote in 1973: "Most of all, however, I thank the seventeen women whose stories are in this book. They gave of themselves, so that others could learn.

I am grateful to have had the experience of knowing such people. If I care very much for all of them, it is *because* I came to know them. But why should understanding stop with those we know? Surely the eighteenth person, and the nineteenth, and the twentieth . . . thousand, would be similarly noteworthy and unique. My debt to these particular women is great, because they have reinforced my convictions that people are good and that the only concerns which deeply matter to human beings are, indeed, the human concerns."

Katrina Maxtone-Graham
April 1987

Postscript:

In May of 1987, the Supreme Court declined to review my suit against Burtchaell.

And now two years later, the Supreme Court's decision in the (unrelated) case of *Webster v. Reproductive Health Services* suggests that the issues settled by *Roe v. Wade* in 1973 are not so settled as was thought.

Alas, again.

Katrina Maxtone-Graham
July 1989

PREGNANT BY MISTAKE

THE STORIES OF SEVENTEEN WOMEN

ANTONIA

Interviewed in February 1971

ANTONIA: I was thirty-seven and I had three children, age ten, thirteen, and fifteen. And I had *always* used a diaphragm. I'd asked our family doctor about the pill. This was about five years ago, and I guess this was just when the pill started getting pretty much used. But my family doctor wouldn't give me the pill. My husband and I had always talked about, if I would ever get pregnant without wanting to, we would get an abortion. And we just hoped to God it wouldn't happen because we didn't know *where* we would get one.

So one day when it happened— You know, I was two days late, and I had already been feeling kind of tired; I looked in the mirror, and my face was puffed up, and I just thought, "My God, I'm pregnant!" I can't see how it happened, but it happened.

Now I started thinking back. And it may have to do with having intercourse twice—you know—like Saturday night and Sunday morning. And no doctor ever tells you about that! I've always been *very* conscientious about the diaphragm, always using enough stuff on it and so forth. And this was the only thing that I could think of that happened. Now I know that the diaphragm is not infallible, because we've had several people to our office who became pregnant. But for me, it had been. For sixteen years. I mean I used it ever since I was married, and my children were planned.

KATRINIA: Is there really no chance that you left it in the drawer?

ANTONIA: Absolutely none; none whatsoever. I never—I —I mean if I—if I didn't have any of that jelly left, I just would tell my husband, "Sorry," you know, "I can't do it." I never took a chance. *Never.* And he feels just the same way; he wouldn't want to take a chance, either. He just wouldn't.

And, well, that's what happened.

I made an appointment with my family doctor and I saw him I guess when I was—oh I don't know—five days over-time, or something. And I am never late; and my breasts were kind of tender. I mean I was pretty sure that I was pregnant. Although I was still thinking "It can't be, it can't be." Because I—as I said, I used the diaphragm.

So I went to the family doctor and he examined me and he says, "Oh, I don't think you're pregnant, you don't look pregnant." And I said "Well, can't you give me a test?"

He's not a gynecologist; he was a GP; but he gave me a little vial with instructions, and you had to use it in a certain way and fill it up and send it by mail in the early morning. So the next morning I did that, and I ran into him in the post office. [*laughter*] And I have never run into him *ever,* you know, except that one morning. And we kind of smiled at each other.

Then in the afternoon he called me and he says he has bad news for me—because it was pretty obvious that I didn't want a pregnancy—so I said, "Good God," you know, "Well, thank you." And I hang up the phone and I call my husband right away at work. And we didn't know where to go, we didn't know what to do.

The doctor was scared; because he knew I was going to

try to do something, and he wasn't going to get involved. My husband calls him the next day and says, "I want to talk to you." And the doctor says, "There's no need to talk to me; I can't do anything for you." He didn't even want to give me a sleeping medicine; he wanted to have *nothing* to do with it. He actually refused to see me after that. And he was the one that wouldn't give me the pill because I was overweight and because he didn't really believe in it yet. And he had said the diaphragm was just fine. So I—I felt at least he could have been more sympathetic.

Then we just started talking around and asking. And, at that time—five years ago—I didn't know anybody. Now, I know *dozens* of people who've had abortions. And especially when people hear you're in this kind of work, they tell you things. But at that time it was different. There are at least ten people that I know now had had abortions before I did, for one reason or another. And I never knew about it. You know, nobody ever discusses it. It's very sad. And I'm just the opposite: if I feel absolutely certain I'm doing the right thing, I want everybody to know about it! Now some people will say that this is another defensive mechanism, you know, "justifying yourself" and all this and that. Maybe it is; it could be. Except that we had already made up our minds, beforehand, that if I would get pregnant this is what we would do. I mean there was absolutely no question in our mind; not even one. And we had nothing against abortion, as long as it was done early enough; and we have three children, they're taken good care of, we've been saving money to send them to college, you know. And they have music lessons, and they turned out to be very nice kids, and we're proud of them.

Well. So I started thinking. Now my husband's connected with a university, so I said to him, "Well, why don't you try the doctors connected with the university?"

And so he went for a check-up himself, and he kind of mentioned to the doctor, you know, "My wife is pregnant."

"Oh, congratulations!" the doctor said. And my husband said, "Well, we are not very happy about it." The doctor said, "So—yeah—that's how it is." You know.

And then I said, "We know another surgeon there; go and make an appointment with him." And he did. And we think of another doctor that we know personally, and I said, "Go, go, go ask him out for lunch and see if he can know something." He actually came up with the name of an illegal practitioner, this personal friend. Our friend was a Swiss doctor; he wasn't a practitioner here, he was just in research. But we had felt maybe he would know somebody. And he found out via, via, via, so many people—you know—about a doctor with a Spanish name, a Puerto Rican, who lived I think in Philadelphia. And we tried to get in touch with this man. And I checked his name; I looked with a friend of mine to find whether he was listed, and yes, he was a member of the AMA. So he was a doctor, but—

KATRINA: This was to have an *il*legal—?

ANTONIA: Illegal. Yes. Well, it wasn't legal in most cases. And this is five years ago. 1966. But at least he was a doctor. But every time we tried to get him on the phone, he was never there. Maybe that's his policy, you know; there's always a nurse that answers the phone, you know, a receptionist.

So then I had a neighbor who's a woman psychiatrist, and I thought, "Well, I'll go to her; at least she'll be sympathetic, I think, and maybe she can advise me."

She didn't advise me, except she said one thing: she said, "If you want an abortion, it gets done in the big hospitals." She said the higher up you go, the better chance you have. That's the advice she gave me. But she couldn't help me. Still, she gave me moral support. Really, all the way through. And the fact that she is a psychiatrist, and that she is a woman, and that she, as a matter of fact, *herself* had a fourth pregnancy that she didn't want— It was a threatened miscarriage and the doctor told her, "If you don't want this baby, go jump in the hay or something."— And she did miscarry. So she actively did that. Well, she probably would have miscarried anyway. But she made damn sure that she did.

KATRINA: So she'd already experienced exactly what you were going through?

ANTONIA: Yes, except that her children were still small. I think if my youngest child had been two I'm not sure I would have gone through the trouble. I would have felt it doesn't make that much difference whether you have three, or four. As long as all the kids are messing up the house anyway, you know, and you have to be home anyway, and they have playmates, and stuff like that.

It's not that I would have been against abortion then; I never was. But I think your whole life situation plays a big, big part. Because our whole life-style would have been changed. I mean, you buy new furniture—and this all sounds very materialistic, but that's not just it. It's your whole way of life. You know, you get involved in things. I was taking violin lessons, and I was taking courses, and I finally—you know—was out of the mess. I'm not a very good housekeeper; I was brought up in Europe with a lot of servants, and I—it just—it would just have changed my life completely; and not the way I wanted it. Well, I was thirty-seven; I was healthy, and pretty young; but my husband is seven years older than I am, so he was forty-four at the time. So, you know, we were just not willing.

Well, this woman psychiatrist was very sympathetic, and so I would go see her, you know, every other Friday or so, and tell her what was happening.

KATRINA: How much time had transpired by then?

ANTONIA: Well, I finally managed to get the abortion; I think I was almost ten weeks pregnant.

It—it took me all that time.

KATRINA: She suggested you try to go high up in a hospital. And so—? Did you drop the Philadelphia illegal abortionist?

ANTONIA: Well, no, we . . . well, I was really scared, you know, I was really scared about an illegal set-up. My woman psychiatrist friend and I agreed that I could not afford to risk getting hurt or getting killed; that it was more important that I be healthy and alive to my husband and family, than that I have an abortion. If that was the choice, you know, I would certainly not endanger my life. But we did make sure this man was a doctor. Then we tried to get in touch with him and we couldn't. And we just didn't know what to do. Finally, we got another lead, and we kind of dropped him. But I still kept his address for many years. [*pause*] That's funny!

And then . . . what did I do then? Oh yes. Then my husband went to a surgeon, a regular surgeon at the university, and just explained it to him, and the surgeon was very sympathetic. He said, "Let me call my colleagues at so-and-so Hospital." Actually, he called the director of the hospital, a very big hospital. The director—who in fact is an old sourpuss—was out of town that day. So the surgeon said, "Okay, then give me the second doctor who's in command." And that was doctor so-and-so. The surgeon talked to this other guy for three minutes, "I've got a colleague here, and wife's thirty-seven." Just, you know, straightforward, "She wants an abortion." "Okay," he tells my husband, "you now have an appointment."

And so I have an appointment the next Thursday, and my husband comes home absolutely beaming. "Why, you see," says my husband, "you belong to a great university and they take care of you," and all this and that. And I . . . [*laughs*] I was really impressed, you know!

But it wasn't that easy, actually.

I was very . . . I remember how nervous I was. And they never make it clear what's legal and what's illegal. And whether you're really doing something that's a little secretive, and that you should keep your mouth shut about it.

And I hate that.

Especially, since I wasn't sure I was getting an abortion, I didn't feel that I should tell my children until I could really be sure. I'm very much against keeping secrets; and now they know all about it. They took it very matter-of-factly. I mean, they know I work in this group anyway; and they accepted it right away. I told my oldest when she went to college, and she accepted it. It has nothing to do with her, after all.

KATRINA: Not before? You didn't tell them . . . ?

ANTONIA: Well, she was fifteen, she was in high school when it happened. I wasn't sure whether she could keep quiet about it in the high school. And I didn't think it was fair— actually—to her. You know, that she might have to either do battle, or defend me, or anything. Because I had an idea that it might. . . . You know, kids might make trouble for her, as soon as she started telling them.

KATRINA: Do you think that was the climate of the times? Do you think that if she were fifteen today . . . ?

ANTONIA: I think it's still— Well, today my whole out-look has changed, because so many things have changed also. But if you think that you're the only one doing such a thing, and the whole society is against it—then that's the feeling you have. And a lot of people still feel that way. Even women who have legal abortions for German measles, they don't discuss it with their friends. They just keep it a little secret. You know, it's just one of those little things that you don't discuss. And it's very sad. I think that's changing a lot though, because now every newspaper you open up, there's something about abortion. It took me a while to be comfortable talking about it; no doubt about that.

KATRINA: Because of the social restraints? Or because of how you felt . . . ?

ANTONIA: Oh no, not because of how I felt. All, *all* my close friends knew about it. You know, every one of them. [*laughs*] I mean I had five close friends and I would—on Monday I would go to see this one, on Tuesday I'm going —you know—and they'd build me up and give me coffee.

The most terrible thing was the uncertainty—not knowing.

And my husband was kind of worried about me, too, and he says, "Well, what if you don't manage to have an abortion? What are you going to do then?" And I said, "Well, of course I'll make the best of it and I'll take care of it." And he looked so relieved! I—I don't know what he thought I would try to do, you know! But I certainly wouldn't have jumped off the roof or something! Because we had already agreed I wasn't going to do that. No, no use in that.

Well, I did end up in the waiting room of this obstetrician who was the number-two man of the hospital, and who said that he "had done some operations like that," and "All you do is, you have to talk to a psychiatrist." But he never really *explained*. It was always kind of—I never— He said, "Well, you know, I have rules." But I didn't know what rules he was bound by, you know. So I never really knew whether he approved of the laws or disapproved of the laws. And I also didn't really know what the law *was,* and I just kind of assumed that it was kind of slightly illegal anyway. I find that a lot of people still feel that way. I remember so well how I felt; and it never even occurred to me to go and look it up in lawbooks or something. And now, of course, I would. I mean the experience has taught me an awful lot, you know.

Also I didn't know if I was supposed to be grateful or—if he was doing me a favor. It turns out that he did do me a favor. Even though I didn't know him. But, you know, he spent an awful lot of time with me. Actually, I think he identified with us because his family set-up was exactly like ours, you see, older kids—teenagers. And he certainly had nothing against abortions. Though he said he hated to do them.

KATRINA: He hated to do them for what reason?

ANTONIA: Well it's just an unpleasant job, he said.

KATRINA: Meaning in the surgical sense he hated to do it? Or because of the emotional aspects . . . ?

ANTONIA: There are lots of doctors like that. I mean, there is another doctor, who actually belongs to our organization, and he says he hates to do it; he says he'd rather prevent it. I agree, absolutely! But what can you do?

Actually, he didn't charge me for the operation, and that bothered me. But we were charged for the hospital, and there were just "surgical expenses." He didn't want to be paid because—just in case of the slight chance that some legal things might follow—then he could say that he didn't get paid for it. And that's all. It was to make it obvious that he did it for my physical health, that he didn't do it to make money. And that he wasn't getting any profit. So that he could not be accused—ever.

Well, you can be sure—figuring it out—that under those circumstances that doctor cannot perform many abortions. I mean he cannot just go give people free abortions, you know. He couldn't afford to.

So then I thought, but why is he singling me out—you know—for such great treatment? It was so very confusing, and I never quite dared to ask him.

KATRINA: Do you think it's perhaps because not that many people reached his office?

ANTONIA: Oh, lots of people reach him. He just turns them down.

KATRINA: Then why *did* he do it?

ANTONIA: I think it was probably a personal—well—spark, or something.

KATRINA: The people that he turns down— Do you suppose that they are also married women with grown families? Or—?

ANTONIA: Well, I think he is certainly more sympathetic toward those. But, you know, he cannot do an abortion without the complete knowledge and agreement of the director and all the people concerned with the hospital. You know, he still needs a committee to agree. But he happened to be the head of the committee, I think. [*laughter*] So if he wants to push it, he can. You see, he was in a position to push, but I still don't know why he pushed *my* case, because I had no medical reasons and I had no psychiatric reasons; although I wasn't sure about that. You are supposed to have psychiatric reasons, you know, but that wasn't made clear, either.

He said to me, "Well, you'll have to see two psychiatrists," and I said, "What for?" And he said, "Just tell them," you know, "Just talk to them." I said, "What do I tell them?" and he said, "Same thing you tell me." And I had the slight feeling that if you are a little bit mixed up, you know, that maybe they'll do it for that reason. But I said to my husband, "I'm not going to say that I'm mixed up, or that I'm going to become suicidal, or God knows what." I said, "I'll have that on my record." [*laughs*] You know, I'm a very suspicious person.

KATRINA: Did you feel he didn't help you enough before you went to see the psychiatrists . . . ?

ANTONIA: He did spend an awful lot of time with me—that I must certainly point out. And that's why I spend a lot of time when I counsel, because that's the thing that helped me most, that he did listen to me. And he was absolutely convinced that I wanted this abortion, and that it would be very bad for me if I didn't get it. That, he was certainly— I convinced him of that. Yet I was always completely honest. I told him, "I'm not going to jump out of the window. That's not in my nature; you might as well know it. I'm not going to do it. And if I don't manage to have an abortion I'll certainly try to be a good mother to that child. But, it's not my wish to do so."

And so I went to the first psychiatrist, and it turned out that the guy was Catholic. And I was suspicious again; I thought maybe the doctor does it on purpose; you know, and that this guy would try to talk me out of it. But he didn't. He was a very nice psychiatrist, and he was very sweet, and very, very kind.

But he didn't ask me any questions, and I was kind of at a loss what I was supposed to do there. The guy said to me, "Well, you're very depressed." I said, "Yes, I am." And I thought I might as well say something, so I said, "Well, when I was a child I used to have migraine headaches, and I know that's a sign of depression and so forth." I said, "But I haven't had any headaches in twenty years, you know, so I don't think that counts for anything." And then I said, "Except last year," I said, "we were in Michigan for a year." Maybe I was a little excited, 'cause I said, "Sometimes my eyes would bother me a little bit, just like when I was a child and I used to have migraine headaches." And he translated it into that I had been depressed for a whole year just because of my eyes were bothering me. But I said, "But I never have those headaches anymore. Any my eyes bothering me, you know, it would go away after ten minutes, and it didn't happen very often. I just thought I'd bring it up, because I—" You know. I don't know if I have problems or don't have problems. I'm not, you know. . . . Well, anyway, he says, "It seems to me you have been depressed for a year." So having been depressed for a year would help me to get an abortion. If I said I had not been depressed for a year I might jeopardize my chances. I mean I really felt like a lawyer almost! And yet I'm not going to just say, "Yes, I've been depressed for a year." So what I said to him was, "Well if you say so, it must be so, but I haven't been aware of it." [*laughter*] I was very pleased with myself.

So he wrote his report. He didn't make any recommendations; all he did was, he said, "I have seen Mrs. G. and she seems very depressed." (And I *was* very depressed.) "It seems to me she's been depressed for a whole year." And that was all the obstetrician needed. Then the obstetrician makes the decision; the psychiatrist doesn't; all the psychiatrist has to do is give an objective statement about my—you know, mental state. And since he is a Catholic and he— I don't know how he feels about abortions, but he didn't do it to help me. You see? He wasn't just saying something to help me get an abortion. Like some psychiatrists do. You know, some psychiatrists. . . .

KATRINA: Well, was he or wasn't he?

ANTONIA: No, I don't think so. Because he said it. He said, "What do you think? You think I like to see—just get twenty-five dollars and then help people to get an abortion?" No; he really felt that I was depressed. Well—I—I sincerely believed so, too, you know. But not the whole year; just those last three months! But if he thinks I've been depressed for a whole year, that's fine with me, too. You know, we'll take care of that afterward.

And I guess that's just what the obstetrician wanted, you see. Because the obstetrician had enough insight to know that I really was depressed. And if he gets a letter from a Catholic psychiatrist saying that I am really very severely depressed—then this is absolutely medically so. That actually makes my case stronger, if you can call it that. Well, at that time, of course, I wasn't really sure *what* was going on.

Then I had to go to the other psychiatrist. He happened to be the psychiatrist at the hospital, and I heard from my girlfriend that he was a sweet old guy. You know, "It's just a rubber stamp, and just go to him, and he'll okay it, and that's all there is to it."

But by golly this guy didn't! He started talking to me and we talked about all kinds of things, you know, but he twisted everything I said. First of all I said, "Gosh," I said, "I was just so mad when I got pregnant, because I've always used a diaphragm." And somehow I said I was always kind of a little bit afraid that this was going to happen. You know, I said, "I was always afraid that I would get pregnant." And then he said, "Well, why were you afraid of getting pregnant?" I said, "I'm not afraid of getting pregnant, I'm afraid of getting—" You know. He'd say, "What do you *mean* by that?" And I'd say, "Well, I have three children, and I had very easy deliveries and easy pregnancies. You know, it's not —" He—he made me look like I was some kind of a so-and-so, you know, who was scared to get pregnant. That wasn't the case. It wasn't the pregnancy that I was concerned with, it was having another *child* at that age. And he just, he just wouldn't. . . . Well, at that point I didn't realize what he was doing. He said a few other things to me. Then at the end, he said, "No, I still don't know why you want an abortion." I said, "My God, that should be crystal clear to you!"

Then—I had brought my husband—then my husband talked to him. My husband is a scientist; he's very straightforward and very exact. My husband said, "If I had wanted another child I would have had it ten years ago!"

And this psychiatrist also said, "Well, how would you feel, if you have an abortion, and some time in the future you lose one of your children?" You know what my husband said to that? He said, "Well, that's why we have *three* children rather than two!" [*laughter*] My husband was really beautiful. That's exactly how it is, you know.

So this doctor saw us both, and nothing was agreed at the end. So I said to him, "What are you going to tell the obstetrician?" He said he didn't know yet.

And that's not all. You know what else he asked my husband? He asked if I would regularly go out and buy clothes for myself! You know, he kind of insinuated that I was a strong-willed woman who always wanted my way; and did I go out a lot and buy clothes? So my husband told him, "Oh no, she sews all her own." [*laughter*] And stuff like that.

KATRINA: To me that sounds sort of nasty. . . .

ANTONIA: Yes. To me, too. And wait until you hear what happened then!

We called our obstetrician and asked him what the story was, and had he heard from this second psychiatrist. No, he hadn't heard from him. The next day I called again, "What happened? Have you heard from him?" "No, he is out of town for three days," he said. "Well, will you let me know when you hear from him?" And in the meantime my kids were home and I never knew. . . . I said, "Please don't call in the afternoon." Because at that point I really didn't want my kids to get mixed up with it. So whenever I got a phone call, or I had to make one, I'd go to the drugstore, go to my neighbor, and all this business. And every time the phone rang, "Oh my God," you know, "This must be him," you know. It was really nerve-wracking; it really was. I—I still don't see how I did it. . . .

KATRINA: You were afraid you couldn't get to the phone without the children being around?

ANTONIA: Yes; well, because we only have one phone and it's right in the living room; you know, it's not very private.

But anyway, this was the situation. And so finally I called the obstetrician's office again and I said, "I want another appointment with the obstetrician." We insisted on having another appointment with him. And then the obstetrician told us, well, yes, he had finally gotten hold of the psychiatrist. The psychiatrist had never called him, but the obstetrician finally got hold of him. The story was that the psychiatrist felt that "Mrs. G. was a serious psychological case, and an operation wasn't going to solve her problems."

And I was just so furious I just—I just couldn't believe it. Because I was almost ten weeks by that time. I had shot all my chances for other things. I—I had just been counting on getting this abortion in a hospital, and I really felt the obstetrician wouldn't hold me on the line that long if there wasn't a chance that I— To tell somebody after, you know, seven weeks of counseling and talking—and then at ten weeks tell her, "You can't have it here"! You know, you can't go anywhere else at that point. And then I felt maybe we had been too naive in not trying other channels, too. Because we didn't. This—this had seemed like a very good lead, you know.

And it seemed that the obstetrician was very embarrassed, too; because he had really been counting on doing it. And he hadn't counted on this psychiatrist not giving his permission. . . .

KATRINA: Did you ever begin to wonder if you *were* . . . ?

ANTONIA: Oh, of course.

KATRINA: . . . as crazy as they were saying you were?

ANTONIA: Of course, of course. But fortunately I have a lot of friends. So I would go, and my friends would say, "Oh, there's nothing the matter with you," you know. And my husband, actually, is not very emotional; he never doubted my sanity, but he should have known—I mean he should certainly have encouraged me more by telling me that I—that I was all right. He never did. But he took it for granted that I was, you know. One psychiatrist asked him if he'd ever been concerned about me, and he said, "No." Then he got home and I was mad at him, "because he's never concerned about me!" [*laughter*] You know, I mean everything gets kind of twisted.

So finally we got this news that it was off, that the obstetrician wasn't going to do it in the hospital. We got home and I was really depressed then. And then I said, "Well, I'm going to see another psychiatrist."

We have a neighbor who is a psychiatrist. It turned out that he was against abortions. He is changed now; he is actually one of the people in that organization to change the law on abortions. It's very funny. But at that time, he told me, "Don't do it," he said to me. "You can afford to build another room to your house." And he says, "You may become suicidal." I said, "What?" "Yes, you may become suicidal. Eighty percent of the women that I see that had abortions, become suicidal." And my husband said, "Eighty percent? Where do you get your figures?" He answered, "I see them in the hospital all the time." So then my husband said, "Well, goodness, how could you know that's eighty percent? Because all the ones that don't end up in the hospital are the ones you don't see! And how do you know?"

Well, I look at this man and I smile; I said, "Well, even if it's true—even if it's true what you say, I'm *absolutely* positive

that I'll be one of the twenty percent that doesn't." That's—
that kind of security I did have. But it certainly didn't help
very much to have to hear, "And even if you don't become
suicidal, you'll be very depressed; and for years on end you'll
remember the date of your operation; and every year you'll
be thinking of that. . . .

"And besides," this guy said, "The director of your hospital will never agree to it." That was the last thing he said to
me. By that time I was ten weeks pregnant.

KATRINA: And the director of the hospital was the "sourpuss" you originally mentioned? This makes a third person
who had to agree to it?

ANTONIA: Right. The two psychiatrists and— Well, the last
psychiatrist—who talked about the suicidal stuff—he had
nothing to do with the case. But the first two psychiatrists.
. . . The first one said I was depressed and had been depressed for a year; and the second one said I was a serious
psychiatric case, and that an operation wasn't going to solve
my problems. So I said, "I don't expect the operation to solve
my problems—only *one.*" What it would do to a child to be
born to a psychiatric mother—you know—*that* he never
even discussed. Besides, he didn't tell us that I was sick; he
told it behind my back to the obstetrician, which I think is a
dirty trick to do to anybody.

So we went home, my husband and I; we talked through
the whole night, and finally I said to my husband, "Go call
the psychiatrist again and give him hell for not telling us.
You say to him, 'I'm worried about my wife. If my wife is so
sick I want to know about it and you better tell it to me. We
have to talk about, you know, medication or whatever; you
know—or treatment. I want to know what kind of treatment
is indicated.' "

My husband tried to get in touch with that doctor. You
know, he wouldn't answer the phone! And he was never

there and this secretary answered and just— You just couldn't get through to him. So I said, "Okay, I'll make a new appointment, I'll go there myself and—" My husband said, "Really? you want to do this?" So I said, "Sure. What do I have to lose? If I can't do anything I'll certainly give him hell, you know, for doing such a dirty trick on me." And what kind of a doctor is he? You know, a psychiatrist that tells you that you're so sick, and then he doesn't want to see you! He doesn't even tell *you* that you're sick, he tells it to someone else.

So I called the secretary. She wouldn't give me an appointment, and she said, "I'll call you back." And I told her, "Don't call me in the afternoon." And sure enough, she called in the afternoon, "This is Doctor S.'s secretary." She got my daughter on the phone and my daughter said, "Oh, you have to call Doctor S., and who is he?"

So I said, "Doctor who?" "Doctor S." "God," I said, "I never heard of him." "Well, call him right back then." I said, "No, why should I?" And I hate the phone, so I mean I had a perfect excuse. I said, "If it's important he'll call again."

So I went to the neighbor's and called him back, you know, [*laughter*] and all this aggravation. So I called him back, and I got the secretary, and she said, "Doctor is too busy to see you. He will advise you to go to another psychiatrist."

So I said to my husband, "Okay, this is it. Now we call the obstetrician." My case had been closed, you know; the obstetrician had said he wouldn't do it. But I said, "We're going to reopen the case. You call—" You know, I had all the ideas, and my husband did all the dirty work!

So he called the obstetrician and said, "I want you to know what happened to my wife. She called the psychiatrist and she is so sick and he refuses to see her or to help her. This is unprofessional behavior," my husband said, "I demand to see another psychiatrist." And the obstetrician, you know, he was already— He was really a very nice sweet guy.

And he felt embarrassed by the whole thing anyway, because he had more or less promised he would do it, you know, and he felt terribly bad, he really did. And that's maybe the reason why he did it, after all, because he did have some push. "Okay," he said, "Go see another psychiatrist." So my husband asked, "Which psychiatrist?" Because in the beginning the obstetrician had made it clear he only wanted me to see psychiatrists that *he* would send me to. Because otherwise any woman with two friends who are psychiatrists could present herself with two letters and say, "I want an abortion." They wanted to prevent that, you see.

But the obstetrician agreed that this woman psychiatrist —my friend, you know—would be agreeable to him. And she had already said from the beginning that she would be willing to write a letter—if he would accept it. So then she wrote a very nice letter. And that was all in one weekend that this happened, that I saw the doctor, you know, about the suicidal, and the telephone calls with this other psychiatrist. So Monday my husband called the obstetrician and the obstetrician said, "Okay," he said, "Tell your wife to stop worrying, and I'll operate on Thursday."

Before, the obstetrician had said he could not accept this woman psychiatrist's letter. They try to keep it within the hospital. I think that's to protect themselves, because they really feel that they can't do more than a certain amount. Now they're doing more and more. But it was certainly, certainly, a pretty terrible experience.

Well, I got in the hospital. The nurse asked me when my last period was and I wasn't sure because it was three months before, you know, and I— Suddenly I started thinking, "My God, maybe I shouldn't tell her." Because I wasn't sure, you know, how open it was. And it turned out that I was signed in as having bleeding. And many people, when they have heavy bleeding, they have a D&C; this is a standard thing. So she said, "Are you going to have a D&C?" I said, "Yes." "And you've been bleeding?" I said, "Yes." Of course I hadn't been, in about three months. That was the *problem*. [*laughter*] So it was kind of funny.

But I did make a point of making sure that I wasn't going to be depressed afterward, being so forewarned. Well, I'm very vague on dates, all the time, so I hadn't looked on the calendar. I hadn't the slightest idea what date it was, so that the next year I couldn't possible worry about the date. It was so funny. And I still, you know, I still really don't quite know which date it was. Of course, later on we got the bill of the hospital, and so I suppose I could figure back what date it was. But you know it still doesn't mean—the date doesn't mean a thing to me.

And I went to the hairdresser and I shaved my legs and took a long bath. And I brought a nice big piece of soap, you know, a real nice-smelling piece of soap. And I brought my nicest perfume, you know. And I felt so happy in that hospital. God, I can't tell you. I felt such peace.

But the funny thing was, that night the anesthetist came in to explain about the operation the next day and what kind of medication he would use, so that I wouldn't be frightened. And there was a woman in my room who had a really—a regular D&C because she had been bleeding. You know, she was forty-two, or something. So I'd already heard what her symptoms were, you see. Well, this anesthetist wanted to know about my symptoms. Of course [*laughs*], I didn't really know what my symptoms were supposed to be. But I just said, "Oh, you know, it wasn't that bad. [*laughs*] I guess it wasn't that bad!"

And, of course, the next day he found out what it was all about, probably, when the operation was taking place. But I wasn't quite sure; so I told the obstetrician the next day. I said, "Good God, that anesthetist came by and asked about my symptoms, you know, and I—I didn't know what my symptoms were supposed to be." And he said, "Don't worry about it, it doesn't matter." He was very reassuring. So obviously the whole hospital knows about it. I mean everyone who has to do with the operation. They probably choose nurses that are not against abortions. I mean they certainly know when they take an anesthetist—and it's certainly not done in a secret way. Except they don't advertise it, either.

KATRINA: But if the anesthetist could have said something to let you know he was in on it—

ANTONIA: Well, no, it was just not important. Whatever this obstetrician does is—is completely aboveboard, so nobody questions it. And that I wasn't sure of, you know. It was just that the obstetrician should have reassured me more about that point, you know.

I—and then I thought, "My God, then is he doing me a favor? And why is he doing me a favor?" You know. That, I couldn't understand either. Whether he feels so loyal to the school that all colleagues should be helped, or what—I couldn't understand that. Or whether he felt that— Well, he did say one thing: he said once, that if I'd had one on the town and had come home drunk, or gone out with another man, he wouldn't have done it.

So he was moralizing, in a way. But since I was such an upright, you know, responsible diaphragm user, and all this and that, you know—

KATRINA: Yes, you'd done everything that medicine had to offer.

ANTONIA: Right, right, that's what he said. He said, "As medicine doesn't have any better ways of protecting you, I feel we are responsible to help you." That's what he said, as a matter of fact.

But then, you know, then you're excluding the people— I mean, you know, irresponsible people make the worst parents. If you're saying that the people who are so responsible should be helped, then you're in a way saying that the irresponsible people should be forced to have children. And they make the worst parents.

Well, these are all things that I've been thinking of recently. I used to be pretty rigid in my thinking, until it happened to me. And I realize how easy it is to get pregnant, *even* for people who are very careful and knowledgeable. But most people don't realize that. Most people still are very rigid about those things. And I have learned so much by having this accident happen to me.

KATRINA: Were you depressed or anything afterward?

ANTONIA: No. No, because one thing I tell you: the obstetrician insisted that I see that Catholic psychiatrist afterward. The obstetrician wanted me to see that psychiatrist once more, just to make sure that I was all right.

So two or three weeks after the abortion, I went to see the psychiatrist, and he was still very sweet and very nice and very kind. He really was a kind man. So I talked to him for an hour, and I said, "Well, I'm so glad that I did it. I really believe we did the right thing." You know, "And I'm so glad we persevered," and so forth. Then we started talking. I make wall-hangings, so I— You know, I had made one for the obstetrician because I felt I had to pay him some way. A case of whiskey didn't appeal to me; so I made a wall-hanging. I spent twelve days working from nine o'clock in the morning until eleven o'clock at night, and it was a gorgeous, big, wall-hanging. He loved it. But I took it along to the psychiatrist to show it to him, and also another one that I had already made. I said, "You said to me that I was depressed, you know. And I agree that I was depressed. But I'm not usually depressed; I'm actually a kind of an outgoing and cheerful person." And I said, "I brought some wall-hangings." So I held it in front of me and said, "This is the real me." [*laughs*] You know. And he loved them. "Oh, that's beautiful!" and all this, that, and the other. Well, I felt that this way I could show him, you know.

And also, when I came to him the very first time— That was another thing: I felt that I wasn't just doing it for me; I felt it was a decision for the whole family. I mean it had to do with the whole family, and the fact that we have children. So—I also make my own Christmas cards—and I brought one of those . . . . We all play musical instruments, so I had a picture of each child playing something, and it was all made up in a nice card. My husband doesn't play anything, but he was conducting [*laughter*] with a pencil. He had just written a book and his book was on the music-stand upside down, you see, and that was a very nice Christmas card and everybody loved it. So I said "Okay," I said, "Here, look at it; that's the kind of family we are." You know. I wanted him to get an over-all impression; not just about me.

KATRINA: Did you discuss whether or not you were depressed for a year? Did you discuss that then?

ANTONIA: No. Well, I said, "I still don't see how you could *ever* figure out—" And he said it was all because of my eyes. "And that's the only thing?" I asked. And he said yes. And it maybe frightens you to think that a psychiatrist will make a snap judgment like that. But of course the judgment helped me to get my abortion. Still, it didn't make me very happy! But I *was* very depressed after I got pregnant. I really was, I couldn't do anything. I just couldn't do anything, you know. The only thing that I managed to do was to make a jumper for myself. And I felt this was to keep up hope; because if I managed to get an abortion, I would be able to wear it; and otherwise I wouldn't. [*laughs*] I better hurry up and make it! So it was very funny.

But I had—I felt absolute peace afterward. I just felt *so* happy. Well, I already felt happy that Monday, when the obstetrician told me he would do it. As a matter of fact, I drove my children to music lessons and I missed two exits on the highway, because I was just sitting there kind of smiling to myself—the great thing that I was going to achieve. I mean all those stories about women getting depressed— Maybe some women do get depressed. I have an idea that if it's your first pregnancy you have different feelings about a first pregnancy than if you already have children. And if you have an unhappy love affair and all those things. But I didn't have that; it was absolutely . . . . So I went to see the psychiatrist; I showed him my wall-hangings. "Well," he says, "It is obvious that you don't need a psychiatrist." So I said, "Thank you very much and goodbye." [*laughter*]

And then I started working for Planned Parenthood and then Planned Parenthood got involved in counseling. At first I couldn't . . . I'm a very private person I guess, in a way; and I hate to—you know—intrude on other people's things. At first, I really hated to ask personal questions. But I still felt it was my duty to do so, you know. And I have been doing it. And now I feel really confident about it, and I feel that very often, I do—really—relieve a lot of their anxieties; although I have no professional training. Well, I was planning to become a doctor a long time ago, but I quit.

The nicest thing is, actually, that *because* of the counseling I've done, instead of helping other people I've helped myself even more. Because, when you realize that you have such contact with people, you get such insight, and you learn so much. The more people you talk to—and so many different people and they have so many different views. And the funny thing is that a lot of things that I didn't know— Like, for instance, black mothers from the ghetto—there's always the stereotyped idea, you know, "They're lazy and they don't want to work," and all this. God, I've counseled several, and I was as scared as they were. [*laughs*] Because I didn't realize I would be able to get through. And I've had the most *marvelous* encounters that way, and I've learned *so* much, you know, from that.

And the last thing is that I'm so comfortable with my own children; because I talk about sex like you can't imagine, really. It's a very comfortable subject. Well, I make cracks and we make jokes, you know, and my husband gets embarrassed sometimes, but still. Some people are just absolutely shocked when their kids mention *anything* about sex. And I've learned so much by just hearing about the young people and how they feel and how they think. And many of them are responsible adults. As a matter of fact, they're very nice people, and they're very responsible, and very sensitive. So I can discuss things with my children. As a matter of fact, I have a twenty-year-old daughter; she wrote a paper on abortion last month in college. If I get a very special case in, we discuss it sometimes. Of course I never use names or anything. "Just explain to me what would you have done? What do you think of such a case?" You know.

And of course I don't advertise abortions, I advertise contraceptives. But it still—it should be available. And most of the people are just caught, just plain caught by a combination of things: circumstances, some ignorance, some fear; you know, embarrassment, and all that kind of thing. And I think that's what we really should get after.

It's not only birth control, you see; it's the whole way of — I've heard of a girl who has been on the pill for two years and has refused to sleep with a single boy. Why is she on the pill? Well, just so that she knows for herself, you know, that she really *has* a choice. And so far she hasn't wanted to and she isn't going to. Now the opposite exists also, of girls who go off the pill because they say it makes them too damn available. And then they get pregnant. You see, now there is an awful lot of ambiguity in those things, and I think it's very important that we should teach our children, boys and girls, that they *do* have a choice. And that the choice is *theirs*. But that they should have all the information before they make the choices. It's personal responsibility; and this I value very highly. And I'm willing to let a kid make mistakes on his own, you know; and I'm still willing to help him.

KATRINA: How do you respond to the attitude of saying to a young person, "Here's your equipment; go ahead out and—"

ANTONIA: Oh no; that's not giving them a choice. That's not giving them a choice. I think it's very important— There are many girls who feel that now there is the pill they've got to go to bed with every boy. And that's just as bad as the old rule of saying—you know—you should never do it. That's not—that's not choice.

And, you know, there's an awful lot of pressure on the girl. And on the boy, too—on the boy. You know, I had a neighbor once, who said to me, "I'm so glad that I have only boys and no girls, because now I don't have to worry." I said, "Damn you, woman, you have to worry more! Because it's worse to hurt someone else!" "Oh," she said, "Oh, I didn't mean it that way." But it's amazing how many educated and supposedly, you know, knowledgeable people still have such old-fashioned ideas. My daughter once said, "Mom, will you please not slop your Koromex jelly on the bathmat." You know. And I was embarrassed. Now it wouldn't embarrass me, but at that time it embarrassed me, and I, "Yah, yah, yah—" But now it doesn't embarrass me anymore. And that's what I have gained. And I talk to other kids, too; and to mothers. I get invited everywhere, invited in the college houses to talk to tutors, and stuff like that. And I have no professional training. It's pretty much fun when psychiatrists call you and ask you for advice, you know. [*laughter*] It's really great.

And I didn't seek it; you know, it's just come. I didn't seek it. But I kind of slowly got involved. I guess that happens to a lot of women who have abortions—they just feel that they have to help other women.

One thing that I also want to point out is that I—I did do a lot of thinking, naturally, afterward. You know, especially, why did the doctor do it, and how did I manage it? It was really such a *great—victory* on my part, I felt. That I had all on my own convinced some, you know, big-shot doctor, to do this for me. He must have seen great value in me, you know; and I was never that self-assured about my own capabilities or anything. "My gosh, I really did this. Now," you know, "if I can do this, then I can do anything." That's the funny thing—that I had that gain that I never really saw or expected. That I *convinced* people to do things. Obviously the doctor wasn't that eager to do it, you know. But obviously I convinced him. Not only that, he did it for free. So obviously he must have felt that it was worth doing. And then I realized how fond I was of my own children. Of course I was already aware how fond I was of them. But, you know, when you get all this, you feel like people are kind of accusing you, that you're either "not a good mother" or you're a, you know, "a selfish so-and-so," and "you're awful," and all these things that they were trying to convince me that I was, you know, in all different ways. And I realized that I wasn't—that I really wasn't. That I was a nice mother, with really great kids. And the fact that you can go through a crisis like this with your husband, you know, and come through—with flying colors, really. Because it's quite an experience. It's really nerve-racking.

And I did several things afterward. I started playing the violin again; and I'm now giving concerts for small groups, which is something I never did before. I never had the guts, you know. And now I think, "My God! Why not?" And I lost twenty pounds, which is something I never did before, either. And I started counseling at Planned Parenthood. So there were three things. Oh, and I also made more wall-hangings and I exhibited them.

Really, you know, it has *affected* me to *such* an extent. I feel if *I* can— I was always afraid, I guess, of not succeeding or something. And now I feel I can do things on my own. You know. And I have exhibited wall-hangings at several exhibitions.

KATRINA: If it had been easier for you to get your abortion, is it possible that you might not have felt—?

ANTONIA: Oh; I don't know. I would still— Well, even if an abortion is very easy, you still do a lot of thinking. You know. It can't be helped; I mean you do. You do take stock of yourself. Because you really have to make a decision. And so you do think about the man you live with. And about the children. Are you going to tell them? How is your relationship with everybody? Who is going to know about it? And then you start thinking: if you really, really make a decision that you don't want another child *because* you are going to do other things or you want to do other things—well, then you really feel it's your duty to *do* those other things. You know; otherwise why did I do this thing? You know. And from one thing comes another. I didn't do it all at the same time. Just, "Now I should try this. Now I should try that."

And the fact that I'm really very comfortable with my children now. Not that I wasn't comfortable before; but I think I'm more, much more comfortable. Well, I think I am more comfortable *myself*, about sex, and about being willing to talk about that.

I'm now involved in a seminar at one of the universities, and we discuss adolescence. And they're all educated women, and I'm not; I quit pretty early, when I came to this country. But sometimes I say things that they don't dare to say. We talk about sexual encounters—you know—talk about young people, and this and that. The matter came up, how some students at colleges—some girls—feel that they've got to go to bed with the boy they go out with because this is what's expected. And this is being a cog in a — As one speaker said once, "Being a cog in a new machine is just as bad as being a cog in an old machine."

And this brings it right back to having a choice. I think having an abortion should be the woman's choice; you know, it's *her* decision, she carries the child. And if she doesn't consider it killing, then how can someone else tell her that it is? Especially people who never had children themselves—like a lot of men, you know! [*laughter*] How can they judge? They tell you you're so selfish when you don't want a child. Well, God, let them try it! Even if you want them, it's still a lot of work. I mean, it takes a lot out of you even if you *willingly* do it. It really bothers me how they feel you can *force* someone to go through with it; and even worse, you know, to have unmarried girls go through with it and then give it up for adoption. How—how can you be so cruel?

Now they're crying, you know, offices are crying because there are not enough babies for adoption, because people are having more abortions. But all the girls that I have talked to who have given up babies for adoption, they say they *never* want to go through that again. *Never*. And looking— looking at kids that would be the age of their children— Ay! My God!

SAMANTHA

Interviewed in February 1971

SAMANTHA: Mine was really very straightforward. I had a loop, which was absolutely fine, I thought. And indeed it was fine for seven months, eight months. And then, lo and behold, it wasn't. I kind of waited and thought, "This is very peculiar." You know, to begin with, I really didn't take too much notice of it. I discussed it with a friend of mine and she said, "Oh, that's one of your favorite fantasies." I said, "No, I'm absolutely certain I'm right this time." That was only about four days after my period should have come. Then a week after that I realized I really hadn't miscalculated. So, panic-stricken, I went to the doctor and I said, "This can't be true, can it?" And he said, "Oh yes, indeed, it can."

KATRINA: Had your loop fallen out?

SAMANTHA: No, this was the thing that was extraordinary. My loop was fine, the strings were all there, everything was fine. That was why I just didn't, really—to begin with— didn't think I could believe it.

So anyway, he said, "There's nothing I can do for you. You have to wait until you're at least two weeks—" or something, I don't remember the number exactly "—overdue." I was really upset over that. And I was very upset by his reaction to it, too. Which was, you know, "Never mind, dear lady. I'll do something, when it comes to it."

But then his office did go to an *enormous* amount of trouble, they really did. They sent me to a hospital that has one of these, you know, immediate pregnancy testings, which you do with blood instead of urine. So I went toddling down there, but I was late for the test and they couldn't run it that day. They couldn't do it on the next day when they ran the test, because it was a Thursday, and that was Thanksgiving. So then I still had to wait a week anyway.

By then I was convinced, absolutely and totally convinced, I was pregnant. I mean I really didn't need a machine to tell me. Because all the symptoms were totally . . . I've never *been* pregnant before, but they were the same as having a period only much exaggerated.

The man who was involved, obviously rather naturally, didn't wish to believe it. And the only other person I told about it was this friend of mine. Her attitude to it was, "Well, you're always fantasizing over this anyway—as to what you're going to do, when, and if, it happens to you—and now you're just doing the same thing because your *head* is muddled." Which I didn't . . . my head wasn't that muddled at the time.

KATRINA: Do you think you had worried about it more than other people do?

SAMANTHA: I just don't know. Possibly. Because I had always taken great precautions never to *be* pregnant. And on any occasion in which I had *possibly* slipped up, I'd always reacted in absolute *terror* that I might be pregnant. And I was really very, very careful. I'd been on the pill for a while, at one time, and—prior to that—had always used a diaphragm. Also, I'm thirty-one. So that by this time I should, you know, fairly much know how to do these kinds of things.

And I think another thing, with the loop, is that when you first have it in, you're not convinced as to how it works or anything, so you . . . the first two or three months that I had the loop, I got very worried about it. But, I mean, my periods were always regular, twenty-eight, twenty-eight, twenty-eight. And then, when this happened, it really *was* a surprise to me.

Anyway, I was convinced. And ultimately, you know, I was told that I was indeed pregnant. And that really came almost as a relief, because that, at least, meant that now everybody would—"everybody" being the man and this other person—would now believe me, and we could get on with *doing* something about it.

The New Hampshire doctor obviously didn't want to do anything about it, because they don't in New Hampshire. And so he just gives you the name of some other doctor, in New York, to whom you go.

KATRINA: Was this before abortions became legal in New York?

SAMANTHA: No, this was last November. In fact, I had the abortion in December, the beginning of December. So New York was pretty free. And we had some discussion, at the beginning, of "do it all properly and nicely through a hospital." But that seemed to involve so many people. And my real feeling was that I didn't want to involve anyone except the people who already knew about it. These were: the doctor, this friend, and the man. I just didn't want to sort of go through going into hospital, and then being in hospital for two days. And it also meant finding some excuse for being away from work, and all that kind of rigmarole. Whereas, as it was, all I had to say was, "Now I'm going to be away on Monday." I think I stayed away two days. But that was mainly not because I was in any physical pain, but just because I, you know, needed the time to recuperate mentally.

So what I did was simply call and talk to this New York doctor's nurse. And it was amazing, because I said, "How long will I have to wait?" And she said, "Would you like to come tomorrow?" I was so flabbergasted I said, "W-w-well *no!* I can't come tomorrow because there's nobody to drive me down, and I don't want to drive myself." She said, "Oh, you could drive yourself." Well, I don't frankly think I could have done, as a matter of fact, but that's neither here nor there. She said, "You can drive yourself back again, too." I don't know. I didn't much feel like driving anywhere. I think it's exhausting. Because of the emotional tension rather than anything physical. And, of course, you can hemorrhage. (I didn't in the least, and I bled only very slightly.) But I sort of said to the nurse, "How long am I going to stay there?" She said, "Oh, you won't need to stay more than half an hour." I couldn't really believe this and I thought, "My God! they're going to throw me out!" She said, "But you can stay the whole day if you'd like." So then I felt better.

My friend drove me down, what would be two days later. And the really worst time of looking . . . looking *forward* to? [*laughs*] the abortion, was the two days between the time the appointment was made and the time when I actually *had* the abortion. I don't know why that should be the worst time. Maybe because it was the time when I most began to realize that I had conceived a child. Also, in a strange kind of way—which is odd since this was completely unwanted and a mistake and everything—I was really very interested in the sort of physiological changes that go on in your body. It was very fascinating, and, furthermore, being as old as I am, I guess I very naturally wanted to have a child. Which I didn't in the least accept until forty-eight hours before it was to be taken away from me.

And then everything became very real, and I got a tremendous amount of feeling of absolute loathing of the man.

And I don't really feel that way about him at all. I didn't want to marry him, he didn't want to marry me, and we'd *decided* that. It had been under discussion, but we had decided it before this had come up. And even when this came up, it didn't make me change my mind about wanting to marry him. But I certainly began to think I wanted the *child.* In a sort of biological way, not in a sensible sort of way. I mean, if I sat down and thought about it: the difficulties of raising a child without a father, of living one's own life as a single woman, and also trying to live one's life as a good parent—it seemed to me generally mutually incompatible Particularly if you're the wage-earner, because then the child doesn't really have a mother, and it doesn't have a father either.

So I very much felt that, you know, on an intellectual level, this was a really stupid thing to do. And I think a lot of women of my age discuss, you know, "Shall we adopt a child?" "It'd be so nice to have a child." But when you come right down to it, it's hard on the child. Not to mention on yourself. And it's really unfair to the child, I think. It's bad enough for divorced women to try and bring up children, and there the child at least has a father figure in the background.

So I . . . on a purely intellectual level, I didn't *want* the child, didn't want to have it, didn't want to keep it. And there was no question of keeping it. I mean it was a decision that had been much *mulled* over, and *discussed,* before the actual question arose. And when it did arise, I realized I still felt the same way. That even though you don't want to do this thing to yourself, you—you don't change your mind on the purely emotional basis. That because you are pregnant, "you therefore must keep the child because it's a life." I don't think I really saw it as a *life* in the sense that I was, you know, sort of committing a murder. I certainly did *not* see it that way. At all.

But I did very much feel that I *wanted* the child in a *bio-*

logical kind of way. And this became . . . only became real those last two days. Thank *God* I didn't have very long to mull it over. You know, I was very lucky in that from the time that I knew I was pregnant—I mean, that I was *"proved* to be pregnant" as opposed to "knew I was pregnant" [*laughter*]—was very brief. So I was very, very lucky. I didn't have to sit around and wait for psychiatrists to tell me that I was . . . you know, to write on a piece of paper that I'd go crazy if I had a child, or anything like that.

And the reason this interest, this wanting to have a child, didn't come up until the appointment was fixed was, I think, basically because— Well, to a large extent, I tried not to deal with it. In order to remain as pleasant as possible to everybody who was around me and not to start bursting into tears all over the place. I think that I just repressed it, very very much, and attempted to . . . simply go on leading my life as I had been leading it prior to this.

Even though, you know, I found that a lot of the things that one did— All of a sudden, I couldn't for instance drink, at all. Because I just felt frightfully sick. And then I realized all these kinds of funny things that started happening to me. Also the fact that I went around perennially feeling slightly queasy. And these things were sort of interesting, and very biological. But I *tried* not to think about them, I think, or be interested in them. Because I knew I couldn't go on with it.

When the appointment was fixed, then it became very, very emotional and very, very hard for me to contend with. And then I really built up an enormous amount of resentment toward the man. And I think part of that was that although, you know, I *was* and *am* tremendously fond of him and probably always will be—I just could kick him, could kill him, for doing . . . for having "done this to me." You know, this very real stupid thing: *he* has no responsibility for it, *he* doesn't have to go through with it. And at that point I started to be very unpleasant to him. And, you know, we sat around and cried over the whole thing, both of us together.

Then, thank God, he went away. He decided to go home to do some work.

But he was very good and very supportive. And I think that makes a tremendous difference. Again, I was lucky, and it was a long-established relationship. It wasn't a sort of one-night stand or something awful like that.

And, you know, it was certainly something *I* hadn't. . . . You know, I hadn't even made a *mistake*. And I felt it was very unfair that it should happen to *me*. When the doctor did the abortion on me I said, "You will find the loop and it is *there*." He said, "It's still there?" And I said, "Yes, it is." He said, "Never mind, we'll find it if it is." And indeed it was, it was still sitting there. So, you know, it was something that I felt was very external to me. It didn't have anything to do with me. I had no subconscious desire to have a child or *any*thing. It was just something really terribly unfortunate, and I felt *this* very much. And I think I felt the whole world was kicking me in the teeth for something that I really had nothing to do with.

But, short of abstinence, this is something of a chance you take. Of course, I certainly won't have another loop! The gynecologist and I discussed it after, when I went for a check-up. He talked about the dangers of being on the pill, but then he said, "I frankly think you should go back on the pill." And he gave me a prescription which I still have and have *not* had filled. And I'm using a diaphragm. Based on the fact that I really have very mixed emotions about the pill, and always have had, even when I was on it. Not about its contraceptive ability, but about its other—you know—peripheral medical problems. And that was why I was so *thrilled* when I had a loop, because it was simply marvelous: it was a mechanical thing, it didn't affect you in any way, physically, or mentally, or anything else. And it was, as far as I could tell, absolutely superb. *Well . . . !*

The man who did the operation was exceedingly kind and considerate and—you know, I was very tense and unhappy and was sort of sitting there on the table crying. And so he said, "How did this happen?" I guess he looked at my age and thought, "My God! How could anybody of that age be so stupid as to not be using any kind of contraceptive device?" He said, "Weren't you using any protection?" And I said, "Of course I was! I didn't want to do this to myself." To which he said, "Well, I won't perform the abortion if you don't want to have it." And I said, "That's, that's— No," I said, "I have to have it. I don't want to have it, but I have to have it." So he said, "Why?" I told him why I felt I had to have it. And he said, "Well, all right, you seem to have made up your mind. But you don't seem very happy about it." And he talked and was very kind.

He gave me some sort of nice shot that made me practically go to sleep. And the whole process was perfectly . . . inasmuch as something like that can be pleasant! He was very gentle, it didn't hurt, and I had a D&C, not a suction. He evidently does—at least from this particular New Hampshire GYN—three or four a week. In New York, in his own office. He and his nurse were talking about it afterward and he said, about doing D&Cs in the office—as opposed to doing them in a hospital or a clinic—"First of all, you don't give the patient anesthesia." Which terrified me, the idea of not having an anesthetic. But he gave me the shot and I felt *absolutely* no pain whatsoever, except for a local, which was an instantaneous pinprick. You know, he gave me the shot in my arm to begin with. Just so that I wouldn't kick him in the face, I think, since I was so nervous. It was some kind of tranquilizer where everything starts going around in circles. But it was infinitely preferable to what I was feeling. And the whole operation took, I think, twenty-five minutes. I was very fortunate. I think I may have been eight . . . maybe *just* eight weeks pregnant. So I was very lucky. I mean, you know, it's probably not really very pregnant at all. [*laughs*] Well . . . !

I felt . . . I was very tense, but I felt no pain except once, and he said, "Is that hurting?" and I said, "No, but I know it's going to." And it didn't. Then I was completely sort of shell-shocked and I cried a lot afterward. But this was the emotional thing of, you know, sort of sitting there and saying, "I want it back, I want it back, I want it back."

KATRINA: You did say that?

SAMANTHA: Yes. Very much so. That was very definitely how I felt. After the operation was finished, I did feel very emotional about it—very much did, you know, regret what I'd done. I was very tense and very unhappy, and I went out and—I sat around in the examining room for quite a time. And then I got up and went and sort of lay down in the changing room. And I just sat there and—and sulked for a bit. Then I thought, well, you know, if I get out of here, it would be much better. So I went to the doctor and talked to him for a while. And the only pain I had was these incredible pains in my stomach, grabbing pains in my stomach. I told him this, and he said, "Well you seem to be having [*pause*] afterbirth pains."

And I got home about eight o'clock that night, and went to bed. I just kind of lay there in a stupor. But mostly I think I was still terribly upset. When I got into the car for the drive back, my friend said to me, "How do you feel?" Really meaning, I think, how do you feel physically. And I said, "All I feel is I want it *back*." There was a long silence. And then I started to talk about it. And I said, "You know, it's an amazing thing, I don't feel any *pain*. Besides the stomachache. But," I said, "that's *all*." So she said, "Well you're terribly *lucky*, because *I* felt the most incredible pain. It hurt the whole time it was being done."

And she'd evidently had a really very bad time. And she hadn't told me this. Although I fairly much knew what she hadn't told me. But I think I was *exceedingly* lucky, and he must have been very, very good and very, very gentle. The irony of the whole thing was that they were playing Christmas carols, would you *believe?* [*laughs*] on the Muzak. And apparently, just when I went in there, the Muzak got turned up very high, and she thought, "Ooh, she's *screaming.*" It wasn't this at all. It's just that suddenly—it was an ad or something—and it went booming up, you know, about ten decibels.

He was very, very kind and sort of . . . he had a very *nice* manner, you know, and was not in the least bit *frightening* about the whole thing. I don't know how old he was, maybe in his forties, I should think.

KATRINA: Would the man have married you? Or is that irrelevant?

SAMANTHA: Oo-ou! [*pause*] That's . . . no, it's not irrelevant, I don't think, because we had— The man and I have known each other for five years now. He's younger than I am but that's . . . well, that *is* irrelevant. Except in that he's not the kind of person who feels any need to settle down, in the sense of getting married. Although we *had* discussed *prior* to this, whether or not we wanted to get married, and whether or not we should get married, and what on earth we were going to do with this relationship. Because it couldn't really continue just meandering along like this. I was sufficiently old that I should really look for another relationship if this were the case. One shouldn't sort of let oneself settle into a pair of old shoes "because there was nothing else to *do.*" In fact, we had just about split, just about at the time my pregnancy came up.

No, it's not irrelevant. At that point he would not have married me because he wouldn't have married me on that basis. Which he has since said afterward. Because we discussed it, fairly recently, actually, as to our reaction to the whole thing. We hadn't talked about it at all, at the time. But we just happened to discuss it, and I said, "You, you flatly refused to consider marrying me! Even when I brought it up in a very emotional moment. Though fortunately you knew I didn't mean it, on a long-term basis." And he said, "Well, under those circumstances it was no *way* to marry you. It was forcing us both and we both would have regretted it. And under those circumstances I wouldn't have considered it." But I mean we *had* considered it previously and really had come to the conclusion that it wasn't the right thing for either of us.

And I think he also felt . . . he was *hurt* by the way I behaved, he said, because I didn't sort of really take him into it, and I didn't feel that he was. . . . I mean, to say that he wasn't supportive is not true because he was, terribly. But my feeling, I think, stemmed mostly from resentment. You know, that he wasn't the person who conceived the child, he wasn't the person who had to have the abortion, and *as* such could not possibly understand what I was going through. So, the closer it came, the nastier I got.

KATRINA: You didn't ask him to drive you down? Or you wouldn't have wanted him there? Or was it just more natural to ask your girlfriend?

SAMANTHA: He said he would drive— When I'd arranged the appointment, he asked when it was. I told him and I said that this girl would be free to drive me down. I added, sort of kiddingly, "I didn't think you were really up for a nice drive to New York." There were other reasons that I didn't ask him, and one was that I was attempting to remain very considerate of him. I don't know why. But I thought that was the best way to deal with it. I didn't admit to having any resentment until afterward. [*laughter*] Because I really didn't want to. I felt that it was unfair on him because it . . . I didn't feel it was *his* fault *either*. And so I didn't want to admit to having such a nasty feeling as resentment. I was "too nice." Well, afterward I realized that that was kind of stupid. It was better to admit it and just not see him for a while 'til it passed. Which is what we did.

He said, you know, "I *will* drive you down if you want." And I said, "Well, honestly, unless something happens to her, I really don't want you to." I said, "I have a very strong feeling that you should be working, you have exams to pass, you're behind in your work anyway. I just don't think *you* should be doing it, first of all. Furthermore, I don't really think I would want you. I would rather have somebody there who's been through it, who knows what it's like. And if I feel like screaming from New York to Manchester, I can. And if anything happens to me, like I have a monstrous hemorrhage, she'll know what to do." I said, "What would you do with me?" [*laughs*] "I mean you can't take me to the men's room, and you can't go to the ladies' room, and it's all very —you know—very difficult."

KATRINA: You mentioned that you felt upset, after you got back. Did you experience depression then?

SAMANTHA: Was I depressed? I was very depressed. I really was. The first three or four days, I wasn't, because I was very controlled. After about four or five days it began to get terrible. The time when it would *hit* me was—for some reason, I don't know why, perhaps one just feels lowest at that time of day—was around six o'clock in the evening. And from six until about ten, no matter *who* I was with, I was absolutely desperately miserable. And I'd sort of sit there in complete silence, I wouldn't eat, I wouldn't drink, I wouldn't do anything.

KATRINA: And were you thinking, "I want it back?" Or . . . ?

SAMANTHA: I was just thinking how *thoroughly* depressing the whole thing was. Not that I wanted it back. But that it brought home to me the fact that I had found it very difficult to hold on to any continuing relationship. That I was thirty-one years old and had not managed to get married. Not because I hadn't had the opportunity, but because I had never felt that any relationship I'd entered into was one that was ever going to *last* very long. I mean, I somehow, when faced with it lasting very long, would turn around and run. Or else any relationship I wanted to have last was always abolished by the other side. Which leads one to believe that it's—it's more oneself who's doing it. It's a matter of a sort of terrible cycle of choice. And all of those kinds of things were brought home to me, very much *more,* and I was very depressed.

The people who knew . . . actually there was *nobody* who knew about it, except this friend and the man. But what I could always do, since I have enough other friends, was call somebody and say, "Can I come for dinner?" or something like that. So I didn't have to sit and bemoan my fate by myself.

And I *was* terribly depressed. And I told the doctor, whereupon he prescribed twelve dollars' worth of librium, which calmed my nerves, but made me more depressed. [*laughs*] Which I resented terribly because I resented the twelve dollars going, frankly.

KATRINA: What did the abortion—I'm sorry, I'm changing the subject—what did the abortion cost you in New York?

SAMANTHA: Three hundred. In cash. So, you know, he's making a nice little on-the-side money. And he's making it perfectly honorably. I don't know what it costs in a hospital, but I suppose probably more than that. And then you've got the hospital charges and everything else. And also, you're probably anesthetized and you *feel* like hell. I don't know what other people have paid. I would have thought this wasn't unreasonable. And I would say to anyone who does have a D&C, that it's really *emotionally* less cost to have it done in an office. Because in a hospital you have to involve so many people in it. In an office, you involve only the doctor, really, and the nurse. And I mean they both know what you've come for. So you don't sort of . . . there's no emotional cost. He isn't going to come in and say, "What are you doing here?" And poke a finger at you and say, "You are immoral." Because if he felt that way he wouldn't be doing it.

KATRINA: You were talking—and I interrupted earlier—about the depression experience afterward.

SAMANTHA: The depression experience afterward, I don't think you can judge me on that. Because I had this depression. Well then, that went on for about ten days. Then one of the girls that I lived with got very ill, and subsequently died, almost within three days of being ill. And I had all that to deal with, on top of the abortion. And I really went nearly out of my head at that point. I really felt terribly depressed. I couldn't sleep. People were nagging at me the whole time to do this, do that, "What do you think we should do with this?" "Oh, isn't it the most terrible tragedy?" And then they'd call up and ask you all sorts of terrible gory details, and you would have to respond sympathetically and be kind to them.

And at this point I really kind of dismissed the abortion thing from my mind, because I just did not have time to deal with it. I had, you know, a very real problem to deal with. And I was having a hard time keeping my head going. I think my depression then was really much more geared toward the whole situation in my apartment than it was to the abortion.

I, you know, I—I think about the abortion *now*. And I have . . . [*pause. sigh*] It's not something I've really talked about in any way. At all. Except to these two people.

KATRINA: Do you still not talk to anybody?

SAMANTHA: No. No—I don't want to. I feel it's a very exceedingly personal thing. I—I think really because I feel illness is that way. Like when this girl became ill: first she had had chicken pox, and it had been almost a joke. I think of illness as being a very private thing, and I guess I feel that to some extent the two are the same. I'm very old-fashioned in that I'm not particularly open about who I'm making love with, or how, or where, or anything like that. And I think this is probably . . . the reason that I didn't talk about the abortion was all part of this.

And . . . there was another reason: that the more you talk about something, the less easy it is to get over it. Because there are *more* people who know about it, and there are *more* people who say to you, "How are you feeling? Are you feeling better? Was it a terrible experience?" It was a private experience to me. And if it was unpleasant, then, you know, it's not something you want to keep going over. Because there's nothing you can do about it. You've *done* it, and, you know—

It *wasn't* because it was an abortion. It wasn't because I'm *embarrassed* because I *had* an abortion. I'm *not*. I mean I had to have the abortion.

And when I left work to come here today, I said, "I'm going to the doctor." And that was that. Because, again, it is a very personal subject. It's something that is very personal to me and, you know, I—I don't particularly discuss it.

KATRINA: Why were you willing to come to talk? I'm surprised that— Well: Why?

SAMANTHA: Why? Because . . . I answered very spontaneously, actually. The girl who's coming this afternoon is the one who drove me down to New York. She's a friend of one of the girls who works at Pregnancy Counseling Service in

Boston. The girl at Pregnancy Counseling Service said, "Do you know anyone else?" And so my friend said, "Well, I do." And the girl at Pregnancy Counseling Service said, "If you think she'd be willing to do it, call her up, and ask her." She didn't ask who it was, or anything like that.

So my friend called me up and said, "Would you be willing to talk about it?" And I said very spontaneously, "Yes." Then I thought about it. And I thought, "I don't really want to talk about it at all!" And then I thought about it some more and I thought, "Well I *do*, because it's important. This is a subject that should come into the open, and should be something that is a decision that is made *not* by some fink over there in city hall. 'Cause it's none of his business! It is *my* business, and my *doctor's* business, and possibly the man involved. And if I'm over the age of fifteen, and if I get . . . if something terrible happens to me when I'm fifteen and I get pregnant, I *should* be able to get an abortion. No *child* of fifteen should be having a baby! And it should be *made* so that this is the way it happens." Because I think I felt very self-conscious about it. I didn't want to have to deal with it. And I'm very thankful that the New York laws have been changed sufficiently so that I could just get into a car and go to New York. Because had I had to contend with the New Hampshire thing I would have felt like a social outcast. I would have been *embarrassed,* and made much more unhappy. And the reason I was willing to talk about it is because I feel that it's very important. That people like me shouldn't be made to go through undiluted hell. Because of a *fluke* that's happened. And particularly since I really *don't* think people regard abortions as a means of . . . as a substitute for contraception. I mean, I can't imagine women just blithely going off. . . . It's a *ridiculous* idea!

BETSEY

Interviewed in February 1971

BETSEY: Let's see. Mine was a couple of years ago. It was not a legal abortion, so my experience will be different than someone now, hopefully; no one needs to have illegal abortions. But it was a good abortion; it was safe. I had a D&C.

At the time, I was living just outside of Saint Louis, going to school, and made a connection through friends of friends. Luckily I talked with a girl who had had an abortion through the same people about a year before, and she told me—step by step—what would happen. So, in a way, it was in place of—say—had I been to Pregnancy Counseling Service.

KATRINA: How did you know about this girl's abortion? Had she already told you? Or . . . ?

BETSEY: I didn't know her at all, but a friend of hers— I was living in the same building with a friend of hers who said, "Oh, my friend, so-and-so, had an abortion a year ago. Call her up and ask her where she had it."

And she was—she didn't know me from—from anybody. I called her up, and she said, "Oh! Well! how far along are you?" and was really warm and friendly and took it very naturally, and just—you know—gave me instructions on how to get it.

What you had to do was go to a doctor's office. I think he was called a dermatologist or something. It was in a building with lots of other doctors' offices; very straight; there were, you know, women with children sitting in the waiting room, this sort of thing. And you go and you tell him you want an abortion. He checks, you know, examines you to make sure you're pregnant. (I'd already had it confirmed before, also.) And then he asks you your name, your address, and if you have five hundred dollars—which was the price. I didn't have five hundred dollars at the time, so he said, "Well, when you get the money, call me back. We can arrange it any time you have the money."

And so then I was. . . . It was very important to me not to tell my parents. I could have told my parents. I think they would have, you know, helped me go through the abortion and everything, had they felt it was safe. But I couldn't worry about pulling them through as well as pulling me through, emotionally. It was very important. I think—you know, when I think back, it was a pretty crucial point in my life. The fact that I did manage on my own, that I made all the arrangements myself, that I didn't go to my parents and say, "Give me money, give me support, give me —" You know, "Get me through this."

KATRINA: How old were you?

BETSEY: I was twenty-one. [*laughs*] Old enough that I *should* have been able to go through it alone! But I—I always had kind of gone to my parents before. [*pause*]

So it really meant a lot to me *not* to have to go to them. And it was kind of really *chance:* I had a little bit of money saved up just from— My parents were always good, you know, gave me more money than I really needed for clothes and things. So I had some money just in a bank. And then I was running around trying— Like I had maybe two or three friends who knew, and we were going to sell all my clothes and my record player and this sort of thing. I think at the time you *make* money the biggest problem, so you don't worry about your health, and what you're . . . what's actually, you know—the more serious parts. It was easier just to worry about how you were going to get the money together. It kind of helps you block out—you know—worries. I wasn't nervous before I had it. My roommates were terrified; but they didn't let me know.

What finally happened was, my boyfriend . . . like he was good, you know, we went through it together, and he paid half and everything. But there was—there'd never been any question of us really staying together. We were very fond of each other, this sort of thing, but it wasn't— We were on a special program from school; there were twelve of us living all together in an apartment hotel and doing special studies together for one term; and it was pretty understood that when we split up and went back to school, it'd be over. But he wrote to his mother and just said he needed money; he didn't say why, he didn't say what. He hadn't seen her in about three years. She lived in Hawaii. And she sent him five hundred dollars! So, it was just like it came from the sky. She had been working for about three years and had saved up money. And she'd been planning to send it to him. So she just decided this would be a good time, since he said he needed some money. He paid for the whole thing at the time, and then I paid him back, two hundred and fifty dollars. So I didn't have to tell my parents, which was very important to me at the time.

It was actually a very positive experience for me, the whole thing.

KATRINA: Why did you get pregnant? You were not using a contraceptive?

BETSEY: I was using foam. It's not rated that high. Well, there was one time that I can remember that we had intercourse twice in the same night and didn't use the foam again. Which is not using it correctly. So it's possible that that's the time I got pregnant. And that if I had—you know—put the foam in correctly, I wouldn't have gotten pregnant. Perhaps. I did have a prescription for pills which I was planning to start taking my next period. So I had already been to the gynecologist. I was probably just pregnant when I went to the gynecologist for the pills.

And I went back to him when I didn't get my period. And he gave me what I imagine was gestest, which is a dose of progesterone which will bring down your period if it's going to come. It didn't, and I knew I was pregnant. And he was . . . he was really great. He was very understanding. He, you know, said— You know, before he even— In fact he was too fatherly; he made me feel *awful.* You know, he was too nice about it. He said that . . . he said, you know, before he even examined me he wanted me to know that he . . . that I was *the same girl*—that he really thought I was *nice,* and all this; and "not to feel I was bad because I got pregnant" and . . . sort of thing. And it made me feel just awful, 'cause I was thinking all this, "I *am* bad! I *am* bad!"

KATRINA: Had you and the boy talked about it, before: "What if I become pregnant?"

BETSEY: No. Because I was using—I figured I was using the contraceptive; I was going to go on the pill; I really . . . and I asked the doctor when I got the prescription for the pill, "Will I be okay if I keep on using the foam?" He said yes, he thought I would be. So I just figured I'd be okay. And I'd gotten by without using anything, other times; but this is the first time I'd ever slept with anybody regularly.

KATRINA: But you really weren't worried about getting pregnant, then?

BETSEY: Well, kind of ambivalent. I think in a way I wanted to get pregnant. And . . . [*long pause*]

KATRINA: Why?

BETSEY: Sort of as self-punishment. I was in kind of a "down" time. And also just great curiosity about it. I find it very reassuring to know that I'm fertile. You know, 'cause I don't plan to have children for a number of years. And my cousins had all had trouble having children and— I just find it very reassuring simply to know that I can.

I wish I hadn't had to go through that, to feel this way. But on the whole it was not a bad experience. It was very positive in a great number of ways.

KATRINA: Did you discuss with the boy that you might marry each other?

BETSEY: No, that was never in the picture. When I was missing my period for a couple of weeks, we were getting pretty worried. And he was also going through with a friend—a close friend of his had gotten a girl pregnant and they *were* getting married, and he was very happy about that and didn't want them to get an abortion. And then he was faced with this situation. He's Catholic, not practicing, but brought up Catholic. But I think a lot of that just simply fell by the wayside when he was confronted with the situation. I mean there wasn't ever really any doubt, in either of our minds, that abortion was the solution. I'd thought, a long time before, that if I ever got pregnant I would definitely get an abortion. So it wasn't a hard decision for me. It was simply a question of where, and how, and when.

KATRINA: Was the doctor an MD?

BETSEY: I have no idea. He was very young. He might have been an intern or somebody. He obviously knew what he was doing. What his actual qualifications were, I don't know.

You see now, it wasn't the dermatologist doctor that I went to see for an appointment that actually did my abortion. No, that's only the first step in—in how you go through it. Doctor Dermatologist was just the connection. He probably was a very aboveboard doctor. And so in this way I didn't know name, address, anything—not even fictitious names—of the people who actually did the abortion for me. And he had referred to them simply as "these people." So when we got back from his office, I didn't know where I was going to get the money. I figured I'd probably end up having to call my parents. Well, we got the letter from my boyfriend's mother. We had the money. So I called him—the Contact-Doctor-Dermatologist—and said, "I've got the money." He said, "Okay; you'll be getting a phone call within the next day or so." They had my name and address and phone number and everything.

So the next day I just went about my business as usual; I couldn't think of anything else to do. Actually, I functioned pretty well. I went to all my classes. I . . . just every once in a while, I'd cry. When I was alone and sitting down. But I was thinking of the details of simply getting through. You know, I was so preoccupied with the money, with this, that—getting everything arranged. Because I realized that if I didn't, I was going to have to confront my parents with a baby. I thought a lot about what I'd do if I had a baby and I just— To me, the *difficult* thing would be to have a child and give it up. Like, I don't think I could do that. I think I would definitely want to keep my baby. And I live in a small town. It would mean going home to my parents who would

—would help me but it—it would crush my grandparents. And definitely everyone in the town would talk. This sort of thing. I don't know how I would be supporting myself; probably to this day I would be depending on my parents, I don't know. And this was an especially crucial time for me *not* to go back and rely on my parents for help. It would have meant not being able to finish college. It would have meant a lot of things. I don't know whether— They probably would have encouraged me to give the child up. Although I think they would have supported me in whatever I, you know, finally decided to do.

But I—I definitely did not want to give a child up. At all. And I've worked with children a lot and I really like children, and it really—you know I have fantasies of—I really want to have children. I think it would be extremely painful for me to go through carrying a child, because at this time —I was seven weeks pregnant—and I really. . . . A funny thing: once I got the arrangements made, I really looked in the mirror and tried to imagine that there was a child in there. I just, with every stretch of my imagination, tried to make myself believe. And I—I do believe there was a child there. And I, you know, *I'm sorry! I didn't want to* . . . to kill it. And I think I did. But I—I also—you know, I can't honestly say I regret it at all. You know, when you're confronted with a situation like that, you can't—you can't wish for a possibility that isn't there. That is, that I had never, you know, become pregnant.

KATRINA: Did your parents know that you were sleeping with someone? That you weren't a virgin?

BETSEY: Yes.

KATRINA: They knew, because you told them? Or they guessed it? Or . . . ?

BETSEY: Well, when I came home, like afterward, I think I told my mother that I was sleeping with the guy. I didn't tell her anything about the pregnancy, or the abortion, or anything.

KATRINA: So if you had had to call them, it wouldn't have been the blow of telling them that their little girl wasn't a virgin?

BETSEY: No. Actually, I think my mother thought I lost my virginity before I did! Because I had a very steady boyfriend at home and we were together *all* the time. We went together for a year and a half, but we just didn't know anything about birth control. And I knew that if I got pregnant by him we would end up getting married. And that terrified me. We weren't at all ready for marriage. And all he would say about it was, "Well, we'll get married. It will be okay." And I knew it wouldn't be. And it would be me who would drop out of school, and me who. . . . The only contraception I knew about was rubbers, and he wouldn't use them. We'd read all these books, you know, about different things you could get, but we didn't know how to get them or anything. So we just never slept together. But I'm sure my mother thought we *were* sleeping together. And it wouldn't have— That wasn't the motive in not turning to my parents, not at all. They would have—they would have been understanding. It would have been very hard for them, though, because although they want to be open about sex, they really aren't. In a lot of ways. It still hurts my father very much that I sleep with guys, even though I'm twenty-three. He doesn't try to tell me not to; but I can just sense, talking to him— I don't *try* to just sit down and tell them about it, but it's . . . you know, it's obvious, just the way I live.

KATRINA: It does point out a sort of double standard; in other words: it's not so bad if you sleep with a guy, but it is bad if you get pregnant.

BETSEY: Yes.

KATRINA: And yet the two go hand in hand; so it shouldn't be—

BETSEY: Well, it's easier to pretend that you don't, if you don't get pregnant—is all.

And they're very aware that they have these double-standard feelings. Maybe they don't want to, but they still do; and they're pretty good about admitting it. My father said that he doesn't want my brothers and me to have the sex hang-ups that he has, or had. 'Cause he really thinks sex is dirty, and he admits it. He doesn't want to, you know; but when you've gone through fifty years of thinking sex is dirty, you can't just change your mind. You can change your mind but you can't really, you know, change your feelings.

KATRINA: To get back—

BETSEY: Okay; so I got the phone call, Friday night. He said —let's see—"Miss Wex, we understand you have a problem." (He wouldn't refer to what sort of a problem.) I said, "Yes." And they gave me directions to some coffee shop connected with some motel. There's a section like just on the outside of Saint Louis that's just full of motels and hotels and coffee shops and places like that, very—they're all exactly alike. Very anonymous sorts of places. I didn't know how I was going to get down there. I didn't know where it was. But I took the directions down.

KATRINA: And you had to carry five hundred dollars in cash?

BETSEY: Yes.

KATRINA: Did that frighten you?

BETSEY: No. It was kind of exciting. Well, Toby'd gone to the bank and he just had it in a sealed envelope. So I didn't really get to see it.

I thought I'd have to take a cab there, but it turned out my roommate's boyfriend drove me down. My boyfriend had to go to a seminar that night, so he just cut out and—

KATRINA: Did you feel that to be inconsiderate? Or . . . ? *Could* he have gotten out of it?

BETSEY: Well, I didn't know what else he could do, really, because he couldn't go with me, and so he might as well not miss a seminar. He couldn't be at the abortion with me; they told me to come alone. And it was my thing. Like he was willing to support me emotionally—he went down to the first doctor with me. But when I had—when they called my name, you know, I had to get up and walk across there and go in myself. And face the doctor and—by that time I realized it was my—my trip—it was my thing. So it—it bothered me—but it was just typical of the whole relationship. Like he was concerned, he paid half, he cared how things came out. But he wasn't deeply, deeply concerned, either. That was just the nature of the whole relationship. Like it didn't surprise me, it didn't really hurt me, that much.

And he was scared, too, he was scared. Probably more scared than me, really. I mean he hadn't— I don't think he'd given it that much thought. Like I'd at least thought out what I would do if I ever got pregnant. I mean it was something I'd made a decision about. And when it came up I knew what I would do. But I think he was still going through a lot of panic about the whole situation. Also there wasn't that much *he* could do and there were things *I* could do about it.

KATRINA: In retrospect, do you think it would help men if they had some counseling in these kinds of situations?

BETSEY: Yes, I think men should— Well, you know, like the sign we have up in P.C.S. [*laughter*] It's a little blatant: "Would you be more concerned if it were *you* that got pregnant?" But I would just like, all the way through, to see men be more concerned, not only about *not* having children, but *having* children. Doing more about raising children, as well. I think they should take equal responsibility for birth control. I think that's something that people should talk out when they're going to sleep together.

So, anyway, my roommate and her boyfriend took me there. And just dropped me off. [*pause*] At the coffee shop. And I sat there. They'd asked me what I was going to wear, and I'd—I'd made all these thoughts about what-should-I-wear. But when they phoned me and said, "What are you going to wear?" I just looked down (and as a matter of fact, I had this skirt on, I think, or something) and I just— "I guess I'm wearing a brown skirt. And I have blonde hair. And a brown coat or something, or red coat," or whatever it was. I just sort of looked down and saw what I had on and so that's what I was wearing. I went to the coffee shop and I sat there, and I sat maybe about half an hour and . . . I ordered a cup of coffee, and an English muffin I guess, and finally this guy came. He was young, with slicked-back hair. He didn't look too greasy, but you know, kind of—almost. And he was, he was pretty nice, he was kind of brusque. He wanted to know if I was Betsey. I said yes, and then he said, "You shouldn't have eaten." And I thought, "Why didn't they tell me this?" But I figured, you know, what the hell? [*laughs*] I throw up, I throw up. Like it isn't— You know, I've had flu before and it wouldn't be that bad a thing.

And then we—he paid for my check and he took a couple cups of tea to go. Then we went out, got in his car, and just drove around. He asked if I'd brought any Kotex and I said "No! Nobody told me to bring Kotex." And—and then I realized, when he said this, that I was going to bleed. And that was the first time I actually thought about what was going to happen to me. I hadn't really thought it out. I hadn't sort of let myself think about it before. And I, you know, I wished that they'd told me these things.

Then we went to . . . we drove around and we ended up behind a motel which was— You know, I had no idea where we were. This was actually very well thought out. It was a part of Saint Louis that just all looks the same. You just drive around and you get— You drive up behind a motel that looks like the behind of every motel you've ever seen. You can't see the front, you don't know what the name of it is, and you go through the back, by the back stairs, and you go into the room. Which is just a typical Holiday-Inn-type room. They had plastic spread out over the two beds, and the television was going.

The guy who actually did the abortion was young; he was *really* nice, and he put me at ease right away. I liked him very much. I was much less nervous than when I go to the dentist. Or to a hospital. I just . . . I really had confidence in him. He wasn't at all like the one who picked me up in the car. I mean the other was nice but he was very brusque. And businesslike, you know, just "this was another case." Whereas the guy who actually did the abortion was really *pleasant*. He seemed to have more education, probably. He really, really put me at ease. Like I had the impression from Doctor Dermatologist that they were going to count the money before they'd even look at me. But he just took the sealed envelope. And the assistant took it in the bathroom and counted it while they were getting me ready. I suppose "discreet" isn't the word—I mean they took five hundred dollars from me for twenty minutes—but it was that they did me a service. Like at that point I didn't begrudge them the money at all. Because they didn't . . . they didn't treat me nearly as degradingly as a lot of doctors do—to women every day. And they didn't make me go through the rigmarole of: why-I-wanted-an-abortion. They didn't question it. If I had the money, they'd do it. They didn't give me any. . . . Like I would have felt really bad going through what women have to do in Massachusetts to get a legal abortion. You know, going to two psychiatrists and convincing them they're crazy and they're going to jump out of windows, or this, that, and the other.

And I wasn't crazy. I just had made a decision. And they never questioned that. He asked me where I went to school, what I did. He apologized for the fact that I had to take my dress off. You know, he said, "I don't want to embarrass you, but you have to take your skirt off." And I was really kind of impressed that he thought of . . . with the fact that he didn't want to embarrass me.

Since I've been doing abortion counseling I have tried really hard to think if they gave me an injection or some kind of an anesthetic. Because it didn't hurt. But I don't honestly know if they gave me anything. And I don't know what they do if a woman makes a lot of noise— Whether they have to like buy the two rooms next door, or something, and turn the televisions on. Because, I mean I thought I was very calm about the whole thing. I was nervous. But I don't know what kind of precautions they have to take.

It was—it was uncomfortable. And I felt crampy some-times, like you would with menstrual cramps. I'm sure they did a D&C, 'cause he explained to me, you know, pretty much what he was doing: that he was enlarging the opening to the uterus and that he was going to scrape it out. And I could feel them scraping, and stuff. It took maybe twenty minutes, and he . . . you know, he was very reassuring. He asked me questions. I was watching the television and he asked me some questions about the guy, asked me when I thought I conceived. Which is something I hadn't really stopped to think about. And I had never counted up when the baby would come. Which I think was a real protection de-vice to keep from— I had never counted during the whole time I was worried about being pregnant. I had never counted ahead to find out when the baby would have come.

I remember the date of the abortion. It was distinct, 'cause it was November 22, which is the anniversary of when Kennedy was killed. And when we were going down in the car, on the way down there, they were talking about Kennedy on the radio, and that sort of stuck in my mind.

KATRINA: Do you remember the date that the child would have been born?

BETSEY: It was in July.

KATRINA: Do you think about it, in July?

BETSEY: The first July I did. I don't anymore. Well [laughs] there's only been two of 'em! The first July, I did. I thought about it. I thought about where I'd be then instead of . . . a counselor in a summer camp in Maine. Well, I really had faith by that time that had I had to go through and have the child, somehow it would have worked out. But I was definitely glad that I was where I was.

KATRINA: When the abortion was finished, did you feel a sense of relief? Did you feel depressed? Did you feel regret, "I wish I had it back?"

BETSEY: Oh no! No. He . . . I asked him some questions, and he let me look at it afterward. And he was very — He had one of these lights—you know—strapped around his head, and he kind of shined it down and let me look at everything that he had scraped out. And it was . . . it didn't look like anything. Which I think was what he was trying to show me. And he was very patient. He let me look at it as long as I wanted to. And it was . . . he pointed out to me which part was the fetus. It was, you know, just some white material. And the rest was blood—as it would be for a natu-

ral menstrual period. And not nearly as much blood, actually.

And then there was—like the money was ten dollars
short. And so I was really embarrassed. At that time I was
very grateful to them. So I started, you know, fumbling . . .
it was really comical. I started fumbling around—with these
people I had just paid five . . . you know, four hundred and
ninety dollars to—trying to find ten dollars to give them
more. And all I could get was a bunch of quarters, which I
dropped on the floor. And he picked it up and gave me my
quarters back.

So it was all kind of silly, really. At least he didn't grab
the quarters and put 'em in his pocket either—which is sort
of the impression you have of criminal abortionists. And I
think, probably, that he very sincerely believed that women
should have abortions and should have safe ones, if they
want them.

He gave me pills, antibiotics to take, about two or three
different types of pills. Then the assistant drove me back to
the coffee shop where I'd been picked up, and my friends—
When he first came to the coffee shop to pick me up, he said,
"Do you have someone to pick you up afterward?" And I
said, "Well, how long will it take?" He said, "About half an
hour." So he waited while I called my friends right then and
said, "Come back and get me in half an hour at the same
place." And so they were there when I . . . when he brought
me back.

You see, my friends had left me, just left me alone in the
coffee shop. That was . . . [pause] Well, I made up fantasies. You know, like I was a spy waiting for the connection
and—

I mean, it wasn't too bad, because that girl had told me
about it. I'm sure if I didn't know that she had gone through
it, that she didn't feel bad about the experience, that it wasn't
scary, that the people were nice—this sort of thing—if I
didn't know that, and if I hadn't talked to her, I would have

been terrified. But she told me about how they tell you to go someplace and then they meet you and then they take you somewhere and then they do it, and that they're nice and that it isn't awful, and there's nothing bad about the operation, it doesn't hurt, and they take you back—and I knew all this. She was really a marvelous help. Oh, if I . . . !

And I talked with her afterward also. I *wanted* to talk about it, I didn't feel horrible about it, I just wanted to talk about it. And it was really good to sit down and talk with her. I had never met her before, just talked with her on the phone. But she came to visit her friend and we talked for about an hour, just kind of exchanging experiences; and I felt good about it.

KATRINA: In the weeks after, the next two days, the next ten days, what were your feelings, as you remember?

BETSEY: The next few days: well, right after the abortion they told me to stay in bed for two days. They called me the next day like two or three times to make sure that I was home and in bed. And they were very concerned. They said, "You may *feel* fine, but if you get up and walk around you may start hemorrhaging. And that's going to get us in a lot of trouble and you don't want that, either." I think he said that to scare me. 'Cause I definitely wanted to get up and go around. I didn't want people to know I was sick. But, I rested for a weekend.

I realize now that I probably should have gone and had a check-up afterward. I never did. I guess . . . I guess I was very lucky. It was an early pregnancy. And the people I went to knew what they were doing, which is not the case with people I've talked to since.

KATRINA: Do you think they would have helped you, if you had had trouble?

BETSEY: I did know just from talking with people about abortion that, had I had any trouble, I could simply go to a hospital and that I was not under any obligation to tell them where I had gone. I never would have revealed where I'd gone, because I was very grateful to these people. I felt that it was a tremendous risk to them to keep on doing this, and that, if I could afford it, it was really worth it to me.

KATRINA: I guess I'm trying to find out: were you depressed? Or if you weren't, how *un*depressed . . . ?

BETSEY: I was never depressed— Well, let's see—

KATRINA: Or unhappy, or whatever word—

BETSEY: I wouldn't say I was never depressed. I wasn't depressed immediately. I think I felt good the next time I went home to my parents, knowing that I *had* taken care of a rather major event in my life entirely on my own. Nobody called up those doctors for me. Nobody, you know, went down there and sat in the coffee shop with me, or anything. And I—I felt good about that. I felt that at least if I had made the mistake to get pregnant, I had, you know, done something about it. And I also felt that I *was* using contraceptives, and that it was a contraceptive failure.

I did get very depressed around toward Christmastime. I didn't get directly depressed about the abortion. I was very depressed about school. And I felt very pressured, and I cried a lot, and this sort of thing. I felt very trapped—that other people were demanding a lot of things of me. Whereas, actually, during the abortion experience, I was the one who was controlling things. But I felt all these people were demanding papers of me, and demanding this, that, and the other. And I guess it had been a lot of strain. Like I wasn't up to—to thinking about papers and this sort of stuff. And it was a strain to have to keep going through the façade of being more concerned with just school and daily things.

I also was very depressed the next term. You know— when the relationship with the guy broke off. Afterward. Whether I felt closer to him because of what had happened, I don't know.

KATRINA: It broke off for what reason?

BETSEY: I think it was inevitable. See, we were living in the group together for just one fifteen-week term. Then we went back to our own schools. Well, the guy went to the same school I did, but we were living in different places and, you know, here we'd been seeing each other every single day, and now we see each other maybe once a week. And he gets all involved in lots of things he's doing. And there was never . . . it was always understood that we'd split apart. But when it actually happened, I—I missed him a lot. And I was very lonely. I really wanted to tell my friends I was living with then, about the abortion experience. But they didn't know anything about it, and I just didn't . . . I thought better not to tell as many people.

KATRINA: Why?

BETSEY: Well, I don't think they would understand the positive aspects of it. That it was a very positive experience for me. I think they would just feel like they had to feel sorry for me that I'd gone through this terrible thing. I don't think they could understand, really, what it was for me. And just from talking with them before—at least a couple of them— the idea of abortion would have disturbed them very much. Also as a service to the guy. I don't think he wanted people to know at school that we had even particularly been sleeping together, let alone gotten pregnant and had an abortion.

I just think it's a certain matter of discretion that you don't go running around telling people everybody you slept with, and that you got pregnant, and had an abortion. It— Not that I'm ashamed of it, but it's—it's a personal thing, also. And I wish that at the time I'd had some, you know, some group I could have gone to, that. . . . Just a year or so later, I was in a women's group here in Boston, and it helped me very much to be able to talk. A Women's Lib group. And it helped me very much to talk about my experience with people who didn't know me then, who didn't know any of the other people involved. It wasn't like they're going to go and see this guy and say, "Oh yeah, you're the one who got her pregnant." Which I wouldn't want people that I see every day at school—you know, back at school—to know that. 'Cause it was just something that happened between us *then*.

KATRINA: And how is your life now? What are your feelings now, about parenthood, marriage—?

BETSEY: Well I'm not . . . as I get older it becomes actually less important to get married immediately. I still think it's something I probably will do.

I really value parenthood. And yet I really want to—to get more secure about myself before I enter into anything. I think I would like to be—to be married, to have children— You know, everybody says, "Well, I'll just have a love-child," this sort of thing. But that isn't really ideal. If I don't ever get married I might, you know, consider a single-parent adoption. Because I do like children, and I've done a lot of work with them, I enjoy being around them, I like to read books about children, and I think I would really enjoy having a child. But I feel at this point that it's more important to—to work out really with *myself*. And I don't have a steady relationship with a guy at the moment. I don't want to—it's not important to me to go around *looking* for one, you know. I kind of just have *faith* that this sort of thing will happen, probably. And if it doesn't, well—

I'd say the abortion, if anything, has lessened my anxieties —in all phases of living. I think it's made me probably really value parenthood. A lot. But I think the fact that I do know I'm fertile and will be able to have children—of course it's not a hundred percent—but the feeling that I was pregnant is very reassuring to me in a way. And it makes it easier for me to not be concerned that I'm not in a position to have children now at all. And that I probably won't be for the next . . . for a matter of years. Also, I don't feel bad about adopting children, either, if I don't ever have my own children. Though I'm still at the stage where I would like to have a child. And go through the experience of being pregnant with it. You know, all the way through. But I don't feel deprived in any way by having let that child go.

I don't say not in *any* way, but not in a way that really depresses me, or really upsets me. I think it's *unfortunate* to get pregnant and have an abortion—as opposed to knowing about birth control, and using it.

And I think I have just twinges of guilt that it *was* such a positive—in some ways, such a positive experience.

KATRINA: Oh?

BETSEY: I don't know.

KATRINA: Why?

BETSEY: 'Cause I feel it wasn't . . . kind of wasn't fair to that child.

I mean it *wasn't* a child. It was a white blob. But, you know, I can see— I just wonder if I *should* feel so positive. [*pause*] But, well, if it had to happen, it's definitely best I find it a positive experience!

ALLISON

Interviewed in February 1971

ALLISON: My reasons for talking to you are somewhat different from the issue of *legalizing* abortion. I mean, I do feel very strongly about that; I feel it's essential. But I also feel very strongly that being an unwed mother shouldn't be such a terrible social stigma. I mean, that's really my feeling about it.

I had three abortions, a long time ago, and I feel that if this were to happen to me now, that the issue that I would personally be confronted with would be: great resentment that society was pushing me into feeling that I had to get rid of the child because I was not married. And that is the only problem that I would have, in deciding to have an abortion. Feeling that I was being pushed by society's values around me, by the social stigma, not to have a child because I am not married.

This is the sort of thing that I think desperately needs to be broken down. I mean, I don't think that being unmarried should be the basis for deciding to have a child, or deciding not to have a child. And I feel that the more people talk about it openly, and the more people are frank about it, the sooner this problem will be gotten over with. Obviously, if abortion is legalized, this is one of the things that will happen. I hope.

The issue seems to me, personally, the issue of getting pregnant and being unmarried, not the issue of whether one has an abortion. That's an entirely other problem. I mean for me it is. They are not the same. I feel that society *makes* them the same. That's all.

KATRINA: How do you answer the argument of, "but every child needs a father"?

ALLISON: Well, I'm not sure. I think that's one of the things that should be considered in having a child. Absolutely. But I don't think that it's the primary issue. The primary issue is whether you are ready to bring a child into the world and want to. With or without a man. And I think a lot of it depends upon the environment a woman lives in, whether it's possible. I think it's ideal to have two parents in some form. But I certainly don't think that it makes for a healthy child just because it has a father and a mother!

I also know, personally, that were I to decide to be pregnant without being married, I would have to consider the fact that I'd have tremendous anxiety about it. Which would then reflect upon the child. So that, too, is part of the issue of: "What about if a child doesn't have a father?" I mean the issue is far more: "How does the mother feel about that? And how is she going to treat her child? And how is she going to transmit this to her child?"

KATRINA: It's an interesting concept.
You've had three abortions.

ALLISON: Three abortions!
The first one was—um—six, I guess six months after I graduated from college. Which was when I'd just turned twenty-two, and my father had just died just prior to that, and I was a very unhappy girl.
I was living in New York then, and I was very involved

with a man whom I disliked intensely; it was a very bad relationship; it went on and on and on for a long time. This was a man who, besides everything else, was physically repulsive to me. It was a very sick relationship, and I was a very unhappy person. And at the time that I got pregnant my immediate response was one of utter disgust. I mean a physical kind of repulsion. I just wanted to get rid of it in the fastest possible way. And I really didn't care about the danger that I was—I mean I had no sense of reality about the *danger* of having an abortion. What I wanted was just to get the fastest possible thing. And so within a period of about two weeks, I, and the man that I was with, found somebody who was a real butcher and who asked, I think, for six hundred dollars in cash.

I went to see him on a Wednesday and then had it done on a Friday. I had no anesthetic. It was done in a one-room office on West Seventeenth Street, after hours. And I had absolutely no sense of reality about what I was doing. The only thing that was real to me was that I didn't want my mother to find out. And that I wanted to get rid of it as if it had never happened. But I think that my attitude toward it was more connected with my being a very unhappy person at the time. In fact, I think, a very emotionally unstable person.

KATRINA: How was the man about it?

ALLISON: You mean the man that I was involved with? He felt terribly guilty and, I felt, was very irresponsible about it. He wasn't really. I mean he was very actively involved in the whole thing. But there was never any question whatsoever about whether I should have the child.

And I was very childlike myself. So it seemed like such an impossibility. I had no sense, really, of the fact that I was pregnant with a child. It was much more as if I had a growth, or a tumor that I just wanted to get rid of, and I didn't want anybody to know about it because it was so "disgusting." This was basically because of my bad involvement with him, I think. And it was *awful*.

KATRINA: Did you ever imagine what it would have been like if you had had the child?

ALLISON: I never considered it.

KATRINA: Did you know it was going to be possible to get an abortion?

ALLISON: Yes. I knew that ultimately, if I really had to, I could go to my family, and then go through legal channels, which would take a great deal of time. I mean, I sort of had a very unrealistic idea of the fact that "money will buy anything," and "therefore I can go home to Mommy and she'll take care of it." But that would have been such a devastating experience.

Besides, it didn't have anything to do with the realistic factors of who there was available, or how it might be done. My family doctor, to whom I did go—that was how I found out whether I was pregnant—had said, well, he wanted me to "get in touch with my mother," and he'd like my mother to "take me somewhere." And somewhere seemed to be something like Mexico, or something like that.

KATRINA: But you had a sense of security that you would terminate the pregnancy? That it would work out?

ALLISON: Yes, I never—I never questioned it. My concern was not letting my mother know. Or my mother's friends.

And finding the money. And finding the money without my mother was a very complicated procedure. The man that I was involved with had no money whatsoever.

Incidentally, I borrowed the money from a very old friend who had a lot of money. He met me on a street corner on

Third Avenue and Forty-second Street and handed me the cash. And I said something like, "Well, I'll pay you back a little bit every month." And he said, "Please don't. Just put it in a savings account and send it to me when you have enough." I didn't tell him what it was for. And I never sent it to him! And I still think about that. Now he had a great deal of money; I always used to rationalize and say, "Well, you know, he doesn't need the money; and if I sent him six hundred dollars today it wouldn't have nearly as much meaning to him as it does to me." But it's one of the things that I sort of think, that when I finally grow up, I will pay that debt. But it was much more an indication of the fact that I really wasn't ready to take care of myself, and didn't want to.

Anyway, I had this very impulsive, compulsive need to do it immediately. And I got the name of this doctor through the man that had been my advisor at college. He had been my counselor, and I called him up, and he gave me the name. He said another student had gone, and he gave me her name, too. And he said—I'll never forget—he said, "She's fine. In fact she said it was just like having a tooth pulled. So don't worry about it. He's very good and he's very nice."

And indeed he was nice, incidentally. But he got panicked, because I got very tense and was in a great deal of pain and making a lot of noise. And I remember him saying to me, "Quiet, other people will hear." And then I was absolutely getting terribly frightened at the kind of sordidness of it. Of going in with— It was winter, and I had boots on that were covered with salt and snow. And I remember him saying, "Just climb up on the table." And I was thinking to myself, you know, "Isn't he going to give me a dressing-gown or something to put on?" But the idea was just expediency. That was my concern, and obviously it was his.

And the other thing—which frightened the hell out of me—was that while he was doing it he was talking the whole time, really I think to divert me and to relax himself, and he kept saying, "Are you sure you're only eight weeks pregnant?" or whatever it was. And I had these terrible fantasies of an arm coming out, and a leg, you know. And I kept saying, "Maybe it's twins." I had these terrible fantasies. . . . The only time that it became a really harsh reality is when I was there on the table, in pain. And he kept saying, "You're much more than eight weeks pregnant, you must have just had a false period, you must have just been spotting," etcetera. And that was really one of the worst—that was the only time that I really had any sense of "an abortion" in the sense of "killing an embryo."

And then afterward I was so relieved emotionally, that it was nothing relative to how I'd felt before. I really—I was concerned *still* about being "found out" by my mother. And I did get an infection, and had a high fever, and my own family doctor treated me with antibiotics. As a matter of fact, the doctor who had done it called me at home the next day to ask me if I was all right. Which at the time I took as something very nice. I thought it was "sweet" of him. The man that I was involved with said, "Oh, he was just calling to cover himself because you had so much trouble and he put you in such pain."

KATRINA: What did he mean, "to cover himself"?

ALLISON: To make sure I wasn't going to go and report him. I had his name. I mean, it *was* his name because that is where he had a practice and there was a plaque on the door.

KATRINA: So he was a doctor, practicing another kind of medicine?

ALLISON: Maybe he was practicing gynecology; I really don't even know. It was very dark and he did have a small waiting room and a tiny, tiny office. In which there was a desk and a sink and a screen and a table—with stirrups.

And it was terribly dark. That's the main thing I remember about it.

KATRINA: But he was *that* unsterile about it, and was a doctor?

ALLISON: Yes. And he had nobody there. And it took about forty-five minutes and I was screaming from the time I went in till the time I went out.

Well, see, I didn't know. I really was so naïve about it. I mean I never—I *assumed* it would be that sordid. And this was in 1961. Things *were* that sordid in 1961.

And "nice girls didn't get pregnant." I mean it's one thing that "nice girls" may have been sleeping with men, but people didn't know about it. But, you know, there was a great stigma to getting pregnant. The whole concept of getting caught meant admitting that you had some kind of sex life. Which "nice girls" didn't do.

I mean I do think it's very different now. Not only am I older—therefore I think I would react with more maturity —but I think that the whole world—I mean, nobody *questions* the fact that women have sexual involvements and sexual drives and, you know, take the chance every day of getting pregnant.

KATRINA: Did you use birth control?

ALLISON: I had a diaphragm, which I didn't use, which I would use very lackadaisically. And the reason I didn't use it was that—I mean there were a lot of reasons. The reason, ultimately, was because I was very self-destructive. But the reason at *that* time seemed to me that if I used my diaphragm I would be *admitting* to a kind of "lack of spontaneity." You know, that if I didn't use a diaphragm, it was *his* fault, "he forced me." You know, "I didn't *plan* it ahead of time." I didn't take any responsibility for it, you see.

KATRINA: How can other girls avoid the same problem? I mean, I believe this thought is fairly common: "If I use a diaphragm I'm being unspontaneous."

ALLISON: Well, you see, that's—using a diaphragm when you're married is very different. It's not that problem of "waiting to be seduced." And admitting you're waiting to be seduced, you know. I mean, I think obviously people who are at that level—which I hope I'll never be at again!—shouldn't be entrusted with something like a diaphragm. I mean, one of the advantages of pills is the obvious thing that when your head is clear in the morning you drink your orange juice and you take a pill. Regardless of all the other disadvantages.

I wouldn't trust myself *today* with a diaphragm. I really wouldn't. But that's more because I just dislike it, and because it's uncomfortable to worry about, and it's not always comfortable physically, and it's ugly.

Now I have a loop, an IUD—despite its shortcomings. I mean, I'm well aware that it isn't perfect. I had a long talk with Doctor N. about it—the gynecologist who put it in—and his feelings were that to entrust me with a diaphragm would be worse, because of my history. Although I do feel that I'm out of the woods in terms of my emotional state. He feels that the diaphragm would be a very bad idea; and that I did already take the pill for years. And he's, at this time, very opposed to the pill. I mean he doesn't really advise the pill either. He *really* advises a diaphragm. But in cases like me he's very willing to admit that. . . .

KATRINA: Then you're following your doctor's advice? You're not being—?

ALLISON: Right. [*laughs*] I'm not using an IUD because it's less effective than a diaphragm. I'm using it because it's more effective than a diaphragm for me. For me, personally,

I'm absolutely sure it is. I really am. I mean I hope that I would never get myself into this situation again. I don't think I need to, in the realest sense of need to.

So, after this first abortion, I was relieved, and then sick. And I felt I was paying my debt. I also felt that this was what happened to people. I thought I was lucky to be alive. But my concern at the time of having it was not whether I lived or not, my concern was getting rid of it.

KATRINA: Then afterward, the next two weeks, or three weeks, or six weeks, were you depressed? Were you elated and relieved? What were your—?

ALLISON: I was relieved, and somewhat anxious that I would still be found out. Because I was very involved in my family—in my mother.

KATRINA: Did you drop the fellow then?

ALLISON: Oh, I tried! And it got worse. I went on and on with him for a long time. And the second time I was pregnant I was pregnant by him again.

That time my response was very much the same, but it was also one of, "That's it. I want out now."

KATRINA: Of the relationship?

ALLISON: Yes. And this was a year and a half *later,* believe it or not! And again I was supposedly using a diaphragm. But that abortion was not a bad experience. I mean it still wasn't comfortable; I was in pain.

KATRINA: You got pregnant the second time, because you didn't use your diaphragm?

ALLISON: I'd been using contraceptive jelly. Without a diaphragm. [*laughing*] And I'd been advised not to do so! In fact, it seems to me that it said in the directions, "Do not consider this a safe contraceptive" or something like that. "Use it *with* a diaphragm." So *again* it was purely a matter of being in a very psychologically disturbed state.

KATRINA: So the set-up, and the reasons for getting pregnant were similar to the first?

ALLISON: Absolutely. Absolutely.

KATRINA: And then what?

ALLISON: I was actually panicked, because I thought I was using up my chances.

KATRINA: This time you were afraid of the danger?

ALLISON: Yes, right. And so we found. . . . A very good friend of Larry's—who was the man—knew a girl who had had an abortion through a man who was from maybe South America. He was here doing a residency at one of the big New York hospitals. He was Head Resident in Gynecology —which sounded pretty classy to me compared to the other situation! Also, it was at a time when residents still didn't make very much money and it seemed to make sense to me: that he was doing it on the side because he believed it was right, and because he needed the money. I wasn't near as upset about it, and it was done somehow in a much more professional manner. By which I mean I went and met him, and he was terribly nice. And he and the girl that Larry knew drove me down to—maybe New Jersey. Believe it or not I don't know where it was! It may have been New Jersey. It was someplace going on the New Jersey turnpike toward Pennsylvania. And it was all kind of a social event. Which I didn't quite understand. Larry didn't come; they asked him not to come. And the girl was sort of there as a girl to comfort me. Also she was a very good friend of the doctor.

And we went down, and there was an actual kind of clinic set-up that looked like doctors used it during the day and they rented it at night, or something like that. And we met another doctor there who was waiting for us. And they just kind of joked about the fact that on the way back I could have something to eat, and stuff like that. They hadn't wanted me to eat anything on the way down, and they'd given me a sleeping pill so I'd sort of rested in the car. I didn't sleep, but I wasn't very anxious.

Then my doctor gave me something that, in retrospect, looks as if it should have been something like sodium pentothal, because he injected it into my arm. But I was not knocked out, and I was in pain. Although I think that had a lot to do with resistance, because they couldn't give me so much that they really would completely knock me out. And I just kept screaming, "Is it almost over?" The issue was to get me up on my feet as soon as possible to drive me back home. Then I slept all the way home in the car, and was fine. There was some mild discussion about whether I wanted to stay at the doctor's apartment in New York. But I kept saying, "No, I just want to go home." Because, again, I just wanted to act as if it had never happened.

KATRINA: Were you afraid, this time, of your mother finding out?

ALLISON: I would have been terribly upset if she had; but that wasn't my primary concern at that point. My primary concern was that I was enraged at Larry, who was the man, that he'd "done" this to me again. And I wanted out of that relationship. Which I finally did get out of. After almost three years.

And I felt all right. And I felt very lucky. But I really felt,

"I can never do this to myself again. I have to be terribly careful."

Then, soon after that, I got married—in a very bad marriage. This was all following the same kind of unhappy time of my life. I stayed married for five months, and at the end of that, got divorced. I moved out here to California, and I got very sick, believe it or not, with a venereal infection which was never one hundred percent diagnosed! And— kind of hit bottom. I was sent to Doctor N. and I was in the hospital for five weeks, being pumped full of penicillin, and seeing a psychiatrist. And got over it. And I kind of came out into the sunlight, really!

And the *first* thing I did was sleep with somebody on a one-night stand, and got pregnant.

Much to Doctor N.'s amazement! He thought I could never get pregnant after my history and whatever kind of venereal infection it was. It was probably gonorrhea, but it's very difficult to be sure because of the strains now, which are all very mixed.

KATRINA: But you were in the hospital for the infection?

ALLISON: Yes, I was—

KATRINA: You weren't in the hospital because of your psychological—?

ALLISON: No. [*laughing*] My psychological state was just finally *exposed*. And the psychiatrist that I was seeing happened to be at that same hospital. I'd just begun to see him, as a matter of fact, just prior to my going to the hospital— to getting sick.

Anyway, I got pregnant and there just seemed to be no question about the fact that—there was never any issue with my psychiatrist or with Doctor N. about whether I should have an abortion or not. Doctor N. was thrilled that I could get pregnant! I mean, here I was, a great medical *triumph.* He really didn't think that after the infection I'd stand much of a chance of getting pregnant. So it was this very bizarre situation.

KATRINA: Were you thrilled, too, in a way?

ALLISON: Yes, sure; and that's exactly what I was doing! I was trying to find out whether I could, in a very immature way. Sure.

Anyway, Doctor N. immediately said that he was perfectly willing to do an abortion, as long as my psychiatrist was connected in some way with the Women's Hospital, which he was. And I was sent to have a second psychiatrist's signature. My own psychiatrist felt that the immediate issue was to deal with my being pregnant. And the secondary issue—which might take years, and which indeed it did—was to find out why I got pregnant and why I kept doing this to myself. But he was not in the least bit moral about it. I mean he said, "Look, let's deal with the immediacy of this. Who are we going to call? And how do you do it? And how much is it going to cost?" and all. He was great. And so was Doctor N.

I had to go to see another psychiatrist, which was the only sort of sordid part about it. I walked into the man's office and he sat there saying to me, "Well, of course, you're a very depressed person." And I kept saying, "Well, really, I'm not now. I used to be." And he kept saying, "Well, you wouldn't have gotten yourself pregnant, right?" And then he'd say, "You probably, as a matter of fact, wouldn't even want to live if you had this child?" And he kept saying this and writing it down when I'd say yes. And in fact at one point, when I kept saying, "No, I'm really not, I'm fine," he finally said, "Look, you'll have to do better than this."

KATRINA: So it was a sham?

ALLISON: Yes it was. And everybody admitted it. And then I went to the Women's Hospital and was there for two days. And I was treated like any other patient. The only part that was sort of bizarre is that they put you in the sort of labor room: the room where women are just about to go in to deliver, you know. And when you come out, you're in a recovery room with women who have just given birth. And this was a very bizarre feeling. You're sort of lying in the bed looking around in your drugged state, kind of waiting for somebody to say, "What did *you* have?"

That was in 1964, and again there is a big difference between now and seven years ago. I think that now I wouldn't just sit back and take that. Now, if I were to go through this, I would find out about those sorts of things before I went through it. But at that time I sort of thought, "Well, that's the breaks of the game. I'm paying—again." You know, "Otherwise this has been perfectly pleasant, the nurses aren't making me feel uncomfortable." And they were all very polite about calling it a D&C. And I sort of really felt that they thought I really *was* having a D&C; and the only person who *really* knew was Doctor N.

I mean that wasn't so terrible. It was just bizarre to me. But I think to other women, it could be *awful*.

Again I was so relieved to be over it, and to have been treated well otherwise. And that I hadn't been in pain! That was just spectacular to me.

KATRINA: Was the guy involved anyone you ever saw again?

ALLISON: Never, and I never told him. Again, there was absolutely no question about my not having the child.

[*laughing*] And from then on it was uphill.

KATRINA: But I'm thinking back—to what you were saying earlier about a single woman having a child.

ALLISON: Well, now it's not the same— Also I feel, now, that I'm thirty-two—which I wasn't then. I have much more of a sense personally in my life of being able to do whatever I want. I mean I don't have the same problems that—I do *deeply*, but I mean as far as coping with them, I don't have the same problems of having to lead the life that my mother leads.

But I still—I still never considered the possibility of having a child. I also really didn't love the man in any sense and I didn't want to have his child. I'm involved with somebody now, living with somebody who's a marvelous, marvelous boy, who's a lot younger than I am and who— It would just be ludicrous if he were to get married. And I'm not particularly into marrying him, or getting married right now, either. But if I were to become pregnant by him, I think that I'd be very happy and thrilled at the idea of having a child, because he's a beautiful person. And he's exactly the kind of man whose child I would like to have. And I would be indeed very, very torn, because the *possibility* of having the child is now very real to me.

KATRINA: Are you considering this?

ALLISON: No, I'm really not, because I really think it would be just terribly difficult. But were I to become pregnant by mistake, were my IUD not to work, I would not so readily just say, "Well the first thing to do this morning is to find somebody who will do an abortion." Which is what my attitude has been in the past.

No, I—I've, as a matter of fact, *often* thought about *adopting* a child. And I always find it very ironic that society now will accept *that*. I mean, Pearl Buck wasn't a whore in 1920 because she adopted twenty little children. You know. I mean, I always found that sort of wild.

KATRINA: Yes, I hadn't thought about that: it's all right to adopt one, but if you have it naturally. . . .

ALLISON: Right. Well, it's a little bizarre if you adopt one and you're not married! But now you can, which you couldn't before. Of course I think you get a kind of—you're really low status in terms of preference. You're not high on the blue-eyed-blonde baby list.

KATRINA: Yes, it helps those children who might otherwise not find. . . .

ALLISON: Yes. Absolutely.
I was adopted myself so I have very . . .

KATRINA: Shake.

ALLISON: Oh, *really?*

KATRINA: Yes.

ALLISON: My God!

KATRINA: I'd love to talk about it . . .

ALLISON: Yes! Yes!

KATRINA: But first I think we ought to finish about your abortion—

ALLISON: Well, that was it. And I can certainly say that if I get pregnant again, it's not going to be my fault. Whereas I really do believe that I brought those others on myself.
I think the reason was also— It's interesting that I haven't said it until now in the interview—but I think that my *get-*

ting pregnant three times—Which is a little exorbitant! I think that a lot of my psycho—my being as fucked-up as I was, especially on this subject, was very connected with being able to do something that my mother was not able to do. And a lot of the conflicts that I had with my mother are embodied in this very issue of being a woman, as exemplified by being able to produce, reproduce. And my terrible fear of her finding out—you know, above and beyond a normal fear— I think was also connected with "doing her in." I was able to do something that she couldn't do.

And the other thing was: there was always this terrible fear that I would do exactly what my "fantasy mother"— which is what I call my biological mother or whatever—had done. That I was just acting out what my idea of the "really *good* mother"— You know, who's completely unreal to me. That I would be kind of following, in some kind of a—like expiating the devil by doing the same thing yourself.

KATRINA: Yes, the adoption aspect is. . . .

ALLISON: Well, it's also why I'm *here!* I mean, why my concern about this is very *great*. It's also why I was involved in getting pregnant, as I say.

KATRINA: It must also have affected your decision, I would think, in not giving the child up. Which was, after all, an alternative that was open to you: having the child and giving it up—

ALLISON: Oh my God! I couldn't even consider doing that! I mean if I were to have a child—! I mean I have absolutely no intention of giving it up!

I mean I don't— I really have never stopped to think whether I'm saying, in that, "Because I don't think adoption is a good thing." I mean, I don't think I'm saying that. I'm simply saying that I feel the child would be rightfully mine, and that I would feel very cheated. I really don't have strong feelings that when a woman is first pregnant that there's any kind of reality about a "human being" inside of her. I think that she *makes* it real if she so chooses. I mean I see pregnancy very much as a purely physical state, that's not unrelated to any other physical state. Growing something inside of you—it's no different than a plant, you know. And I really feel that the thing that makes it real is the choice to *have* the child. And the choice to have the child is the choice to be a mother, it's not "to give it up." I mean, this is terribly real to me.

KATRINA: Yes. I now realize you said several times that you would adopt a child.

ALLISON: Oh yes, sure. But that's only because that seems like a much greater possibility to me; in that I'm not married and am not at this point choosing to *be* married. And that there are a great many children up for adoption. I mean I don't think it's the child's fault, that it's been given up. I mean, I really feel very strongly that mothers should not give up children, for their *own* sake.

KATRINA: And for the child's sake?

[*long pause*]

ALLISON: Well, after everything I've said it's going to sound very contradictory, but I—I'm not sure it is. I—I don't think it makes that much difference to the child. I think how the adoptive parents handle it is what makes the difference.
Well, I suppose— I mean, yes it *did* make a difference. But the differences, you know, were— I mean I feel that the hassles I've had with my parents have been very much the hassles that everybody has with their parents. And I think that were my mother to have actually had a child, that child

would have had very much the same problems with her as I do. Because she's a very kooky lady. Now there is an issue —that I really deeply believe—that part of her kookiness was her inability, was exacerbated by her inability to have children. But I—I mean I had a home and parents like every other kid on the block.

I may— I *used* it, often, for sympathy outside of home. I mean it was like— Even at points when I was very young, I would walk up to people and say, "My name is Allison Trimbley, and I'm adopted." I mean, instead of saying, "I'm Allison Trimbley, and I live on Green Oak Road," or whatever. I mean I would *define* myself—in the hopes that they would say, "Oh! isn't it wonderful!" or "Isn't that cute!" or something like that. [*laughs*]— Which would indicate a certain amount of problems that I had with it!

But I really don't feel giving up a child for adoption in terms of the child, is bad. I feel as a *woman* that it's absolutely unfair and ludicrous. I think at times there are very real reasons for a woman not to keep a child, but then she shouldn't have *had* it! She should have had an *abortion!* If she couldn't be a mother then she shouldn't have— I mean, in addition to everything else, why bring more people into the world? Which is no longer a question.

KATRINA: Yes, right. And it's only in the past few years that this idea. . . .

ALLISON: Well, every doctor would say to you, "Either get married, or have the child and give it up for adoption." Those were the only two legal options.

KATRINA: What do you think your future is going to be?

ALLISON: Well, I've just graduated from engineering school as a civil engineer, as a matter of fact, just two days— yesterday . . . I mean I just finished finally—I just got a

handshake saying, "You've done it." And what I really—
my fantasy is to continue working as a civil engineer up until the point where I can have my own practice. Or be so
marketable that I can work when I want to work and make
enough money to survive. And, ideally, to in some— I mean
I certainly feel very strongly that I don't want to be gypped
of the opportunity to be a mother. Whether or not it's biological. I'm beginning to question and worry about the fact
that, you know, if I'm limited in the number of years that I
can bear a child— And, also, be an active healthy mother
with the energy that a mother needs— So one of the obvious
solutions now would be to adopt a child. I mean I certainly
wouldn't turn it down as a possibility. If I definitely decided that I wanted to have a child, and if there were too
many things against my physically bearing a child—which
could be anything from the social issue of not being married, to physically not being able to bear one—then I
would seriously consider adopting one. Also, I think in
terms of adopting a child who is not necessarily an infant,
so that I could continue to work and be professional and
be out in the world—and continue to lead the kind of private independent life that I'm now very used to— And at
the same time have a child. To be a mother is very real to
me, and I certainly have not given it up, at all.

And indeed it *was* when I was pregnant the three times. I
mean it was very real to want to have a child *then*. But not
those children. And those children were defined by my emotional state, and by the man I was involved with, and everything else. I mean it wasn't like I was saying, "I don't ever
want to have a child." It was, "I don't want to have *this*
child." For whatever reasons.

The interesting thing—that you might be interested in:
when I turned twenty-one, which I somehow thought was a
great momentous occasion in my life, I marched over to the
X Adoption Agency, where I'd been adopted from, and said,
with great *guilt,* that I'd been adopted from there in 1938

and that I would like to find out everything there was to find out. I expected them to say to me, "Go home!" Because I'd been told all my life that nobody knew anything and that, you know, I'd been dropped from the heavens. I really just didn't know anything at all. And my parents insisted that they knew nothing, other than the fact that I "come from healthy stock." That was a big thing. Like my mother didn't have diabetes or something. And I'd always sort of get self-conscious if I'd be in a hospital and having a medical record done and they'd say, "Is there any history of heart disease?" and I'd say, "I don't know."

Well, I went and— Imagine my surprise when I found out there was a woman there—a marvelous woman, her name was Alice Mueller—whose full-time job it was to talk to people like me! Isn't that astounding? That's all— She's a social worker and that's what she was there for, to dig out old records and to talk to people who'd been adopted through the agency. I was absolutely astounded. I thought I was the *only* person who'd ever gone back. Because I thought it was *sinful*. Well let me tell you what they did! They made an appointment for me and I got there, and they had a little file on the desk, and I sat across from her; it was all very formal. And she said, "I can tell you absolutely everything I know except your mother's name." And she said, "I don't know your father. I don't know anything about him, your mother wasn't married." And then she proceeded to tell me a story which was just like any other story that I'd made up. That she was thirty-five years old and— I remember her saying to me, "She was obviously a fairly sophisticated woman, because she came to us in a very early stage of pregnancy and wanted to give up the child for adoption legally, and wanted the *best thing* for you." I mean she kept sort of encouraging me about how my mother wanted the "best thing" for me. And then she told me that she had *red* hair! I mean, all kinds of things which were so bizarre. And that—I don't really—she was into music in some way. I mean, there was very little about her.

And then a year or so later I told my own mother that I'd done this—with great guilt. Any my mother said, "Well, I assumed you would, at some point, but you probably didn't find anything out." And I told her what I had found out, and she said, "Well, I could have told you that!" And then she said, "In fact, I have your original birth certificate. Do you want it? Because I can burn it. But I've always kept it because I thought you might want it." Which is a very bizarre thing. And I said, obviously because I was programmed into it, I said, "Why would I want it?"

But then I said, "But what was my name?" And she told me my name! Which was "Virginia Parro"! And then I said, "What kind of a name is Parro?" My mother said with great disgust—my mother is very Anglo-Saxon—my mother said with great disdain, "It's obviously Greek." [*laughter*] And that was the end of that. And then I said after the discussion, "Well, as far as I'm concerned you can burn it, because that's not my name." And that was all.

And as far as I know, that woman is still operating. Her name is Alice Mueller. Well this was 19— It was when I was twenty-one, so it was 1959. I'm sure they have somebody in her role at every big adoption agency.

She said something very interesting, though, which I found very poignant. She said that they make a very strong effort now, with adoptive parents, to tell them practically everything they know; and they encourage the parents to tell the child everything they know. Because it's better than the child thinking that the mother died in childbirth, or that the mother dropped them on a doorstep because she didn't want them. Which are the only two alternatives for a child to understand. It's much better to say to a child, "Your mother wasn't married and wanted you to have two parents."

You know, incidentally, when I did this I had absolutely

no intention—and I still don't—of wanting to go out and find my mother. I mean this is something that people ask me continually, "Well don't you want to go find her? Don't you look for her?" And I don't think I do. I did want to find something out about what I was beginning to sense as my own identity. I kind of, in all senses at the age of twenty-one, was beginning to say, "I no longer flatly accept that everything I am is Mommy and Daddy." You know, "I am something more than that, and I *came* from something more than that. And what did I come from?" But it wasn't that I wanted to specifically go out and find *her* or get any love from her or any response from her. I mean that would just be a nightmare to me.

KATRINA: But didn't you dream of that?

ALLISON: Well, I have dreams of the fact that she's big and warm and loving and that she'd be terribly proud of me.

I think I also just believed my family's story; you know, that I never would be able to find her. And also because there was enough popular kind of communication about adoption by that time, that I knew that the agency would never tell me my mother's name. I mean there were enough movies around about women in agencies saying, "I will lock the name up in the safe, and I will blah, blah—" I don't think I ever thought that I would have to deal with that.

Although I must say, every once in a while I do have fantasies of looking up "Parro" in phone books when I go to a different city.

[*pause to change tape*]

KATRINA: Where were we?

ALLISON: Oh, I know. I was going to tell you about when Joanie Van Platt got married. She had been adopted, and she had a sister who wasn't adopted. It was one of those stories where her mother got pregnant the day after Joanie was adopted. Anyway— And Joanie was always a spectacular girl. And Beth was a big crashing bore. Anyway, when she got married, she stood up at her wedding and she said, "I recognize the fact that it's unusual for the bride to give a toast, but I want very much to toast my parents, and to thank them for the two happiest days in my life. And one is today at this beautiful wedding that they've given me. And the other is the day that they adopted me." And everybody cried and everybody applauded. And I went home, and my parents were there in the living room and I told them this story. And my mother sort of responded in the way you expect one to, "Oh, isn't that dear," or something like that. But my father was enraged. He thought it was very kind of exhibitionist, he thought it was obnoxious, he thought it was rude, he thought it was out of taste. His whole response was, "Well, then obviously the Van Platts weren't very good parents."

I mean his whole response to it was that if she felt that she had to get up and thank her parents at her wedding for the day, effectively, that she was born— I mean what normal person gets up and says, "I'd like to thank my parents for the day I was born, for the night they conceived me?" I mean he just felt that's the level at which a parent was a parent. And if the child had to feel that she had to make a statement like this, then obviously it had not been a successful adoption.

KATRINA: Do you agree with his point of view?

[long pause]

ALLISON: Oh, not really. I think that in some kind of storybook fashion I do, because the ideal adoption would be, you know, something that would be absolutely no different. But it is different. And so why not—why not deal with it?

KATRINA: Yes.

[*pause*]

ALLISON: But I think the main thing for me is that I don't have any sense of my own physical reality. Or sense of being able to reproduce a child as a human being. Because I don't have any sense really of having been born myself. I mean, nobody ever talked about being pregnant with me, or giving birth. You know, I was dropped from the heavens. So that when my brother— Do you have a brother?

KATRINA: Yes. Two brothers.

ALLISON: Adopted?

KATRINA: Yes.

ALLISON: Wow!
   So was mine.
   And when my brother first had—his wife first had a child, I was terribly involved in what the child looked like. Did it look like my brother? And the child was jaundiced and had *black* hair. It now is a very blonde pugnosed beautiful child, but at the time she looked like this little Chinese baby. And I went through this incredible fantasy, as an *adult,* of the fact that my brother really had Chinese blood in his background, and all kinds of things. But, I mean I really thought that he had conquered the devil by having a child.
   And the other thing is, that I *do* spend, still, a lot of time looking at older women. Wondering if that's what I'm going to look like. I mean, I have very little sense really of what I look like. Which was an earlier problem of identity—of not knowing who I was. But I—I do continually say to people, when I see somebody on the street, I'll say, "Do you think that's what I'm going to look like when I *grow up?*"

And I do think that a lot of the problems that I had—that relate, incidentally, to the whole Women's Movement, which I feel very strongly about and am involved in—have to do with the fact that I was *terribly* mercurial and schizophrenic in my appearance, and in my interests, and *terribly* adjustable. So that I was always kind of looking for the thing that I was real—that I really was. And I could always adjust to kind of any situation; so that if anybody were to sit down— Like I'm still panicked—when I went to fill out my passport form two weeks ago and it said, "color eyes"—color of eyes and height and all that. I really had to think, you know, "What do I look like?" And I could very easily change how I look; not so much now that I'm older, but— I really wonder — I don't have any sense of what-I-am-going-to-be-as-an-adult. And I am shocked every once in a while when I hear — I mean, I *am* an adult. I'm thirty-two years old!

CAROLE

Interviewed in February 1971

CAROLE: I went off the pill in May, because of an infection that I'd had for about a year. The doctor said that the pill was contributing to it, with the extra hormones. We were using—let's see, a condom I guess, and that's all. We didn't use foam with it, the way we should have. I wasn't even aware that the foam was as good as it supposedly is. So we just used a condom, and at times we *didn't*. So it wasn't necessarily a failure of the method. It was a pretty stupid thing to do. And I just got pregnant.

KATRINA: You're married?

CAROLE: Yes. I have two children, four and two. And we had decided, long before this, that we didn't want anymore children. I was going to school at night, and I have a garden, and I keep busy, and I just didn't want anymore children.

The first one was a mistake and we found ourselves in the position . . . I was raised in a middle-class family, grandfather's a minister, and abortion just was never a question when I was eighteen and pregnant—so we got married.

KATRINA: You "had to" get married?

CAROLE: More or less. Right, had to get married.

KATRINA: Would you have married anyway?

CAROLE: Eventually. Probably. Yes, that type of thing. We'd been dating for quite a while. I was in school, and he was in school and working. It wasn't really the smartest thing to do to get married. But you know, the situation— There was nothing else to do, so we did.

So she was more or less pushed on us. But the baby, the second baby, was planned. And then we decided no more after that. When this pregnancy came along it was a surprise. But we decided, just with no discussion at all, that this baby wasn't going to be born and raised.

I went to my doctor who, I found out afterward, is very liberal. PCS has been in touch with him for a long time. At first, when I thought I was pregnant, I didn't know what to do because I didn't know his attitude. I didn't really know him that well, and I thought, "How can I get a lab test?" And I found out that I couldn't get a lab test unless it was through a doctor.

So I went to the lab and had the test and told him. And he said, "Well, it is positive." And I just—I just started crying right on the phone and I said, "I—I can't have anymore children."

So he was very nice, he calmed me down, and he said, "Don't worry," and he told me to call Planned Parenthood. They put me in touch with PCS and I came over here and had an appointment—with Beverly—and I was very impressed. It was so informal, and they were so helpful.

I made my New York appointment and there was no problem there. I thought the price was a little high. It was about . . . let's see, it was two-fifty for the doctor and three-fifty for the hospital. So that was six hundred dollars. But we could afford it: my husband has a good job.

We got the money together, and of course nothing could be

said. But he'd said something to his mother and she came over and tried to talk me out of it. You know, "You're taking a life," and this and that. And I said, "I just feel that my life is more important to me right now."

So she couldn't talk me out of it. And I cheerfully went off on the train in the morning and went down and was admitted to the hospital, and didn't— Well, I saw the doctor before I went into the hospital the day before. And I went in and spent the whole day—very bored—in the hospital, hearing people moan and groan, for different reasons, operations and things. And girls would come in with their parents, like sixteen-year-olds, crying, and carrying on. It was not really very pleasant. But they went through the whole pre-op thing with X-rays and lab tests and all the rest of the prep that they go through. And the next morning I waited around, and waited around, and waited around. Finally, I was taken up to the operating room and given the anesthesia. And that was that. I was fully confident, "Hello, Doctor." (I hadn't met the doctor who did the abortion. I'd met his associate when he examined me the day before.) "Hello," you know, "You're sure I'll be able to leave later on this afternoon? I have to get home." "Oh sure, sure."

I woke up about . . . I guess probably three hours later, and I was strapped down to the bed and I had bandages all around me and I had intravenous in my arm. I just went hysterical. I—I couldn't imagine what had happened to me. And I asked . . . I asked the nurse—the nurses kept coming and going—and the nurse said, "I can't tell you what happened." I—I just— All I could think of was cancer or— what had they found, you know, in this whole procedure. The nurses would say, "No, no I can't tell you."

Finally, about six hours later, the doctor showed up. It turned out that he had perforated my uterus and my bowels. And supposedly no one was to blame. It wasn't his fault, it wasn't my fault; my uterus was soft. Be that as it may, I don't know. The doctor, the day before, hadn't said anything about it, and my own doctor in his exam hadn't said anything about it.

So, they had me on narcotics, and I couldn't eat anything. I was on intravenous for about six days. The attention was all right. The nurses were nice and I didn't feel that they had anything against me—the stigma with abortion, or anything like that. It was just a dreadful . . . it was a traumatic experience, it was just the worst thing I've ever gone through in my life.

And my husband, of course, didn't come with me. I was all alone. Well, the doctor called him. I guess he told him that it was, you know, serious. And he told me that I would have died if I weren't in the hospital. You know, if I were in, say, someone's back garage or whatever. And he said that even if I were in his office, I would have been in serious shock by the time I got to the hospital, and things would have been much more serious than they were.

And then he started— He knew I was interested in women and their problems and . . . just the whole Liberation thing. And he started in on me, "Well, you know that this isn't as simple a thing as they try to make it out to be," and blah blah blah. And I said, "Well, no, I guess I can see *that*." [*laughs*]

So, you know, that was it. I spent about ten days in the hospital. And finally I could get up and walk around. They took the stitches out of me, which didn't help much. It seems most of the problem was internal. I couldn't eat anything, I couldn't pass anything. So it was . . . it was really dreadful. And I came home and spent about two more weeks in bed. And, you know, then I was all right.

But, it was just a dreadful thing. I'd never seen the man before, and I didn't have any confidence in him. He treated me like a child when he came in afterward. He wouldn't tell me what had happened, he just said that "we ran into complications." And I pushed and I pushed; I wanted to know what happened. And it was . . . it was just a dreadful thing.

KATRINA: You were in a reputable hospital?

CAROLE: X Hospital in New York City. When I came to PCS it was June—well it was around June fifteenth—and PCS had the word that the hospitals in New York had loosened up a couple of weeks early, because they knew they were safe and that they wouldn't get in trouble.

KATRINA: You didn't want to stay here and do the two psychiatrist . . . ?

CAROLE: No, not in Massachusetts, no.

KATRINA: Why not?

CAROLE: Because I didn't want to demean myself. I didn't think I was insane, and I didn't think I was suicidal. And I just . . . well, I didn't think I could convince a psychiatrist, for one thing. My reasons were probably selfish. I had my own plans for the future, for school, and for other things that I wanted to do. And they just didn't include another child. So I didn't think that I could get to a psychiatrist and convince him. I really don't know how you have to convince them that you need an abortion. And if I did convince him, I didn't think that probably my case would be more worthy than someone else's to a hospital board. I think Beverly explained to me the route that you would have to go in Massachusetts. I was aware of it anyway, because I had seen articles in the newspaper about England, when England was the only thing that people used.

So I didn't think Massachusetts was really a possibility. And I also asked my own doctor. He's the head of the hospital board at the hospital that he's affiliated with, and he said that *his* hospital was out. And the other hospitals were the same way. So what PCS gave you was the New York doctors' names and addresses, and then when you called the doctor, they had an appointment ready.

KATRINA: So it was still illegal then—?

CAROLE: Oh, it was perfectly legal. Even though it was a couple of weeks . . . it was the twenty-fourth of June. So this was like a week before the first of July.

KATRINA: Well, that . . . if you had an abortion in a hospital in New York before July first, and without seeing any psychiatrists, I think that would fall under illegal, wouldn't it?

CAROLE: I guess it would, maybe.
Well, as it turned out, with the extra stay in the hospital and the operation and, you know, there were a couple of other doctors involved . . . I don't even know to this day who did the operating. There were two other doctors, I know, that were called in because it was an emergency. So I don't really know who did it. But anyway, the bill turned out to be like about a thousand dollars more. And of course we wouldn't have paid it; I just wouldn't pay it. And so my husband brought down the Blue Cross Blue Shield forms. And on those, when they filled them out, they said that it was a therapeutic abortion. And for the reason—*this* they must have done to protect themselves—they put "Psychiatric." With no further explanations. So with the emergency and everything, they must have somehow pushed it through with the signatures.

KATRINA: You never saw a psychiatrist who made a statement?

CAROLE: No. No, I never did. No.

KATRINA: Do you think the guy must have been a hack? Or, what are your . . . ?

CAROLE: I don't know.

KATRINA: I mean it's a— You know, you "did all the right things." You were in a hospital and— What *are* your feelings now?

CAROLE: I don't know. Well, my doctor checked for me in his book—I don't know what they call it—of qualifications, doctors and their qualifications. And I don't really remember exactly, but I think that this man had only recently graduated, or finished his training. Even though he was an older man. He was probably fifty-five. And I think that his certification, or whatever, was pending. So in other words he hadn't been, maybe, practicing long enough, or something. But he was in association with another doctor who *was* certified. My doctor checked this for me, beforehand. But, see, the doct. . . . He wasn't the doctor I expected to have do the abortion. It was his associate that I expected to do the abortion. And . . . I was surprised. But I wasn't turned off by the idea, because my own doctor's associate had delivered my first child. So I just figured, you know, one or the other, it didn't make any difference.

So I really don't know—what the story was. But—it's hard to say. I can't say it was his fault; but then again it might have been his fault, you never know.

When I came back, my own doctor— My impression of doctors is, they stick together, and they're very ethical, and they don't say things about their colleagues. But my doctor said, "All I can say is, he must have been a rank amateur."

And that blew my mind. I couldn't believe that he'd said that. He examined me afterward, you know, for a check-up, to make sure everything was okay. Of course he couldn't see the inside of the uterus or anything, but he checked the incision; there was some adhesion in the incision. I guess it's maybe not the best job that could have been done. But in the circumstances, at least I'm still alive. And still functioning. But he thinks that perhaps I wouldn't be able to get pregnant again. Even if I wanted to, I might not be able to have anymore children.

But I just couldn't imagine what would cause him to say anything that harsh about one of his colleagues. He didn't explain to me exactly why he said that. That's one thing that really aggravates me about doctors: they never seem to tell you what they find. I know a little bit about my own body, and I've taken biology courses, zoology courses, so I know what I'm made of. But they just treat you like a child, and I —I—that makes me angry. Of course I was glad he told the truth. It's just that he never elaborated why he said that. At least he could have told me why he said something that harsh about another doctor.

KATRINA: You said earlier, your husband didn't go with you.

CAROLE: No.

KATRINA: You said "Of *course*" he didn't go with you.

CAROLE: Well, he's very busy, he's in business with his father and it's just the two of them, and he just . . . he would have gone with me; he wanted to, and I said, "It's no problem, I'll be home in two days." I'm fairly independent, and I didn't mind going. I have friends in New York, and I just got on the train and went myself. And I had a baby-sitter which I got at the last minute, you know, and he was going to come home at night and relieve the baby-sitter. And I didn't know whether I *could* get a baby-sitter who could stay all day, day and night. This was a younger girl, a high-school girl. So I said, "No problem, I'll go by myself." There was really no need for him to come. I'd had two children, I'd been in and out of the hospital before. So I wasn't really apprehensive about it. And I—I just figured all along that D&C was a simple procedure and there was no cause to be anxious about it.

But he came down after the doctor called him. I had the abortion on Wednesday, and he couldn't really even get away until Saturday. So that wasn't too good either. Well, the people that I knew came to visit me; but I was on narcotics so I was not feeling . . . I wasn't really aware of what was happening, anyway. So it wouldn't have helped much if he had come. But he came Saturday and stayed for the weekend, and then I came home the next Thursday or Friday.

KATRINA: Are you a counselor here?

CAROLE: Yes. The green sheet that they give you after you're interviewed—which is to follow-up the feedback—I sent back, and I told them how angry I was about the whole mistake. And that I thought that— What made me angry was that my own doctor, who's very competent—he's the head obstetrician at the hospital—that he couldn't help me out. Morally he would have, but legally he couldn't. And I know this wouldn't have happened if he had done the abortion. And that's what made me angry. That I had to go and be in someone else's hands, that I knew nothing about, just because I—well—made a mistake and was pregnant.

I told them that I was angry about that, and if there was anything that I could do, come in, answer the phone, or whatever, I would do it. And I would be glad to give some time because I thought I could get this same girl who baby-sat for me—she was very good with the children. So I figured that I could get her a couple of afternoons a week, if they needed help. Then Beverly called and said, you know, how sorry she was about it, and that they would like to have me.

So I came in and I went through the counselor-training. That was last August, and I've been coming in two afternoons a week since then. It's . . . it helps a lot. I can identify with a lot of . . . especially the younger girls, you know, who find themselves pregnant and in school, and don't know whether to get married or whatever. With a lot of people I think that getting married isn't the right answer.

KATRINA: But when a girl comes in, whom you're counseling, mightn't you be reluctant, in a way, to send her off to New York? After what you've been through . . . I mean, how *do* you feel about it?

CAROLE: I just feel that mine was maybe one in—I don't know how many—maybe a million. And it was really probably no one's fault. It was just an accident. And I just feel that even though she has to go to New York, and she's probably half afraid that she's going to get lost, and she's not even met the doctor who— Half of the girls who come in here have never even been to a doctor or had an internal exam. And the whole experience is going to be bad, probably, and not very pleasant. But still, on the whole, I think that it would be less traumatic to—to go down to New York and get lost in the city and feel bewildered and have all these *things* happen to her—would be less traumatic than having a child. So, you know, it's like the lesser of two evils. Massachusetts is out of the question for most of the girls. So New York is—as bad as it is—is still better than—than having a child if you don't want one, or you can't afford one, or . . . whatever your reasons might be. I don't think that anyone's reasons really need to be questioned. If someone is really sincere in—in wanting an abortion. And, with the questionnaire, and just talking, we try and make sure that they are; that they're not being pressured by anyone else. You know, find out if it's their own decision.

KATRINA: And you feel all right, sending them to New York, to a clinic, or to a doctor's office, even though you—in the same situation—might have died?

CAROLE: That's right. That's the way I justify it. But also I've read that there's less danger in having an abortion than in having a child. So, I could have died when I had my second baby, if that's the—you know—the question.

KATRINA: Have you had any regrets about . . . ?

CAROLE: None. No. None. I just . . . I keep so busy, I don't really have time to think about it. We have so much fun with the two children that we have; doing things. And now the baby is two and he's started to be trained. It's just so much more fun now that he's getting a little older. If we had a new baby we would be tied down that much more. We like to do outdoor things and this is impossible with a baby, canoeing, and camping, and things like that. So I just feel that it's better for me, and it's better for the children, and better for my husband.

KATRINA: Was your husband behind you all the time?

CAROLE: Oh yes. Oh yes, 'cause we had talked about this when we had planned the second baby. We decided this was enough. There's not that much room in the world. And there's not that much room for me to do the things that I want to do and children also. We decided that two would be fine. And especially when it was a son, because he did want a son. We were just happy to have *him* and decided that that was all we wanted, and all we needed.

Just a couple of days ago, Beverly told me that a woman called and wanted to talk to someone who would be about due, someone who had had an abortion last year in the springtime. This woman was worried about the traumatic birth—I don't know what they call it—syndrome. And Beverly asked me to talk to her, since it would be about now for me. And I said to myself, "Gee, I've never even thought about that. It would be due right about now." But it just, you know, doesn't enter my mind at all. I did think about it a little then, and I mentioned it to my husband and he said, "Oh no." Then he said "Wait, that *is* true; it would be right about now." But it never really entered my mind before she mentioned it. So I guess it doesn't bother me, you know.

KATRINA: Do you feel any particular sense of relief? In other words, not the negative I've been asking about, but a particularly positive difference? Or is it more matter-of-fact?

CAROLE: I find myself much happier now. I get out of the house two afternoons and two evenings, between PCS and school, so I find myself much happier than I was. And the kids and I have much more fun when I'm home, now that I do get out, and have other interests, and get to talk to people, rather than being stuck home with "Mummy! Mummy!" and dirty diapers all day long. So I—I think the feelings *are* more positive. And the negative feelings just aren't there.

KATRINA: Can you attribute this directly to the abortion? or could it be more everything else?

CAROLE: Well, the school—I was going to school before. But PCS has helped a lot. I've made a lot of friends here, and it is rewarding. Some people just come in, and all they want is a name and address. But some people are really helped by having somebody to talk to. And you feel as if you've maybe done something to help, you know, made somebody smile that day, or whatever. And so *that* I can attribute to the abortion. Just because I probably would have, if I had had an abortion with no complications, come back and sent the green sheet in, and maybe made a contribution, and that would have been the end of it. So, I guess that's one positive result that came out of the whole experience. This coming in here and volunteering, and meeting the friends that I have. So, yes, there is a positive side to it.

KATRINA: I want to ask you a little bit about your first child because it's— That could have been one of the cases you were counseling.

CAROLE: Right.

KATRINA: You could have had an abortion then.

CAROLE: I guess I could have.

KATRINA: But does the fact that she arrived too early—as they say—do you think about it? Or, what—?

CAROLE: Oh, I think about it a lot. I used to think about it more because I— Well, I used to be unhappy, I think, a lot of the time. Because I just would say, "Here I am, only nine-teen, twenty, and I graduated from high school and went one year in college, and I was always a good student, and I had a scholarship." And I just used to think all the time, "What am I doing? I shouldn't be here, I shouldn't be a mother. I had all these other plans, and I never had a chance to carry them through." So I think that if—if I were eighteen now, and pregnant, I *would* have an abortion. But then there was just no question of it, because it was illegal. Well, that was five years ago and I don't know where it was legal. I guess maybe Japan. And I didn't have that money. I—I suppose that from my in-laws and my parents I could have *gotten* that much money, but not without having them know what it was for, and they never would have agreed.

KATRINA: Do you feel guilty that you— You think, "If I were eighteen now and had it to do over again, I probably would have had an abortion." Do you feel, then, *guilty* that you could think such a terrible thing about your child? Which it can sort of be twisted to—

CAROLE: No.

I—I see what you're driving at. Uhm.

She's—she's really terrific. And it would be a shame if —if rather than being Jenny, she were an abortion. But then again, the second one is fine and terrific; and so I could have had her, probably, again. You know, like right now, if I were just getting married now. So, you know, it's a hard thing to talk about, "If everything were different." It's just hypothetical.

Oh, I always wonder what I missed. This is also why I like to counsel younger girls. Because I—I used to more than I do now—but I always wondered what I missed while I was young, and was able to go here and there—and single—and do what I wanted to, and work, or do whatever—travel. Just having a child and settling right down, you always wonder, I think, what you might have done if you hadn't settled down so early. I think that seventeen, eighteen, is too young to decide your whole life with one man and one family. As it is, we've worked it out pretty well I think. He had quite a bit of money saved; we didn't have financial problems. We had known each other for a long time so we knew we were fairly compatible, even though we were only seventeen. So we've worked it out pretty well; but I . . . for most people, and even for myself, it would have been different. But for most people, I think it's too young to decide that big a question. Regardless of the fact that when you're eighteen you think, "Oh, I'm an adult and I can make these decisions." And you *can* make them; but they're not necessarily the right ones. You don't have enough background to—to know if that's exactly what you want. So that's another reason why I don't feel quite so guilty about sending off some sixteen-year-old to New York to have an abortion, rather than to send her off. . . .

I think an abortion is also less traumatic than having a child and giving it up. You would wonder all your life, every little child, "I wonder if that's mine," "What would he or she be like now?" I don't believe that I could ever have a child and give it up. I could have an abortion and forget that, much easier than I could have a child and give it up. Even if I never saw the child, and even if they never told me whether it was a boy or a girl. I would still always wonder. Oh, I wouldn't like to have that on my mind!

KATRINA: Are you using your birth control better now?

CAROLE: Right. Well, I didn't go back on the pill because I do still have the infection. I figured, after *this* I couldn't possibly—you know, after this whole D&C and the whole other business. But I do. So I haven't gone back on the pill. We use a condom and the foam now; and I should finish school in May, and I want to have my tubes tied then. My doctor has agreed to do it for me.

KATRINA: Is that hard to get? Legally?

CAROLE: I guess it depends on the doctor. It's legal. There's no problem as long as you get a doctor who'll consent to do it. But I guess most doctors don't, if you're young. My doctor will, because he knows what I've been through and he knows that I've made up my mind and there's no changing it. Plus I've tried other birth control. I've had a loop, and that didn't work out; I bled all the time. And so —there's not too much left.

KATRINA: Your parents-in-law had tried to talk you out of the abortion. Did they then give you a hard time?

CAROLE: He never spoke to me about it, my father-in-law. He told my mother-in-law that he didn't want her to babysit for the children. My parents and his parents are fairly close to us and they babysit for us quite a bit. And he told her that he just didn't want her to volunteer to babysit while I was in New York, because he didn't want any part of it. And he never mentioned it to me. So that was his part. And her part was, she came over and talked to me. I told her my reasons, and she said she could understand my reasons but she had just always been taught and always believed that this was— well, I don't know, fetucide, or whatever; that it was a life. And I said that I didn't consider it a life, that it was a mistake. And it wouldn't be a life until the baby was born, and I just didn't want the baby to be born. So she—she's a nice woman and she understood my reasons—and she just said, "Well, I guess you've made up your mind." And I said yes.

My mother—I didn't tell my mother; she has problems of her own and I thought, "Well, maybe I'll tell her afterward; sometime we'll just have coffee and I'll explain to her." But as it was, my poor mother had *more* problems, because she called the house while I was away and talked to the baby-sitter; and she thought that I had left my husband. Because at this point I had been gone for a week. She didn't want to interfere, because she had had the same situation one time with my grandfather while she was away one time; and my grandfather had had my father believing that she had run off with another man. And so my poor mother wasn't knowing what happened for about two weeks, until I came home. When I finally talked to her she said, "Ah! I'm relieved it was only an abortion! I thought you had been divorced, and I never knew anything about it."

I never talked about it with my father. I don't know whether she mentioned it to him or not, but I never said anything about it and he never said anything to me about it. He's—he's sort of old-fashioned and this is like, you know "women's problems." So he—he wouldn't say anything about it.

As it was, it worked out fine with my mother because she was relieved that it was—quote—"only an abortion." That it was not something more *serious*—to *her* something more serious: that I up and left my kids and my husband and went off to parts unknown. I think she's right, too. And I was so glad to hear it, because I thought she was going to be vindictive and, you know, "How could you do such a thing?"

But as it was it's . . . I think I've always underestimated my parents anyway. Because at the time I was pregnant, when I was eighteen, I—I was just so *afraid* to even go home. And—and—my boyfriend went over— I was at school, and he went over and told my father that we were going to be married, and I was pregnant. And my father accepted it very well, and he shook his hand, you know—But I was terrified, I figured, "Oh, I don't dare go home! They'll kill me!" And as it was, I—I've always underestimated them.

So, you know, it helped that she said that, too. Because since then I think I've been even closer to her. Because I can open up a little more now and see that she's not quite so old-fashioned as I thought she was all along.

And my mother-in-law, too, when she heard I'd been sick, she said, "Gee," she said, "I wish you had told Ronald to call me and he could have brought the kids over here and made it a little easier." She said, "Oh, you should have let us know that you were, you know, in the hospital and going through this terrible thing like that. Even if we couldn't come down and see you, we could have at least tried to make things easier on Ronald and the kids." And that was . . . I thought it was nice of her to say that, too.

KATRINA: If someone said to you, "Ah, you were just seeking the abortion you never had the first time." How would you react to that comment?

CAROLE: I've never thought of that.

Uhm. I would only say, "I don't know. I'm not a psychiatrist. And this could be." But the reasons I had at the time. . . . Maybe subconsciously that entered into it, but consciously it didn't.

KATRINA: In your counseling, in your knowledge of other people, do you feel that this ever *could* be an accusation?

CAROLE: I don't think so. I think it— Well, [*laughs*] unless you may be a masochist! Which I don't think I am. I don't know why anyone would want to have an abortion, just to have an abortion. No, I think it was just a mistake and it just happened to come up. But this could be, I suppose. I don't know. Now I start to wonder.

KATRINA: Maybe I shouldn't have brought it up. You know, because—

CAROLE: Oh no, it doesn't matter. I just feel so strongly about it, that it wouldn't bother me.

Now there's a bill that's coming up in the legislature, in the Massachusetts legislature, to establish the rights of the fetus. Which is completely absurd. They've never even established the rights of children. Or women. Now how can they justify establishing the ri—? And one of the rights is the right to protect property—something, protect and own, or protect and preserve, or however they have that legal gibberish. But, for the *fetus?* I just think this is absurd. It's—it's amazing to me that they can. . . . They dream up these things. And how a man can even talk about a fetus. They haven't got the *vaguest* notion of what it's like to *carry* a fetus and what goes through your mind. How can they establish the rights of a fetus to own property? It's absurd. They could better be spending their time making sure that the fetus is getting enough vitamins, and that the fetus's home is getting sufficient milk. I mean, rather than establish the fetus's right to life, liberty, and the pursuit of happiness, why not establish its right to be born healthy, and at least have a good start on it? Or its right to be wanted?

ANNIE

ANNIE: I knew I was pregnant. I have two children. Unlike what I did before—I had gone to an obstetrician to confirm the pregnancy—this time I had such negative feelings about the idea of being pregnant, that I went to a laboratory. My husband took the little sample for me. This was seven days after I was late, and the confirmation was done right away.

KATRINA: How old were your children?

ANNIE: My children were eight and six, an eight-year-old girl and a six-year-old boy. We had just moved here from another city.

Maybe I should backtrack a little bit.

I took the pill for five years after my son was born, on the advice of my obstetrician. He said to me, in reference to using a diaphragm, "Oh, you're such a spontaneous person, of course a diaphragm would not work out for you." This really left me, psychologically, with only one alternative— Since I was so spontaneous, the pill was the only thing. And he said, then, that I should not take it for more than two years at a time. But every time I went back to him, he okayed it for two more years.

Then I began to read reports that made me uncomfortable. I did not like the fact that I was taking something which was doing things to my body that I wasn't really sure about. And at that time we thought even about having a third child. With the pressure of the population explosion, and feeling very sensitive to the social situation—that is, of bringing another child into the world—there were a lot of questions to weigh. But we first decided that I should protect my own body. I was at that point frightened that, in fact, I had done something to my body. I stopped using the pill and didn't use anything.

Our thinking evolved then, to hoping that I would get pregnant. We decided we wanted to have another child. Twice before, when I wanted to get pregnant, I did. But this time nothing happened for a year. I began to suspect that I was in that category of women who have become sterile on the pill. I knew that there were women who had taken the pill, and then wanted to have children, and were not able to get pregnant. And here in my mind was the fact that I had taken it for five years.

So, well, we moved, and our lives took on a different form. By this time I was really sure that I was sterile, and that it was no longer an option whether or not I would have another child. But, certainly, in the back of my mind there was also that testing . . . of wondering: What have I done? What has happened to my body? And I realize now that this was a part of my getting pregnant. It only happened after the abortion: that I could really see there had been something to being able to say, "Well, I can get pregnant. I haven't done myself irrevocable harm."

Also, in reference to the move: I had had a job that I really liked where we lived before. It was teaching. It wasn't easy for me to move. But I did. For my husband it meant a new job that he really wanted to do. So, as I had done before, I adjusted myself to the fact that we were moving to another city. But again, in terms of my feelings, I viewed getting pregnant—because I was not using anything—as a solution to a lot of problems. I mean, what else does one do? This was my view. I had worked, I had always enjoyed working, and I love children. Also, I had passed my thirtieth birthday a year before, and here I was, faced with—What am I going to do with my life? That's a very real question to deal with when you've just given up a job that you really like. And I think all of those feelings were tied up with why I got pregnant. I don't know whether one wants to say it was a kind of—almost a hostility toward my husband, almost a subconscious anger that we had left where we were living. Although, in reality, we had discussed all of that. And we had discussed even *not* leaving, because I was so happy in my work. But I think those feelings were tied up: wondering whether I could ever have another child, whether I should accept being over my child-bearing years, dealing with— now that my children were of school age and I had this free time—what I was going to do. It's not that easy to get a job here. The unemployment rate is very high. Teachers are— they have waiting lists a mile long. All of those things, now, looking back, fed into my getting pregnant.

At that time, my involvement in the Women's Movement had been a very peripheral thing. I was sympathetic to it, and I had friends who were involved, but my interest was never really on a personal level. And this fall I received a phone call asking if I would be interested in getting together a women's group. I had more time than I had had in a long time. It sounded good. . . .

KATRINA: This was before you knew you were pregnant?

ANNIE: This was about a month before I knew I was pregnant.

KATRINA: And, just to be clear: it was still possible you might one day have more children?

ANNIE: Yes, oh yes. But now we weren't trying. And I worried about sterility. Again, that wasn't a very defined thing. I'm talking about feelings, now, all of those floating things.

So a group of us started meeting. And it was an amazing clicking of human beings. Most of the women in the group were women who were very much in my situation. I mean, I would describe myself as being happily married. I married young, and a lot of those things I had planned— I had thought I was going to wait until I was twenty-eight before I got married. I met my husband when I was seventeen, and we got married when I was twenty, when I was in college. And we both had never had any sexual relations with anyone else. Or in fact with each other. We didn't have intercourse before we married. That's how it was. We both had a very moralistic background that way.

And we really kind of grew up together. My husband was in seminary when we got married. He's a minister, an ordained minister. We worked in a church, and lived in the inner city for six years. Our life was very much shared by a lot of other people. Our children were born into a community kind of situation. That was another thing that was really interesting: when I tried to deal with the fact that I was pregnant, I realized how isolated I felt from people. I was new here, I was no longer a part of that rich community as I had once been. In the neighborhood that we had lived in, our friends were also having babies, and so we kind of brought up our young children together. Whether they were welfare mothers, or colleagues, or neighbors, I didn't feel isolated. Here I felt very, very trapped. That was one of the things that I really thought about, in considering having a third child.

But anyway, in terms of the group: we met, and as I started to say, most of the other women were in situations similar to mine. They all had a couple of children. They would call their marriages happy; that is: they have hopes, they're working on their marriages, and they affirm those marriages. There are two younger women, in their early twenties. The rest of us are around thirty. And I can't think of one person who came there who had ever been involved in any kind of a militant way, or even strongly, with the Women's Movement. We had all been on the fringe, and very interested. And it just became clear from the very beginning that we could all trust each other, and that we respected each other. We talked about ourselves immediately. Then, after a month—just a month or five weeks of being in this group—I discovered that I was pregnant. I found out on a Monday. It was confirmed that I was pregnant, and I was so upset that I went to bed that night and just slept. I had a terrible feeling of tiredness. My husband and I, we didn't even talk. We were both visibly shaken by the news, and I went to bed.

The next night was my women's meeting. And we decided that I should go ahead to the women's meeting, and that we would—in terms of us dealing with this—that we would deal with it another time. I got to the women's meeting, and somebody turned to me and said, "Annie, you really look concerned, you look worried about something tonight." And suddenly I—it just came out, I just started talking. . . .

And what was amazing was that I somehow was able to speak with the utter confidence—I hope that I can somehow relate this feeling to you—the total confidence that my feelings would not be judged by these people, that they could accept me for whatever I wanted to say about how I felt. And my feelings were very ambivalent. I was saying things like, "I'm pregnant, and I'm so upset about it."

Two women said, "I just want you to know right now that I've had an abortion." One said it, and then the other one, and my response was: how the whole idea of an abortion was just so foreign to me. *Abortion?* This thing that society deals with in such a heavy way that . . . ME? I'm such a *straight! I'm* the person who—

And all of these very, very negative feelings about abortion came out. But what was interesting, what came out was not how *I* felt about abortion, but how I knew society viewed it. And what also came out was how I did not want this pregnancy. I had gotten into this situation and the reasons were beginning to appear. I mean, I wouldn't have been able to guess that my hostile feelings toward my husband for having moved here, or that I was now over thirty—all of those reasons that I mentioned before—that these were at work. But those things began to come out as I was talking. And I began to realize how, for me, it was very very important that I have control over my body and over my life.

Then I started to talk a lot about my two children. And how much getting pregnant and being pregnant with them had meant to me. What it had meant, having them both by natural childbirth. And the next thing that became so obvious to me was the utter respect that I *do* have for human life. How their births were such an affirmation of that. But, to give birth because a sperm and an egg bumped into each other, and not to have the courage to do something about that happening—to go ahead and fulfill a pregnancy that was really so foreign to what my other two pregnancies had been—would be wrong!

I kept talking, and I had the freedom— I didn't worry about whether I was going to sound crazy or like some horribly immoral person. All of those feelings that I really felt, I was able to say to this group of six or eight women.

KATRINA: Your other children had been very planned, or very desired?

ANNIE: Absolutely planned, down to the month. My children were so many months apart, because that's what we had decided. I was very, very lucky that it all worked out the way it did. They were very, very planned. And my pregnancies were marvelous, and my husband went to the classes with me, and natural childbirth, and he was in the delivery room. For us—both of us—those experiences were ones that—that we'll cherish together forever.

And those experiences made it possible for me to really deal with the *un*wanted pregnancy. I had to realize my strengths in that. And this is what the other women helped me to see. I mean, they kept asking me questions. It wasn't them suggesting any course.

Well, that evening ended, and they left with the feeling that I was really freaked out about abortion, that abortion was a totally strange notion to me.

KATRINA: They had the impression that you were very antiabortion?

ANNIE: Anti—in terms of myself—yes. I think I could have dealt with it for anyone else, but for *me*—I never viewed myself as somehow doing anything in that way. I mean I'm a very—I always viewed myself as a very orderly kind of person. By the planning of my children, by—I never thought of myself having to be put in that kind of a position. Society has made this such an extreme thing to do.

KATRINA: After that evening, did you change your point of view?

ANNIE: Well, after that evening, my— Again, my husband and I had not even had a chance to talk to each other about it! I never would have planned it that way. Because my husband and I, we do have our history. Our relationship is such that we talk to *each other* about things. But it was that strange combination of not—of going ahead to the women's meeting.

Then, that night, we did talk. And what was amazing about that, when you consider the timing, was that when we were able to talk to each other, it was one of the most—one of the closest times between us. We were able to talk about it, and there was an amazing sense of calmness on my part. We found we could discuss my being pregnant in a very rational way. It was as if all of the emotional confusion, all of those things that were floating around in my head, I had gotten out. It wasn't that I had mentally made any kind of decision —because, still, we had not talked—but I found myself, with my husband, discussing abortion. Bringing up that whole possibility.

And my husband—his feelings, I should say, were that he was very satisfied with having two children. His inclinations were, like mine, that it's kind of hard, when you've had a very good experience and you love little children, to think about not having anymore. There's that element of, "Gee, that part of my life is over." So even for him it was a possibility of having a third, but he was more inclined not to. His feelings about abortion were certainly not as emotional as mine. Obviously, being a man. And he does not have moralistic feelings about abortion. He also very, very much feels that people ought to be in control of their own bodies. And, interestingly enough, even as my husband of eleven years, he felt that in fact it was *my* decision really, because it was my body. We shared this together. It's not that he— It was a very sensitive situation. He felt a part of it in many ways. Yet he felt that he could support any decision that I made. And he was absolutely responsible for having me really consider the possibility of *having* the child. We talked about that a lot, and about our feelings. And together we realized that we didn't want this, that this was not *us*. That our lives had been such that in fact we were *strong* enough to absorb, and to take the brunt of an abortion.

Of course, it didn't become definite, that night we talked together. We felt this was something that we should really take our time about. It was very early in my pregnancy, and I had time to deal with it.

I don't know how else to put it except to say that our decision was really made on our strengths. For me, it was a matter of having enough confidence in myself as a human being to be able to say: I know that I'll have feelings afterward. How can anybody not? Feeling empty, feeling— But I will cope with these feelings. I don't need to hide from them. I'm pregnant now, but, my God, will I bring a child into the world simply because I am too afraid of having to face my *feelings?* No, we are too strong. We love each other too much. Our children. The whole philosophy of: we affirm life; and so, therefore, we cannot treat it in such a shabby way as to say we are not strong enough to have an abortion. What happened was an error, and I am going to undo it. And undo it out of my feeling of strength.

What I had to deal with, for me, was that terrible weight. I am very conscious, personally, of what society says about abortions. I think that, as I tried to consider all of the reasons for having the child, that child would have been symbolic of all my weaknesses: that I hadn't had the courage to handle it, that it was not what I wanted, and that somehow nine months later this thing had happened because I hadn't been able to do anything about it.

And interestingly enough—also during this time—it was not a decision that we would *never* have anymore children. We absolutely acknowledged that probably our feelings were such that it would be very, very nice to have a third child. But that it was going to be done the way it had been done before. And with those same kinds of feelings.

KATRINA: How long ago was this abortion?

ANNIE: Six or seven weeks ago. It was early December.

And I should say that in terms of me, as a person, psychologically, the afterthoughts—the feelings that I thought I would have—I've had some of them. I think that it's really important to be honest about this. For Christmas, I gave my daughter a stuffed animal. And I did it, knowing, being able to stand there in the store and know that I—for an *eight-year-old?* She loved it! And finding myself during the holidays walking through the baby section, just to kind of put myself through these tests—and realizing why I was doing it. But also realizing, you know, that I was thinking that I *should* have certain feelings, and that I *should* feel all of this. And, in fact, I was very relieved, and very satisfied, and I felt very close to my children and to my husband for what we had done together.

And the only reason I want to be at all secretive about this— And I feel badly about that. I think it's wrong for me to have to be anonymous. I think that's *society*'s hang-up. And that's what I want to work on now— But this secrecy is really in terms of protection of my children. You see, I feel that my children could handle our telling them. What I don't think that they could handle would be the response of people to them, with that information. Their grandparents—there's a whole sector of people who would be very burdened by knowing. I love these people and I accept them for what they are, but their feelings are different.

The other thing I'd like to backtrack on a little bit is that, obviously, when I say all of these things, all of my feelings —those feelings certainly didn't come *out* like that. But those feelings came out of a process of my women's group, in my collective, where they were able to throw back at me the things I was saying about my children, about my pregnancies with them, about having planned their births. These things didn't come out just . . . I mean, it all sounds very neat, now. It wasn't that way, obviously. I was in a very anxious time, and my anxiety was hanging out all over. I couldn't make much sense. And that's where, for me, I view that experience as having been so important. I feel that these people helped me figure those things out.

At one meeting I explored the possibility of going through a legal abortion right here in Rhode Island, which would have meant going to a psychiatrist. But I couldn't have been honest with a psychiatrist. I mean, to go to a psychiatrist to ask for an abortion in a hospital, you have to indicate that you're somewhat crazy, or that you couldn't deal with a child. I could have dealt with that child. I wouldn't have tossed the child out of a third-floor window. And I couldn't say things I didn't believe. Also, the vulnerability of such a position was very distasteful to me. The whole idea of going to a psychiatrist, and then having *him* decide what *I* should do—really I find it absurd. Now I'm not against the psychiatric route. I think, for some women, it's a very important thing. But for me, it would have meant that the psychiatrist was the one in control. And for me, that issue was probably most important.

And my experience in this women's group was that their approach was not at all manipulative. The people just cared for me as a human being, and it didn't matter to them one bit what I did. Whatever I might have decided, they would have supported me. What they were concerned about was me as an individual, and helping me find out what I wanted to do. Never, at any time, did I feel any kind of coercion. Do you know what I mean? It didn't even seem important what these people felt, or thought. There was no sense of judgment, at all. It's difficult to describe. It doesn't happen with very, very many people.

KATRINA: Do you think that in your previous community, where you had such closeness and so many friends, the people would have been as helpful?

ANNIE: No, I don't think so. In terms of the kind of situation we lived in, sharing everything—assets, liabilities, children we were helping out with, meals eaten together—our lives were completely embedded in that church kind of community. It's hard to imagine, but I think that if I had been faced then with this problem, it would have been only a personal thing, only between my husband and me. The decision would not have been made with the others. And the reason, again, is control—that I would have really wanted to do what *we* wanted to do, and not to have it be influenced by all kinds of other things; that is, by people who knew us so well that they just couldn't bear the brunt of it: influenced by feelings that were theirs, their own personal involvement, the suffering to *them.* You see, that's another thing that I found out. People feel very burdened by this. Again, I think what society has done . . . the weight of it, is fantastic.

I heard a newscast on the radio the other day—to give you an example in terms of dealing with my children—with somebody from a church discussing whether one is considered a *murderer.* And my daughter was listening, and she looked at me in a very quizzical way, and she didn't say anything. But I thought, "Just imagine what she is receiving! The *force* of society's judgments!" That's a very very heavy thing in our society.

KATRINA: Is your husband still in the ministry?

ANNIE: No.

KATRINA: How does he feel, theologically speaking?

ANNIE: As I said, I think that for him, the abortion was ultimately the only sensible thing to do, the only *real* thing to do. And I would simply have to reiterate what I already said, that for him it was *affirming* life.

The way both of us feel—to us, *life* is so important. This has occurred to me so many times while I was going through this. I felt, while reading statements— You see, I really tried to put my ideas to the test. I wanted to expose myself, almost, sometimes, in a brutal way, to all of the other arguments. Just to see, because I really— And I found that in many cases the loudest spokesmen *against* abortion are those who are *for* our presence in Vietnam. I can't tell you how many times that analogy has gone through my head. Here we, as a country, are dropping bombs on people, and children are getting killed; and I find that absolutely disgusting. And I will do anything in order to help end that war. *That* to me is destroying human life. We have these laws on abortion that are just absurd, and then there are children who are hungry. After living in the inner city and really seeing how people in *this* country aren't cared for . . . I mean, I really care about life! I think that *that's* what we should be working on.

My view, as I said— To me, it was absolutely a collision between a sperm and an egg, and I don't feel at all that I did away with a human being. Nor does he. The point was that I was able to make a decision as an independent person. I had control over my own life and body. And I think that's really important.

KATRINA: Does your husband feel as good about it, now, as you do?

ANNIE: Absolutely. I'd say the only difference in our feelings, since, has been that afterward I tended to talk about it more than he did. He responded to me, but he did not really initiate talking about it. It frankly was not that big a deal. The big deal was making the decision and getting it over with. Then, after that, we wanted to simply continue our life.

And in terms of still dealing with being thirty-one, still dealing with all of those— No, those things didn't all disappear. And I knew that they wouldn't. But I also knew that by making that decision I was dealing with those things. And it was like proof to myself that I have the strength to really cope with those feelings. And as far as my relationship with my husband, and my relationship with my children— Now, I can so deeply sense the solidity of these relationships. Of course, they were solid before. It would be wrong to paint a picture of tremendous change. It's more solid than maybe it was for a few months, what with the moving, and all that. But I really view this as part of a continuing thing, as just one more important event in our relationship.

Even the whole experience of having gone through that abortion. That's like another whole story. As it was becoming clear that I was leaning toward the New York abortion, two women from the women's group said, "Listen, whatever you decide, you can count on us." They each said it to me individually. "We will drive you down to New York, if that's what you want. Or we'll take care of your kids, if you want your husband to go. Do whatever you want. We want to help in any way, whatever you decide." And that lifted such a weight off my shoulders. I realized that, in fact, half of what I'd got caught up in was having to figure out the whole mechanics of it, having to go through all of the degrading phone calls, the response of receptionists. And what my husband and I really found ourselves feeling was that the children should be cared for by him. That was what we wanted. And I drove down with the two other women, in one day, and came back.

And for my husband it was very, very meaningful to him to be staying with the children while I went with the other women. He just thought that was utterly fantastic. To him, you see, he was responding about two other people caring about *me*. And when you love each other, you share what . . . you share your *lives* with each other. He was so deeply impressed by the care and by the response of the women in the group. Just absolutely fantastic. I mean, to the point of his being really overcome by that. You see, for us those were things we always hoped for, and looked for in the church. And, frankly, *here* . . . I mean, all the things that we had always talked about, all the names that we had for community, and love, and all that. Here, these things were real. They weren't called all of these names, but they—it was happening.

What comes clear from all of this, is how important it is

that it be one's individual decision. How no one can be suggested into it, coerced into it. But that, instead, what's really important is to help people arrive at the decision they want. And this is not always easy. You see, I guess I really do believe that these women helped me do that. And that perhaps my husband and I alone would not have arrived at that. And this is what I really feel very, very warm and very, very good about. I view this as a political experience as well as a personal experience. I say that, because I think that we all have to work toward allowing people to do what they know they must do. We have to allow people to have control over their own lives. And we must support each other in this. I really think that this is important. And I hope that it really comes through.

SANDY

Interviewed in February 1971

SANDY: In the beginning . . . I guess it has a lot to do with my background and how the whole thing came about. First of all, I'm from the Midwest. I come from a small town. I guess we're fourth generation in this town. It's the kind of setting where all my life I've had to be a particular kind of person, because I come from a particular family. And every year when I go home to visit for a week or so, I have to put on this façade and be who they think I am. Go to all the social functions; do all the right things in their eyes.

I also have a very strict mother who once told me, in high school, that should I ever get in trouble, just to keep going, because she never wanted to see me again. And—she means it. It isn't just a threat, because it would mean that the whole family would have to leave that community. And the reputation that we have built up, my grandfather being mayor for eighteen years, my father a prominent banker—this would all be destroyed. And I also have—well, my father is chairman of a state council for Catholic businessmen. And this council is to prevent the legalization of abortion in our state! So he feels—the whole family feels—tremendously strongly about the whole issue of abortion.

So all that really affected my ideas about sex. I went with

a boy from back home for five years and I went through all the trauma of what to do about a sexual relationship. It was tremendously splitting for me because the boy would come in, several times a year; we would have sexual relations; he would go away; I'd go to confession. The Church was very much a part of my feelings about sex. But the priest always asked me, after I had told him that I had had sexual intercourse, "Did you use any protection?" And I would always say no. And then he would say, "Well that's fine!" So long as I didn't use protection I didn't feel it was that bad. At least I hadn't prepared myself to go to bed with the guy that I was going to marry.

KATRINA: It was "fine" because you hadn't prepared yourself for intercourse? Or because you hadn't used birth control?

SANDY: I think it was both, I think it was both. I could not get it into my mind that I was going to go to bed with this guy. But at least when I owned up to my sin, I didn't have the double sin of having used preventatives. I mean, I was really into the Church and what it said. And particularly what it would say about abortion. I mean, birth control was kind of an issue that I hadn't really figured out for myself. But abortion was a very bad thing—to face.

Well, during my senior year in college, I broke my engagement. And as soon as I graduated, I came out here. Which was mind-blowing in itself. I mean, the family just could not believe that I would go East. Nobody's ever gone East. I had never known anybody who'd ever *been* in Connecticut before!

But I came out here and started teaching and it was a lonely first year. You know, you come to a city and all. . . . The school was out in the suburbs, and I started dating one of the fellows who was teaching there. He was sort of a big brother, really. I had all these uptight feelings about a sexual relationship, and I just refused to get involved, for quite some time. And then we did get involved eventually and it was—

KATRINA: You were how old?

SANDY: Oh, I was twenty-one; I'm only twenty-three now. It's only a couple of years ago.

But at the time, I was having hormone problems, and the doctor had put me on some medication which he didn't really tell me too much about. Later, I learned it had sort of acted as a contraceptive device, in that it gave me an overdose of estrogen or something. But with this medication at least I had regular cycles, and he probably should have told me a lot more about it. But anyway, we were getting involved and I decided, "Well, I'm just not going to take these pills any longer." I mean, I thought that they were making me fertile. So I decided just to stop taking them. And almost immediately, I got pregnant.

KATRINA: Why had the doctor not told you about the pills?

SANDY: He didn't think that I needed to know. I asked him, I said, "Why didn't you tell me this?" after I found out I was pregnant. And he said, "Well, I didn't think you needed to know that kind of information." You know, "I didn't know you were having sexual relations with anyone."

And the guy that was—well, who got me pregnant—he had wanted me to take some kind of contraceptive pill. But I had told him that I just could not force myself to do that, because I felt that it was wrong to prepare myself for a sexual relationship. And so all he did was withdraw. Which was the most, you know, unsatisfactory way in the world. And I —I don't understand his reasoning, because he was older. I mean, he should have known what I didn't know. And we were having intercourse fairly regularly—

KATRINA: So you were really kidding yourself to think that you were being "spontaneously seduced"?

SANDY: Oh yes! Yes, well, my attitudes about sex back then, though, were a continual seduction, you know.

But I was just being very deceitful to myself during the whole period. And this really brought it to the point of reality: I'm pregnant! Neither of us was overly surprised at all. We talked about getting married, and that was just a farce. I mean, we were going to split up at anytime. I just couldn't do it that way. And I couldn't say anything to my family.

We were both teaching in the same school; I moved in with him so that when I started getting sick in the morning, at least somebody would be around. We'd get up real early, I'd get sick, then we'd go to school. He taught across the courtyard from me and whenever he saw me leave the room suddenly, he'd come dashing out to see if I was all right. It was just hell, trying to keep up the appearances and at the same time trying to decide what we were going to do. We went to the courthouse one day, but we just couldn't go through with it.

And so, one night, he and a couple of people who lived across the hall from me had gotten together and had talked about an abortion. And this one girl knew of a guy in Pittsburgh.

So Ted brought up the issue; and I was hysterical. I mean, I packed my bags, I said I was leaving; he could face the issue but I wasn't going to stick around. You see, what it would mean would be—should I just pack my bags and leave the school—there might be a lot of gossip. He was from the town that I taught in. His whole family lived there. So he was very uptight about the place, whereas I really didn't care.

And I really was getting . . . becoming very fond of the idea of being pregnant. Very, very fond of the idea. It was the most stabilizing factor that had occurred to me in a couple of years, anyway. And it was something I really, really wanted; and I was just horrified at—at the thought of abortion.

Yet marriage was—ridiculous. I mean, we talked about it, and each time we talked about it, my stomach would just do flip flops. I just could not marry this guy.

But somehow he got me to at least promise him that whatever was decided, we would decide it together. And so, through a very effective campaign that he and these two girls who lived across the hall from me conducted, I was talked into going to Pittsburg.

KATRINA: Did you consider keeping the baby? Or having the baby and giving it up?

SANDY: I considered leaving town. I didn't get beyond the point of having the baby. I thought, possibly, of going to stay with friends of mine who graduated with me. And . . . I just could not face the idea of giving up that baby.

And I really considered abortion wrong. And I still do. I have never said to myself that abortion is the right thing to do.

I think now my attitude is that abortion, in my case, saved my life as my life is. It left me so that I could still communicate with my family. I could still have a job. It didn't totally destroy everything I was. And it was sort of a choice between me and that baby. But I don't feel that it was right. It, in itself, is not a right thing. Contraception is the right thing: to prevent having babies that you don't want. And all these ideas that people put into your head—that the Church puts into your head—about if you don't use contraception you won't sleep with somebody and therefore you won't get pregnant—just don't work too well.

KATRINA: But you are, really, opposed to abortion?

SANDY: I'm opposed to the idea, yes. I think it's necessary in people's lives. I would effectively work toward the legalization of it. But I think people should really think of it as a deep philosophical question, not just something that happens.

I certainly do feel abortions should be legal. And I think that this is a crime—just *horrible*—what's happening with it being illegal! What's happening to so many of my friends. And particularly it affects me now, as a high-school teacher, because I have students who are getting abortions; and my hands are tied. I can't do anything. And they still have a lot of hang-ups about using contraception. Their mothers say it's wrong for them to use contraceptives, so they get pregnant.

KATRINA: If you had kept the baby, would that have meant the end of your relationship with your parents?

SANDY: Exactly.

KATRINA: You would have lost your job, you would have been alone in the world; you'd have never returned home. And *that* was worse— Am I understanding you correctly?

SANDY: Yes. That was worse. But it wasn't really a conscious decision on my part; I felt more coerced by other people. Because I made two trips to Pittsburg. The first trip to Pittsburg, I was almost three months pregnant. Ted went with me, and I was very, very scared and very uptight, and the whole scene with the doctor was very suspicious. He was a doctor who had this extra office—had no nurse—it was only open in the evenings; you had to call ahead of time. And he inserted something into me, a tube of some sort, which I've heard almost always causes infection, the method that he used. I've heard this since, from secretaries who work for doctors. It's fairly common knowledge that this is an infection-producing means of abortion, and it almost always causes complications.

But the first time it did not take effect. It didn't. And we waited a couple of weeks and . . . I was delighted that I had not aborted. I really didn't want to; this was not my decision.

So, of course, the people across the hall and the guy that was involved in this—they pushed me back on the plane. And this time I had to go by myself. And it wasn't what I wanted to do, at all. There I was, alone, and it was in the middle of the afternoon, and nobody was in his office. He came very late, and I sat outside until he arrived. Then he did the exact same thing that he had done before. This time he gave me all these pills. And he gave me several penicillin shots, he didn't say why. And he gave me pills that I should take very regularly so that I would not hemorrhage when I aborted.

And I went back, and stayed with the guy; and I taught, all week, not knowing when it was going to happen.

Friday evening, after almost a whole week of waiting around, Ted went out that evening and he said, "Do you think you'll be all right?" And I said something like, "Everything will be all right, I don't feel any differently."

After he was gone, I started getting these incredible pains on my left side, just shrieking, terrible, terrible pains. And they just kept coming and coming with no regularity whatsoever, and then I started getting what felt like . . . what I would imagine contractions would be like. A very different kind—not just pain, but something that my body was doing. It was getting rid of something, I could tell.

And after several hours of this, I rushed into the bathroom and I just released this . . . blob; I don't know what it was. By then Ted was there, and I told him what had happened. Then I started having a very heavy flow. But it was all right, and I was just tired.

The next day I seemed fine, just tired. We went for a short walk, we went out to dinner. Then I started getting the sharp pains again—just terribly, terribly sharp.

And I went to bed and I thought, "Well, maybe they'll be all right in the morning." And I sat up most of the night with them 'til about three-thirty in the morning. I—I'd have to grab something, you know, when they would come—

KATRINA: Did it make you cry?

SANDY: Yes! Yes, and finally Ted heard this and woke up. And I got up to go to the bathroom and I just . . . like the bottom half of me just dropped out. I was just covered with blood. And he had to grab towels and bundle me up and call an ambulance—well he didn't call an ambulance, he called a cab—and it was difficult getting dressed, and I was flowing very, very heavily. I had all these pads on me, and towels wrapped around me. And he got me into the cab and we went to Hartford Maternity. He had called my doctor, and fortunately my doctor was there. He was the doctor who had given us shots so that we could get married. He had been in on a much happier scene before, and I had not told him anything about this abortion. In fact, he was such a fatherly kind of person that I didn't want to tell him now. I just—I got to the hospital and I told him I had just miscarried. And he said, "Well, it seems like that was rather fortunate."

KATRINA: "Fortunate"?

SANDY: That we did not have to race into getting married; that I had fortunately miscarried on my own. And I never did tell him about the abortion.

So we raced into the hospital, and first they took me to the labor room, because they didn't know what was going on. Then they took off my coat, and obviously I was not delivering. The doctor came up and examined me and he said that I had lost an awful lot of blood, and that if we had waited a couple more hours, I probably would have died.

And at that point I was getting very, very cold, and things were beginning to black out. I lost my hearing; and I don't know— I know Ted talked with him and then they just took me into the operating room and I was freezing. That's all I can remember. I was just freezing to death; I was so cold.

They performed a D&C. I had to spend a whole week in the hospital, which seemed rather unusual just for a miscarriage D&C. But I kept having these pains on my left side. And I should have told the doctor, then, that I had had this illegal abortion, because it *was* an infection. That was what was causing the pains. It was these pains that kept me in the hospital for so long.

And for weeks afterward I had trouble walking, and just getting around. Then it sort of went away. It wasn't until mid-summer that I started getting the pains again. And I went to a doctor. This time I wanted to go to an entirely different office; I didn't want to see the same doctor; I just. could not own up to the fact that I had had this abortion. So I went to this other guy whom I didn't know at all, and he wanted to operate right away. He wanted me to sign this thing saying that—should they find infection or something like that—He told me there was a large mass inside of me the size of a grapefruit, and that it was probably one of my ovaries which was infected. And he said, "Now, I want you to sign this release that we can do a hysterectomy on you."

Well, that terrified me. And so, fortunately, I went to two or three other doctors, and I found out that this guy is known to be a butcher.

This was . . . let's see, I had the abortion the beginning of May—this was now the end of August. I'd had the infection all this time. It was just never gotten rid of, you see.

And so I finally called my family. I did not tell them, of course, the reason; but I told them that I had this infection. I'd had menstrual problems all through college, so my mother's theory was, "Well, now we finally know what the problem is," and she just didn't question any further than that.

So, since I knew that I would be spending about a month recovering after I got home from the hospital, and that this would be difficult if I were by myself, my family talked me into coming home for it. I didn't really know exactly what the operation was going to be. But they thought that they were going to have to remove one ovary, anyway.

And so I decided to go home. I met the doctor, and the only thing that really made me very uptight was I was terrified of telling him the story. Because I know all the nurses in the hospital; I know all the personnel in the hospital; it's a small town, and things like that do get out. I did tell him, but I felt very, very hesitant about it. And I still don't know if it ever got back to my family. I sort of suspect my mother thinks there's something more to this whole thing than what I told her and what the doctor told her.

They put me in the maternity ward when they performed the operation. I had spent a week in the maternity ward out here when I had that D&C, and I guess that's just standard procedure. But at home it was particularly traumatic because there *are* no women my age who are not married and do not have children. That is strange enough in itself. But then to be put in with all these other women who just could not understand anything other than the way they were leading their lives—it was difficult.

Well, in this operation they removed the right ovary and tube, because they were completely infected. There were also signs of infection on the other side, but fortunately that was dormant at the time. The doctor told me there's no way to cure the infection; it's just a matter of keeping it down, keeping yourself healthy. And that I would probably someday have to have a hysterectomy, in the not too distant future, but that I should be able to function normally with this one ovary for some time, as long as I maintained my health.

So I was in the hospital a week, and then a month recuperating at home, on top of which I smashed my foot in a door, and had to stay three more weeks. And it was a drag, being home. There was a tremendous amount of pressure on my family's part to keep me there, not let me go back out East. It was "dangerous" out there, "you don't have the health for it." Just a lot of fears that were coming out, you know, "Look what's happened to you," "You're not well," the whole thing.

But I came back two months later. School had already started, but I did get a job. I had not even applied for a job, because when I realized I was pregnant, I just dropped everything. Now it was a matter of góing back and picking everything up.

KATRINA: Did you come back to the same guy?

SANDY: No. He met me at the airport; and we talked, and that was the last time I saw him.

It was just— What had happened between us, we just weren't prepared for at all. We had no kind of relationship that could handle that sort of thing. And, you know, what could he say? What could I say? He felt just absolutely terrible about what had happened to me.

KATRINA: So he was decent, and nice, and supportive—?

SANDY: Oh, yes!

KATRINA: You have no—?

SANDY: I have no bad feelings at all. Actually, I saw him last spring. I stopped out there in his school district—to get references for a job—and I ran into him. And we talked for hours and hours; it was very good to see him. He was engaged, and it was nice to hear.

KATRINA: But you don't feel he let you down at any point in the whole thing?

SANDY: No. The whole thing was— It was the first time in my life that I had really had to support someone emotionally. He was there, but he was so shaken by this, that I . . . when the chips were really down, I really came through on this. Ted was definitely with me the entire time. But the abortion itself and the trip to the hospital just about did him in. I mean, he was just crushed by the whole thing. That was a terrible experience for him. And he said that for weeks afterward he couldn't sleep. He couldn't, you know, stop thinking about it: how I almost died, and the responsibility that had been on him.

And he told me last spring that it had had a great impact on his life. He felt, when he met this other girl, that he wanted to settle down now; he wanted a family. So, *that* I have no ill feelings about at all.

But I came back and got involved with someone else; and, this time, I did persuade myself to use birth-control pills. I met him several weeks after I returned, which is probably a bad thing, because I was just recovering mentally from all that had happened to me. But we started going out and we became very involved right away. Probably a lot of that was emotional needs that I had at that time. And it was very obvious. I have to have some kind of contraception.

KATRINA: Did you use contraception the first time you had intercourse with him?

SANDY: Oh yes, yes.

KATRINA: You didn't "get seduced," and then get sensible?

SANDY: Right. I had a very different attitude about contraception.

I was relatively healthy all last year. I kept going to the doctor—and every time I would get pains on that same side, I would go back.

But then, this fall, I was moving furniture, and I started — It was a whole day of moving furniture, and I started getting pains on my side. And then I started spot-bleeding the next day. So I just didn't get out of bed; I was absolutely terrified. The guy thought I should have gone to the doctor right away, because he knew the history— Strange, though, I couldn't tell him, almost all of last year, the history behind my operation— But, by this time, he did know what was going on. I waited a week or so, and finally I went to the doctor. Because now I was enrolled in school and I could afford to go to the doctor. At the time it started, I didn't have a job.

Well, the doctor wanted to put me in the hospital right away. He said, "Your other ovary is infected, you have to have the hysterectomy now." And again I said, "No. I'm not going in the hospital, I have to see more doctors." I've just learned this, that you have to go to five or six doctors when they say a hysterectomy.

So I went to this wonderful woman doctor. She was just marvelous. Here I was, bag and baggage, ready to be admitted to have a hysterectomy, and just hysterical about the whole thing. I don't know what brought it on, this second infection. I had been careful with myself. It must have been the moving itself; I have no idea.

But she told me . . . she said, "You know, if you were married and had children, I would operate. But I'm going to try everything else." And she said, "I know the other doctors will think I'm crazy, because obviously you need this; your blood count says that you have a massive infection." So she had me come in every day for shots. And other than that, I spent about a month in bed, trying to get the infection down.

And it hasn't gone away. I've been sort of struggling with it. Every once in a while, it'll flare up and I go back to the hospital, I get more penicillin, I spend another week in bed. And there's nothing that they can do to make it go away. It's just a matter of sort of keeping it under control. Like now, I have to be very, very careful when I have sexual intercourse. Very careful. Because that, in itself, is irritating; I probably shouldn't at all. But the doctor says that, well, that's being sort of unreasonable. But I should be very, very careful and not have sexual intercourse very often. [*pause*] And it hurts when I do.

So I know that it won't be very long before, you know, something will cause the infection to flare up. I went skiing for a week, and I could hardly ski because I was so conscious of falling on that side and hurting that side. So, in a way, I'd like it to be just over with. I've spent since September simply babying myself the whole time. And I know it won't ever be conquered. It's a matter of restraining it long enough so that, should I want to have children. . . . It puts a tremendous pressure on me because I have a very strong desire to have a baby. Yet I'm in no state in life where I can do that sort of thing.

And it's a constant burden to—to be thinking about this all the time.

[*pause*]

KATRINA: It's a devastating story.

SANDY: It's horrible.

KATRINA: You didn't ever mention money. How much did all this cost you?

SANDY: Well, the abortion itself cost four hundred dollars. Plus two trips to Pittsburg. The operation to remove one ovary was a thousand dollars. I don't exactly remember about the D&C. It was very expensive, because the Hartford

Maternity is so expensive; it's expensive just to stay there for a week. The, D&C itself, I don't think was that expensive.

Plus, I go to the doctor at least once a month, if not twice a month. I spend an awful lot of money on medicine, and doctors, all related to this. But I've never added it up. It would be in the thousands, I'm quite sure. Maybe somewhere around three thousand dollars.

Still, the most horrible part is the present and the future. You know, just knowing how much longer I'm going to be able to go on.

I had sexual relations last night, and it sort of hurts to walk today.

It's a tremendous burden for the guy that you're sleeping with, too. I mean, he has to be aware of this.

KATRINA: All this infection, and discomfort, you could get over if you had a hysterectomy?

SANDY: Yes, exactly.

KATRINA: So, in a way, you have to choose between sex and motherhood?

SANDY: Which is a crazy decision!

KATRINA: Do you feel that? I mean, is it my wording or is it yours? Do you feel that yourself?

SANDY: Yes. What I should be doing is totally abstaining right now; I really should. The doctor—this woman doctor —told me that right now I cannot get pregnant. Which is helpful to me. She says, "You have to be taking those pills because if you tried to get pregnant now, the tube is so swollen that you would probably have a tubular pregnancy, and we'd have to operate."

So that is curtailing my desire to get pregnant now. But I

. . . I don't imagine I'll have children, you know. It's just sort of . . . trying to foster false hope, really.

KATRINA: Has the doctor specifically asked you to totally abstain?

SANDY: She tries to avoid being really direct about it. She says it isn't good; and that when I do have sexual relations, it would probably be a good thing if I only slept with one person. Which I do. And that he should be very clean. I mean, he's been very good about that; he never goes to bed with me unless he's just taken a shower. But the whole thing really does affect your sexual relations, because you don't want to let go, because you don't know if you're going to hurt, to find it's painful—

KATRINA: It's come a full circle from not using a contraceptive and "spoiling the spontaneity," to having to take a shower before intercourse. Do you see what I mean?

SANDY: Yes. And be very, very prepared! Really calculating about it.

But I still have mixed feelings about abortion. I still have mixed feelings about the baby that I lost. They're not . . . most of them are not realistic. Because I would not be where I am now, if I had that baby sitting on my lap. I'd be someplace else, much different; and my life would be very different. But it's hard for me to really imagine what that would all be.

I definitely feel that abortion should be legalized, that it's something that— I mean, who was to tell me that I have to go through this kind of agony? And I've run up against so much hostility and ugly feelings about people who have abortions. The way nurses treat you in the hospital, or nurses in doctors' offices, when they find out that you're pregnant and you're not married.

But I think the whole thing really goes back to the idea of contraception. I feel it, so much, working with high-school girls as I do. We've just got to educate ourselves and be realistic. I mean, we're going to go to bed with guys.

KATRINA: Do you feel, in your knowledge of high-school girls, that by offering contraception—by, say, pushing contraception at them—it might push them from virginity into intercourse?

SANDY: I think they're being pushed, now, by their own peers. I really do. I think it's becoming more and more a thing that they have to do. And I've heard a lot of girls complain about it. You know, "I don't feel ready to sleep with him, but everybody says this is what we're supposed to be doing." I think they are being pushed.

But contraception isn't easy for them to get their hands on, and high-school kids don't realize how easily you get pregnant. I didn't know, myself, even at twenty-two. I thought it was something you sort of had to work at. You hear about all these people who have trouble getting pregnant. And for many people it isn't like that at all; it's very, very simple.

I would really like to do some sort of counseling work with high-school girls. It's something that is not effectively put into their health programs in the schools. It's even illegal for us to talk with the girls. Anything I might say now would have to be very hush-hush and behind-the-scenes. I knew one couple, particularly, that I was very close to—both the guy and the girl—and she went through the whole abortion thing. And I really wanted to reach out to her. But I couldn't. Because, legally, I could have been screwed.

KATRINA: You could lose your job?

SANDY: Oh yes!

KATRINA: Did the boy *beg* you to marry him at any point?

SANDY: When I came back East after the operation. When he met me at the airport, he asked me to marry him. You know, totally out of guilt. Just the whole—

KATRINA: This is—this is much *later*.

SANDY: Oh yes. Yes. [*pause*] This is after everything was over. [*pause*]
  I think he was afraid that I couldn't have children, and that he was responsible.
  But he never "insisted." When I told him I was pregnant, we just assumed that somehow we were going to have to work out getting married. I mean we both had Catholic upbringings and that was what you did when you got pregnant. And the idea of abortion didn't come for probably a month after I found out.

KATRINA: But you hadn't gotten married, either!

SANDY: No. Right. There had to be some other answer.
  And I don't think either of us would really have thought of abortion if it hadn't been for those other people involved, the people who lived across the hall.

KATRINA: What would you have done?

SANDY: I don't know.

KATRINA: You weren't thinking of getting married—

SANDY: We were thinking of it; we just could not— We had plans A, B, C, and D: you know, get married and say that we'd been married, get married and I drop out of teaching, get married and we both leave; there were just all kinds of things that we talked about. None of which was satisfactory because we didn't want to get married; we really didn't.

KATRINA: Do you, in retrospect, think you should have married him? Or did you at the time?

SANDY: No, not at all.

KATRINA: Did you feel, as a Catholic, that you couldn't marry him and then divorce him?

SANDY: That never even crossed my mind. I just did not want to spend my life with him; we didn't have that much in common. Actually our relationship was on the verge of splitting up, when I found out that I was pregnant. There was absolutely no regret, whatsoever.

KATRINA: So, though you were coerced into the abortion, it was the only alternative. It was the lesser— Am I right in saying for *you*—?

SANDY: Oh yes!

KATRINA: Although you were pushed into it—

SANDY: I was pushed into it.

KATRINA: Nevertheless you chose abortion above all the other options.

SANDY: Yes. But that's the way I make my decisions mostly. As being pushed into, you know, the least—

KATRINA: But you would still feel honest in yourself, saying that this was the decision that *you* made, as well?

SANDY: Yes; I hate to look at it that way; I still do. I really wish that I had had some other choices, but I didn't. I really didn't.

I wish I had known more about *abortions* and where you can get them. I didn't have to go all the way to Pittsburg, and I certainly didn't have to go to someone like . . . *this* man. Particularly in Pennsylvania, where, with a psychiatric examination, or something like that, you can go into a *hospital*.

And I—I wanted to have that baby. And I think it was a stabilizing influence on me. Up until then I didn't know what direction I was going in; nothing seemed particularly important to me. It was a good biological feeling to know that I was pregnant. I enjoyed the feeling.

KATRINA: To what degree, if any, was the social climate itself . . . ?

SANDY: Well, that was it. Exactly. And my parents, going back home— Mainly my parents.

KATRINA: Yes, your hometown doesn't sound as though you really care about going there—

SANDY: Well, I don't; but still, it's very much a part of me. It's a community. It's my image back there; it's something that I'm very hung up about—maintaining that image.

If everything were different, yes I'd have kept my child and been a single mother. Also, if it were possible for me to support myself and the baby. But I imagine that's the major reason for abortions: because of what society says about being single and having children.

You see, my feeling about the whole thing was social: How can I do it and maintain appearances? I can't, it's impossible. Even while I was in the hospital after I had the

D&C, I was still calling the assistant principal about preparations for a Glee Club picnic that I was in charge of; you know, because I had to keep up appearances! So I dragged myself to the phone, implying that I was calling from home, and that I still wasn't feeling well, and that I'm sure I'll be back Monday morning, and don't worry about me, and tell the kids to read pages thirty-five through forty and I'll be back—you know.

KATRINA: Now do you have regrets? I mean, does it plague you? Do you think, "Oh God, why did I?"

SANDY: Yes it does. The thought of not being able to have children. And I have *not* resolved it, I really haven't. It was very clear that I hadn't when, this fall, I thought I was going to have a hysterectomy. I felt this was a *punishment* for my single sexual life. That this doesn't happen to girls who get married like their mothers say they should, and lead normal lives. And I still have not resolved all of that. I don't know. I mean, I have some rather unpleasant facts to work with. It is a problem, and it is something that I face very often. I'm facing it today, because I'm worried about having slept with someone last night, because it hurts. And I was going to go away with him, but I thought, "No, maybe I'd better stay here and rest."

And it's very hurtful when you see— Particularly at home, where everyone I went to high school with is married and has children, and there's a tremendous stigma against people like me who are not married.

And I want very much to have those children. I found that when I had faced the hysterectomy I began to question my own femininity: Would I still be female? Without ovaries and uterus and everything at twenty-three? Would I still have sexual desire? Was there any point in getting married? These were not rational questions. These were very emotional questions.

But, if I've had regular intercourse, then each day it becomes a little more painful; and then I just have to abstain for a while, and rest. I'm in a very good relationship right now, with this guy who is just really a very good person. We have been talking about getting married; and of course I don't know exactly where his feelings are about this whole thing. Because he's so much a part of it; I mean he's so aware of what's going on.

KATRINA: Are you still a practicing Catholic?

SANDY: No.

I was very strongly Catholic in grade school and high school. I was almost fanatically religious, super-religious. And I was, up until the time that I had the abortion. After the whole thing was over, I felt very repentant, and I wanted to cleanse myself of my sins. And, you know, "God has punished me for this horrible sin." I went to a priest, and he said, "Well, I'm sorry, my dear, but you're excommunicated! You have committed one of the unforgivable sins of the Church and you have to go through the Bishop or the Pope," or something like that. And I said, to hell with it! That's it, and that was the end of my contact, really, with the Church. I mean, that they could say that to me! And of course there was no stigma against the guy who got me pregnant, or the people who suggested the abortion, or the people who performed it. Just me. That was, to me, the most dispassionate thing that the Church could— I mean, what good is the Church, at all?

KATRINA: Have you tried another priest? You might get a more understanding one.

SANDY: Well, since then, I've come to question the whole thing of the Church, the whole thing of God and religion and everything. I've come very far away from it. But I would like, sometime, to talk with other members of the clergy about the Church, and about my feelings about the Church. How useless I feel it is. Just totally useless as a social institution; you know, trying to do something for people. It really is not functioning. I would like to talk about some of these things. But I don't feel that I really want to get back into the Church and into being a practicing Catholic. In fact, the very fact that they reject me, on the point of this abortion, seems ludicrous to me.

KATRINA: How does your family feel about your removal from Catholicism? They must know about that.

SANDY: They know that I'm questioning, and they think that that is disastrous. They're very upset about my questioning everything. I went to Washington, marched in Washington last year while both my brothers were in Vietnam. It's sort of all along the same lines as that—when I talk about my feelings about the Church, and birth control. But as far as they're concerned I still go to church and I'm still a practicing Catholic.

KATRINA: What would you say on the "murdering" issue? As far as you yourself are concerned, do you feel you committed a murder?

SANDY: Yes. Yes, I do. It's a human being. I really do. I think it's a very technical question: which human being is more valuable or has a greater right to live. But that baby, or that young fetus, or whatever it was, was having a tremendous effect on my body. I mean, there it was, growing.

KATRINA: So would a cancerous growth.

SANDY: Yes. But this was not a cancerous growth. This had all the genes and all the potential of being like us. Not just "potential," it was *going to be*. I can't buy the theory that at a certain point that unborn being becomes human.

KATRINA: Could you have, maybe, "killed in self-defense"?

SANDY: Yes, I feel that way.

KATRINA: How does the Church stand on that—outside of abortion issues?

SANDY: Well, that's fine, that's fine.

But the Church has a peculiar, and I think very male chauvinistic, view of women and children: that the child has the right to live over the mother, in the delivery room. That a woman's purpose in this world is to bring in more babies, and that's it. Essentially, that's what the Church says. I mean, I'm sorry, I'm not going to sacrifice my life for someone I don't even know. And that was the one thing that I did feel most strongly after the abortion: that I did save my life, by sacrificing somebody else's.

KATRINA: Why did you agree to talk to me? Why did you want to?

SANDY: Well, I think Women's Lib is the first time that I was able to talk about it and really to admit a lot of this to myself. Women's Lib has really been a beautiful thing as far as my attitudes about women, particularly, are concerned. For the first time in my life, I began to trust other women. You know, I probably could have told this story maybe to a man. But I could never have told it to you, unless I had been involved in Women's Lib.

And since then, I've wanted to do something with what happened to me. I really have. I feel this all the time. I feel very frustrated that I can't blurt it out and say, "Listen, this is what happens!" And it's still going on in me. I would like to have even more direct means of helping. Really. Helping other people, by making my story known. That sounds really corny. But that's the way I feel.

ALEX

ALEX: The fact, that I mentioned on the phone, that I had given up a child for adoption *before* the pregnancy that I aborted—this is significant to you? How much do you want to know?

KATRINA: Is it to you? Significant?

ALEX: Oh, yes! Definitely.
How much background do you want on the pregnancy that was adoptive?

KATRINA: Whatever is relevant to you, personally.

ALEX: Okay. I see.
I'll try to cut this down, because if I gave you everything from the psychological view— As you will learn later, I've had four years of a psychiatrist. All of this has been hashed over.
I was born and brought up in a medium-sized town in the Midwest. I knew, from the very beginning I guess, that my parents were divorced. My mother remarried when I was six. If you want dates I can give them to you. Uhm—finished

high school. Was involved with a fellow who was at a university nearby. I had won a scholarship to a local school; I went there at night. I also worked full-time, in the daytime. That would have begun in September, after my graduation from high school.

The romance was not progressing well. Distance between hometown and his school, and so on. In the spring, a girl friend of mine called and said, "Hey, I'm going out with a fellow. He has a roommate. Would you like to go out?" I didn't know if I should. Because technically I was—at that time "pinned" was the term. But I thought, "Oh, what the hell." So we went. We had a nice time. About a week later she called me and said, "Somebody wants your phone number." And I said, "Who?" The fellow *she* had been out with wanted my phone number. Very ticklish. But of course he couldn't find my name in the phone book because my mother had remarried. He had called all the people in the phone book; nobody knew me. So I told her to give the fellow my number, and he called. That was in March. In April he decided very quickly that he wanted to marry me. It was beginning to be a problem for me. You know, which, and what, and so on.

KATRINA: Were you considering marrying him?

ALEX: I was considering very strongly marrying him. But what was I going to do with the fellow who was away at school? And I knew that was shaky. And what was I going to do about my own future schooling?

Well, to make a long story short, at the time, I said, "Yes, but—" And he said, "I'll ask you again in the summertime." And he did. And—my mother had a lot of upheaval about it. But we were married in the fall.

Now, some things to consider: I was an only child. I never knew my own father. I saw him twice. Very briefly. To put it plainly, I wanted to get out from under my mother. The man in question, whose name is Rees, had finished college. He came from a town nearby. He was working in a responsible position. It was a way out. At that time, I did not know this; I swear by all that's holy, I didn't know it. I didn't even suspect it. I—I thought that I loved him. And I wanted to marry him. I wanted to be married. [*laughs*] Hindsight is an ass's point of view! But in much of my background, and I think in the background of many people, a woman is not really *real* until she gets married. And I mean *gets married*. It's a ritual. It's a kind of validation. "Now I am Mrs. Somebody! I'm real." It's like being able to vote, or opening a charge account.

So we were married. A pleasant, quite lovely wedding. Oddly enough, my parents did not squawk about money. My parents—mother and stepfather—always gave me the impression that we were of restricted means. Now I don't say they have money piled up in the backyard, but they're comfortable. They've saved, they've been judicious.

We lived in the same town, he continued to work where he was, I continued to work where I was. And I was still going to school at night. I did not feel at that point that there was anything wrong with the marriage. We had some little bits of flack from his parents, *I* felt. He adored my mother. He'd fight with her about politics or religion, but he really thought tremendously well of her. So as far as we could tell, as far as everybody else could tell, it was a good marriage. In fact, a rather smashing one. We were interesting people, you know, vital, enthusiastic. We had two jobs, we had two salaries.

We had some hassle, because when we were married, we knew, mutually, that we did not want any children. The neighbors, the relatives, the parents of friends began to question: "When are you going to have a family?" A very classic situation. Rees's mother—actually his stepmother—didn't agree with our philosophy; but she was pretty good about buffering us against her friends, his brothers, and so on. My mother was good about it too, in this period.

There were a couple of times I thought I might be pregnant. And I will tell you that I went through a lot of hell considering it. I wasn't too sure exactly why. But the idea was that I would be absolutely trapped, that my life would end. I never knew any little kids. I never knew any babies, or children. So it was completely foreign to me. And—it scared me. And there would be days, I do recall, when I thought, "My God, if I get pregnant, I swear I'll take my bare hands and—claw it out." I really felt that way. Just [*makes scraping noise*] dig it out.

Rees was outgrowing his work. He had a couple of promotions. We decided that he would look for a job in a very significant large city nearby. He did. When we moved, I had a reasonable amount of regret at leaving a pleasant job, and some schooling, and family, and so on. But I wasn't scared. I wasn't afraid; I didn't feel that I was going to a place of loneliness.

We went. I fell into quite a good job; which I began to like more and more. I got quite involved in it. Rees was traveling all over hell, the whole country really, so that I had a large amount of freedom: to go where I wanted to, to do what I wanted to. I had my own car. I met a couple of girls at work that I liked very much. And my job was such that I had an awful lot of contact with the outside world. I knew a great many people in the outside world, enjoyed being with them, enjoyed doing my work. I would go back home many times on weekends. And we lived in a very nice place. Things were quite good, really. Again, from the outside.

Well, lo and behold, the Company decided to send him East. That nearly blew it. And so for many weeks we went through the question of, should he accept the transfer? And he told me, "If I don't go, the Company will either say 'get out' or else they'll leave me sitting in the local office for the rest of my days." That was around Christmastime. By January, Rees, technically, was already East, living in a motel. And I was supposed to come in March. He was doing his new job; he had made the decision. So the question then became one of timing: When would I leave my job? And my reluctance—almost refusal to go, was to a great extent based on my job. I remember . . . I had a gorgeous office—beautiful windows. And I remember standing at those windows one afternoon and looking out the window—with my back to the door in case anybody came in—and I was just crying very quietly. And I thought, "What is to become of me? Just what is to become of me?"

I hadn't considered staying there without Rees. I don't think that thought really entered my mind. It was so—unusual, unthinkable, so unreal to me—that I would ever say, "No, I'm not going."

My mother at one point said something to me about, "You'd better hang on to that job or one like it. Because the way you're going, that's all you're going to end up with." She has a tendency to, you know, self-fulfilling prophecies.

One day Rees called me. Around about March. And he said, "I've been thinking about it." And he was *gravely* sincere. He said, "If that's what you really want, stay." And this meant stay 'til September, when a very large conference in my business was coming up. So I stayed. For a while I lived with an aunt of his in the suburbs, and then I lived alternately with my two friends there in the city. And come September I finished the conference and went East.

I drove solidly for, well, a day and a half. I got to the New York City apartment at about four o'clock in the afternoon. Rees told me that a Mr. Somebody, an employer I'd been referred to, had called. Well, I called Mr. Somebody back at four-fifteen. I could start work tomorrow. It was very important to us, continuum of employment, not being at loose ends; you know, to be doing something.

I went to the new job. I didn't really like it. I didn't stay there. I went to another place. Then another. It was beginning to be a problem. And I recall, on a Saturday afternoon after Christmas, we were sitting in the apartment, and I suddenly broke into tears. And I said to Rees, "You have no idea how it feels, how miserable it is when you can't find the kind of job that you really want." My whole focus was on work. And I knew that it was on work. What I wanted was to find a job—obviously to replace the other one—where I could find my identity.

Then one day I happened to see a little notice in a magazine about "Volunteers wanted to work with people from foreign countries." Newcomers to the city and so on. Business people, students, whatever. And I went. And lo and behold, they said, "Yes, come in." So now I had another interest. Which was very good because, for one thing, I had never been in New York before and I wanted to go places and see things. I don't mean the Times Square set; I mean the development of interest in museums and art, and just seeing the city. Rees was a stick-in-the-mud of the first water. He wanted to be home watching the television set.

So I found that these people from foreign countries, naturally being new, were interested. So I spent a fair amount of time with them. I took them home to my house, cooked them dinner, learned how to cook their food. My husband was terribly pleased by the whole idea. Most of my students were in business in one way or another, and it was interesting to him to know about the foreign corporate operations; and he could give *them* advice in many cases. It seemed, "Ah! Things are looking up. The job's not that great but I have this other thing that I'm doing. Fine." Also, I didn't know what was happening but, with the visitors, I felt in my bones: "Here are people who respond to me." I think at one point I even said, "They like me." Another kind of what I call self-validation: I *am* somebody.

A job came up in a suburb that meant a hell of a lot of commuting. And I asked Rees if I could take it. And the salary was great. I mentioned the problem of the commuting. He said, "Yes, go ahead." Now this meant that I was on the train two hours a day. But—all right.

So I would come into town when I finished work; I would deal with my foreign visitors—whom I call students really—and go home, sometimes with these visitors, sometimes not. But the point is, I was absent from the home a fair amount of time. I was away from where I *didn't want to be*.

Well, finally one calm Saturday afternoon— [*laughs*] we had all our discussions on Saturday afternoon. So, on that famous Saturday afternoon, I finally, with a reasonable amount of fatigue, said, "Is it time for us to get a divorce?"

And Rees said, "Yes, I guess so."

I said, "Well, when should we do it?"

And I mean just about that calmly. He said, "We don't want to mess up Christmas for everybody. Why don't we make it at the end of the year? It'll be easier for taxes." A famous quote in my life. And it *would* be easier for taxes.

So I went back to the Midwest for Christmas. My mother knew something was going on and she wormed it out of me on the phone before Christmas. Oh, leuuuuh! Upheaval! Upheaval! Upheaval!

KATRINA: You weren't that upset yourself? I mean—?

ALEX: Well, no. At that point I was not that upset, myself. I was tired. Now Rees had said to me, many is the time, "Without me, you can't get along; you can never earn enough to keep yourself." I was making a fairly good salary and I never sat down with pencil and paper and figured it out, but I thought, "Damn it, I can! I will!"

So I went back for Christmas without him. And my mother did all her various dramatic scenes. I didn't really know at that point if she wanted to save the marriage, although to some degree I thought she did—I dare say, because of what the neighbors would think; you know, repeat the divorce pattern—so she screamed and yelled and fussed.

And then my good old mother— And I say this with some

malice, not really at her, but for the situation: my mother drops the news, that famous Christmas season, "Well, your father and I were never married."

You know, I wasn't too surprised. Really wasn't too affected by it. I have subsequently come to believe that she said it then and there in that tone of voice as a punishment —to *me*. You know, "Here you are: your marriage is going to pot, you're getting a divorce. Damn you! Your father and I were never married!" I think, truly, that she meant it as a way of—I say punishing. Slapping me. Spanking me. Beating me. I'm not a psychologist or a psychiatrist so I can't tell you what it does to somebody; but the—putting you down —almost as if in a way it were my *fault* that they were never married. And *of course* it was my fault that this marriage of mine had gone to pot. That was absolutely certain. It was my fault because I could have come East with him immediately. I *could* by that time have had children.

She said to me once, in a very significant moment, "Isn't that something you want to give him?" And although I agreed with the idea that if you love a man, yes, you *do* want to give him a child, or children, I still had this marvelous mechanism inside: "No, I don't. It is not something—" Well, the truth is, I didn't want to give it to *him*. Should we say, now, that I didn't love him? Probably. But I didn't know that. And I felt, in my head, that a marriage could exist without—having children. Without the *desire* to have children. And I thought that all these people running around to fertility clinics were crazy as hoot owls. You know, I felt, "If you want a child, go out and adopt one!" There's no necessary reason for bearing the child. And I got awfully hot and heavy on that. I felt that people were being hypocritical as hell when they would say, "Oh, I'd love to have a baby." Meaning have, deliver, gestation, pregnancy, sperm, egg, all that. I thought, "Well, if you really want a kid—" And I would tell them: "There are lots of kids who need you. Go to an adoption agency and get one!"

KATRINA: Your determination not to have a child—that was forever?

ALEX: It was forever; forever and forever. And the context in which I saw it, is that my marriage would last forever. I never thought of being married to— I thought many times of being widowed. Because my husband had tons of insurance and it would be great. And I knew perfectly well I'd go back to school. That was always very clear in my mind. But I never contemplated that another situation would come up.

KATRINA: And this break-up, this Christmas you're talking about—you'd been married how many years?

ALEX: '55 to '64. Nine years.

KATRINA: You had been married nine years?

ALEX: Oh yes! Yes, it surprises everybody. God, nine years! I was married when I was nineteen. So I was then twenty-eight.

I packed up the household belongings and so on. There were subsequently some very heavy fights. We had a roll-around dishwasher, and one time I rolled it on him. And the divorce that was supposed to be unemotional, businesslike, calm—as most divorces do, I think—got hot and heavy, then. I had taken an apartment in Pennsylvania where my job was, and I left. We made it a point not to see each other, not to have any contact, to deal only through lawyers. Then — Let me think of timing—it took almost a year to get the divorce—

Anyhow, I had moved down to Pennsylvania. I was still in New York for the foreign visitors' situation. I was developing quite a thing with one of my students. And I knew that ultimately the time would come when he would have to go back to his own country. It got to be quite serious. Very serious. To the point that we discussed marriage, the question of cultural conflict, language, me living in a different place, him coming here to stay, the visa problems: we were very much involved in it.

KATRINA: Were you sleeping together?

ALEX: We were sleeping together, using *no* contracept—well, yes, come to think of it, we were. Some of the time. Using rubber condoms. But basically I would say, more than half the time, no contraception.

KATRINA: Was this your first affair outside of marriage?

ALEX: This was my first affair. And I think possibly this is also significant: this was also the first orgasm.

I'd been married nine years. I had traipsed to doctors, the finest in the land. I was healthy as a horse. There was nothing wrong with me. And I tell you I was—I wasn't the hottest little number around, but I was healthy. And I mean this in a positive sense; I wanted a sex life. I don't mean sex as fornication, I mean a love life. A good, heavy love life. My husband was healthy, and vigorous—and a fool. And I did what most women do. I just fooled him. He was flattered and pleased by my interest and vigor in bed. Until such time as I finally had no interest. And then we used to fight about *that*. To the point that occasionally he'd write down when was the last time. [*laughs*] And he probably was right.

KATRINA: So anyway, you started this affair before—after the divorce had . . . ?

ALEX: No, while the divorce was pending. We were physically living apart but I was still legally married.

KATRINA: You didn't start sleeping with him before all this came up?

ALEX: No. I can tell you that I—hindsight again—I'm damned sure I wanted to. We went to lots of places together. There were what I would call "electric feelings" between us. Before, while he knew my husband, while he had been a guest in our house, I was beginning to be aware of them. But I had not acknowledged them. Not verbally and not even to myself. But I tell you that I think *that* acceptance by him, that feeling good toward him, is probably what made me feel —not think, but feel, "Yes, it's the time for a divorce." You know, "Here comes *me* after all this time."

So there I was, commuting back and forth because this fellow lived in New York. And I was—well, you can imagine how women feel if they've had the problem of the delayed orgasm. "My God! At last I'm alive, it *wasn't* me. Hallelujah it wasn't *me*." You know, "I'm real!"

We decided to get sensible about the questions of marriage, country, visa, and so on. He decided—and I to a great extent encouraged him to do this—to go home. To deal with his job there, things like that; and that probably I would come over sometime later.

He went.

The letters got less frequent. The phone calls from overseas got less frequent. There were times that I would write some pretty heavy letters. Basically, "Why don't you write?"

He had a friend here who was in a similar job. In a way we had been assigned to each other. He had said, "Well, you take care of her while I'm gone." And he had said to me, "If you can help him—language and cultural situations—do."

So we started seeing each other as friends. *Always* talking about "the man." And in June, while I was still legally married, while the divorce was pending, I was at this fellow's house one afternoon, and I knew that he liked me. And I think that he liked me as the woman belonging to his very close friend. But lo and behold, we went to bed together. No contraception.

I didn't think too much about it. I regretted it. And I

knew then— It was the first time I ever knew, intellectually, what loneliness was. Because I was alone. I had no husband. My mother was raising hell by letter and phone. And the fact that I felt the pull of the fewer letters, the fewer phone calls. You know. You *feel* these things, in your bones.

Now with his friend, I went to bed twice. It was routine intercourse, sexually; it was friendship and comforting from the standpoint— I mean it was the friendship, the closeness; we *liked* each other; we were friends. It was a—a scene of taking away the aloneness.

That was in June. I was getting ready to go overseas. I was thinking very seriously of quitting my job. I was trying to find out how to break the lease on the apartment in Pennsylvania. And—no menstrual period. No menstrual period for a month. My God! It can't be true.

Now while I had been married, on one or two occasions when the situation came up, I had mentioned to my boss, "If this ever happens to Rees and me, do you know anyone?" He had said, "I could arrange it. But it would have to go distantly through a lot of other people because, of course, if anybody heard about it here— After all, this is a small town." Okay. "Well, then," I thought at that point, "The smart thing to do is for you to go to your boss and tell him." Uhm. But I didn't.

Second month came and went. That was the end of August. I quit my job, closed the apartment and was damn near —well, I was practically on the plane. Now, here comes the significant factor: while I was in Pennsylvania there was a fellow who worked in the same building I did. And I knew that he spent a lot of time in New York. I guess I just got to talking to him because we saw each other in the building. And I told him that I was leaving but I had these people in New York: Would he be interested in taking over my volunteer spot with this group? He said yes, maybe he would. So we went to New York together a couple of times. I was then staying with a girl—woman; technically old enough to be my mother. But she was a widow, and I call her a girl. She was a friend. So I was living with Peggy in her big old house in Pennsylvania. This fellow was very pleasant. Uhm—he was very good-looking. He brought me home from New York on the train a couple of times, walked me to her house, came in, and we had drinks or something, the three of us.

I was beginning to be aware of the fact that I was pregnant. In fact, I'm quite sure that I really had acknowledged it to myself. And I thought very fleetingly about an abortion. *Just fleetingly.* And then I thought, "Well, maybe I can go over to his country and convince him that this child—who will of course be born prematurely—is his." Those thoughts were nebulous. But I figured that this was the only way out. Abortion was—so *unknown* to me, that I did not pursue the matter. I never called anybody. I never asked anybody. You know, I did absolutely nothing. On the subject.

I was—well, on the plane for a connecting flight to the man's country, and I decided to fly to the Midwest to see my mother. She knew where I was going and pretty well why. Though I was smart; I had also lined up two jobs over there.

KATRINA: "Why you were going"? Were you going "to get a father for this baby"?

ALEX: No. I was going to be *with* him. And I did think, "God, this could blow the whole thing." But in my innocence, or inexperience, or whatever, I think I honestly believed I could tell him this was his child. Now that shows you how unreal the whole thing was.

Anyhow, while I was at my mother's and he knew I was there, she came into the garden with a telegram. And I said —she had it in her hand—and I said to her "Well, what do you want to bet I don't go?"

And I opened the cable and it said, "Delay trip." So I got on the phone and I called him. He said, "Some things are coming up. Wait a while." I said, "Look, I have quit my job,

I'm here, I'm on my way, I'm ready." "Well, wait a couple of weeks." I wasn't about to sit on the overseas phone all night, so I said, "All right."

KATRINA: Were you concerned about the pregnancy at this point? Was that a big factor? Or was it in the back of your mind?

ALEX: It was a factor that was then only about two months along. And when you're not very pregnant, I don't think you're very—*as* concerned as you're going to be later on. I didn't *feel* pregnant. I didn't *look* pregnant.

Again, aloneness. I needed somebody. I needed a connection. I called New York. I told this fellow I had been working with, "Look, something's come up. Can you come out here for a while?"

KATRINA: This fellow is now the—the neighbor in your office building? Or the good friend of your—?

ALEX: Neighbor of the office building. Exit father of child. Because he doesn't really *concern* me that much. We're good friends. Nobody knows I'm pregnant. Except me.

So—he couldn't get off work. I said, "Well, I think I'm going to come back East for a while." "Okay, fine. I'll meet you at the airport." He met me at the airport. With my huge overseas trunk [*laughs*] and everything else.

So I didn't really know what to do. And I thought, "You have to do *something*." I was beginning then to feel the pressure: "What the hell am I going to do?" Well, when I feel pressure, obviously what do I do? I went to bed with Jack—the neighbor in the office building.

Uh. [*pause*] I then realized that I was not going to get out of this country. I *knew* that there was no sense going over there, pouncing myself in, messing up both my jobs plus all the people I knew— This is a terribly small world. And I thought: there I'll go, I'll march into the office building, and he'll say, "What the hell are you doing here?" If he sees me coming, maybe he'll run around the corner.

KATRINA: Did you suspect that he was no longer emotionally interested in you?

ALEX: He *was* emotionally interested in me, but the cultural problems, the language problems, his parents' disapproval of an American girl. His job. His bosses. Pressures were getting at him. He does not respond well to pressure.

KATRINA: And did he communicate what was going on in his thoughts?

ALEX: In terse, one-syllable, reluctant, hesitant style, yes. He didn't say it in what I would have considered a manly and honest fashion. But I knew what was happening.

Then I began to see reality: "Damn it. You have to do something. You've got to get yourself in order." Nobody knew about this. I did the smart thing, having left my job: I came into New York, went to a temporary agency and said, "I want to go to work." Work was no difficulty, so I worked here.

In September, maybe late September, I told Jack that I was pregnant. Well, of course, he thought he was the guy who had done it. And I spent hours convincing him, telling him this whole story, "No, you did not do it." He said, "What are you going to do?" I told him that, all things considered, I'd probably go to England. No language barrier. Public medicine—you know, you don't need a lot of money. Have the child. Place it for adoption. And come back. Be perfectly normal for little Alex: "She left her job; bang, she's off to England." Nobody would think anything of it.

Jack thought that was a good idea. Now there came a question of money. Which I subsequently had to borrow from my mother. And never told her why. She sent the check; she sent lots of lectures with it and wrote some rather nasty letters. But nonetheless she sent the check. I had the money. So then I set about the reality.

I talked to the British Consulate. Told the man straight out what the difficulty was and what I wanted to do. And he said, "Yes, it can easily be done." I posed the question, "What about citizenship?" He said, "If you place the child for adoption in England he is a British subject." And I said "What if I register him at the American Embassy?" He said, "Then, technically, he would be an American citizen. But it's most likely the adoptive parents would want him changed to British citizenry."

Well, that began to bother me. It really did. Because I thought, "What in the hell can I give this child?" I had not yet seen a doctor, by the way. Uh—it really bothered me.

And—I think around Thanksgiving, I went to my own physician. I said, "I'm here for a physical." And I said, "One thing you will discover is that I'm growing a wee bit of a pot here, and I'm pregnant." He knew I was divorced. He said, "What are you going to do about the baby?" I told him about England. He thought that was fine and gave me the names of a couple of good hospitals there. I figured I had enough money. So that's when I started investigating with the consulate.

The day after Christmas— These are the most gory details, but I swear they follow a pattern: I had Peggy's car. She was working, I wasn't. I came around the corner where Jack lived, in her car. And here he is in his car with another woman. God damn! And I was—I was furious. You know, "Why? How could he?" and so on. So I went back to Peggy's house. And about an hour later he appeared. He walked in the door. And I said, "Whatever it is, don't worry about it." I knew something was wrong.

So we went for a ride. And he told me a rather classic story. That this girl had been hustling him for a hell of a long time. She lured him into bed sometime in October, *after* he knew me. And *naturally* she was pregnant. [*laughs*]

I guess that's— [*laughs*] Well, I don't know if that's worse — I don't know if that's as bad as it gets— She was pregnant.

He'd gone to bed with her once. During the time that he knew me, and was sleeping with me, and really we had quite a good relationship.

So now we had the problem: she was quite pregnant. She was in a neighboring suburban community . . .

KATRINA: But . . .

ALEX: She was a schoolteacher. She was beginning to show. Her parents . . .

KATRINA: But, wait, she couldn't have been more pregnant than you?

ALEX: Well, no she couldn't, come to think of it. But she was going to get an abortion. Time was of the essence.

So, the question became, "What in hell are we going to do about *her?*" And there was a question of money. She was a schoolteacher; she didn't have much money. Of *course* she couldn't ask her parents for the money. The whole big megilla.

So I called a girl that I had worked with on one of the free-lance jobs. No—I guess, first, we were all looking for abortionists. Sandra was looking for an abortionist. Jack was looking for an abortionist. I was trying to but I didn't know where to look. I didn't know where to look without being caught. The only people that I knew were people that I knew! So—

Sandra got the name of somebody. And—I called the girl, Margo, that I had worked with, because she told me that she knew of somebody. And she gave me the name of a doctor in New Jersey.

Oh, then the question came up about the money. It was *my* money which my *mother* had lent me, that was used for the abortion. Thereby cutting the rug out from under me. Making me totally dependent on my friend Peggy for her house, and she did not yet know I was pregnant. Making me dependent on Jack emotionally, and perhaps to some degree, financially.

KATRINA: Why did you give it to her? Instead of thinking of yourself? Was it your insecurity about going to England? Or was it—some other reason?

ALEX: No. Because at the point that we made the de—that Jack and I made the decision about the money and so on, I knew that the England deal was out. Which I already sort of felt because of the citizenship question. And in all honesty, I didn't want to leave Jack. I was then beginning to realize, "My God, I would be [*hits table with fist*] *all alone.*" And although I'm very good about carrying on professionally—I would be over there all by myself.

KATRINA: You wanted to continue your relationship with Jack?

ALEX: Oh yes. Absolutely. Definitely.

KATRINA: You hoped to marry him? Or—?

ALEX: Ultimately, when I got these messes cleaned up. Probably, most likely so.

KATRINA: Had the two of you talked about it together?

ALEX: Uh—a little. We were both concerned with the problems of one baby, one abortion, lack of money.
So Sandra went and had the abortion with my money.

And I had met her. This kid was scared. I don't know if she was older than I was, I'm not sure. But she was a child and she was scared to death.

She went to the doctor, she had it done. A couple of her friends took her. She came back. Jack called her house that night because she had not yet called to say she was home and safe.

A couple of days later, the guy who had done her abortion was pictured in the *Daily News* with his bottom showing, going out the window of his office. He was a doctor. Who also did abortions. And the *Daily News* had been on a raid with the police and they caught him. Well, it was by the skin of our teeth, oh my God!

KATRINA: And Jack did not have a romantic interest in this woman at this time?

ALEX: No. No.

I think, really, he took her to bed— At least I believed at that— I feel now, of course, that he tended to be irresponsible, or nebulous about sexual involvement with women. But at that time I was not that much aware of this.

KATRINA: You weren't worried about his being more interested in her?

ALEX: No. I was not worried about him being more interested in her. And I was not yet worried about him being more interested in other people. I felt that he had had his succession of women in his life, and I was this particular chapter; and I hoped to go on with it.

So— Sandra had the abortion. That was all well and done. Doctor What's-his-name obviously was out of business. Margo had given me the name of this other guy, which I still had.

KATRINA: Another abortionist?

ALEX: Another abortionist also in New Jersey.

KATRINA: You were beginning to think of an abortion?

ALEX: No, not for me. No, I just had it as extraneous material. It was too late for me to think of abortion. This child was due in March. I got pregnant in June. This was Christmas.

I went back to my own doctor and said, "Look, I've decided to stay here. I don't want to go to England." He said, "That's fine." I said, "I would like to do it as close as possible to natural childbirth. Who should I go to?" And he gave me the name of an obstetrician whom I called.

A word of advice to receptionists in doctors' offices: You may have to ask the questions, but do be cool in your responses. She said, "Is this a gynie visit? Or is this to determine pregnancy?" And I said, "No, it's not a gynie visit, and the pregnancy has been determined. The estimated delivery date is sometime in March." I heard her go "Auck."

KATRINA: Because you had called as Miss So-and-So?

ALEX: No, I think what she was going "Auck" about was the time-factor. That here it was, the first of January, and I was calling about a baby due in March. I called as Miss, but I think that was less startling than the fact that I was *so* pregnant. Because, you know, middle-class, white, Anglo-Saxon people don't stay pregnant that long without seeing an obstetrician. Somehow.

So, I went to see the obstetrician. He said, "All right, I will take care of you. The hospital has a social service department. The gal's name is Miss Lander. She will take care of the other things." We talked about the technical aspects of having a baby. He said to get the book: you know, Grantly Dick Read. And to come back and see him at such-and-such a time.

I was great! I did not look pregnant! I was working! Nobody had the faintest idea that I was pregnant.

KATRINA: You don't sound very *involved* with your pregnancy.

ALEX: At the time when I began to feel some of the kicking, I was aware of the fact that "I liked it." Now I can tell you, it's very simple: I wasn't *alone*. It's a tremendously significant factor. Which you don't know until you've been there. And although I was concerned about Jack, and I was concerned about "I don't really want to go to England because I would be alone"—as the child became more of a reality, I was less alone.

Finally I figured, "I've got to tell Peggy." And this was hard, because her married daughter was having great difficulties with her husband. And one night the daughter took a whole bottle full of aspirin, and I got home and there was a note on the door: "Come to the hospital." She had taken the aspirin. I went to bed that night thinking, "Oh my God, it's a shitty world." I mean, I was in this mess. Jack and Sandra had just gotten out of *that* thing, that I was involved in. And now Peggy's got this mess with her daughter, who has a young baby girl. And "Oh boy!"

And it was beginning to bother me. I talked to Jack an awful lot and I said, "I have got to get out of here. I want to be someplace where it's peaceful and quiet. And since I'm not going to England—" Well, we made the decision. I would move into New York, into the city. So I finally had to tell Peggy. She was not angry. She was not distressed. She said, "My God, I can't believe you're pregnant. You mean all this time—?"

We had a fellow living next door [*laughs*] who was an obstetrician! And I would see him, and he said to me one day in January when I had gone out without my coat on, "Gee, Alex, you've lost a lot of weight." Well, the truth of the matter was, I had lost weight. Chemically I can explain all this to you. I weighed less then and was less rounded *then,* than I am now. Well, we thought this was humorous as hell. But in a way it was shocking. I began to feel the—you know, *"Why* don't you idiots *know? You're* an obstetrician, and *you* don't know? Is the world full of blind people?"

I moved into New York. I got an apartment, a sublet. I began to develop a little bit of swelling and so on. The doctor was a little worried about it, and he had told me I shouldn't work anymore. Well, all right. Jack was providing me with money. He was able—Sandra was able to give it back in pieces. The loan was being paid back. I still had some money in the savings account. I was in modest circumstances, but I was all right.

On a Monday, I went to the doctor, and I had a very high elevated urine specimen. Enough so that he took the test a second time. He really was concerned. I was getting very puffy ankles. He said to me, "Go home. Lie down. Take as little fluid as you possibly can, and come on back Wednesday. Don't do a damn thing." I was in pretoxemia, and he told me so.

Wednesday morning, very early, I woke up, I didn't feel so good. Throughout the course of the morning it was becoming more definite; I felt bad in my middle. Took a shower. And about eleven o'clock I called Jack at the office and while we were on the phone I said, "Oohp, here it comes again!" And I must have sort of passed out. And he kept saying, "Are you there? Are you there?" And I said, "Yeah." And he said, "What's happening?" I said, "Well, every now and then I just, you know, sort of blank out."

He said, "You're in labor?" and I said, "Oh my God it's too soon." He said, "Well, you're in labor. Call the doctor. I don't know when I can get down there. I can't leave; but I'm coming."

I called the doctor's office. The woman said, "Go to the

hospital." And I said, "I can't make it by myself." She said, "Call an ambulance."

I was very calm, I called the operator, I said, "I need an ambulance." She plugged in and a man's voice said, "Something Police," and he asked me the necessary questions.

I got up. Put on a half-slip, no bra. A pair of shoes and a coat. And it was physically difficult then for me to walk, because I felt "I want to be lying down." I was not uncomfortable. It was a new situation.

The buzzer buzzed. I buzzed to let the people in. And I unlatched the door because I really wanted to be lying down. And who came in, but two great big cops. Now I had never seen cops up close. And I, you know, "What are you doing here?" They said, "Whenever a city ambulance is requested, we come."

The operator at one point— She stayed on the line while I talked to the police-telephone man, and when I finished there was no dial tone, and I said, "Are you still there?" And she said, "Yes." I said, "Well, I'm done." And she said, "Yes, but are you all right?" I said, "Yes." She said, "Well, I'll leave the key open until they come." And I said, "Do you always do that?" And she said, "Sure." That was *so nice*.

So the police came. I said to the operator, "Okay, the police are here." Well, by then I was up. And the pressure was tremendous. Finally the ambulance arrived. The cops said, "Do you want us to carry you downstairs?" I said, "If you tip me over we're through; the baby's going to be here." 'Cause then I realized what was happening.

The thought had not yet entered my mind, "something was wrong." I was busy thinking about the matter at hand. They put me in the ambulance. We went to the hospital. The uniformed doorman was there with the wheelchair. Everybody ran. They got me off these stretchers and onto other things and somebody came in to take my name. And she called me Mrs. and I said, "No, Miss." I was very lucid. And one nurse said to me, "Can you stand it if I prep you?" I said, "Oh yes, go ahead." And I was doing all these cooperative things and they were all surprised.

Well, we get up to the delivery room, and everybody's there, ready. My doctor comes in. During a pause I said to him—and I was very clear-headed—I said, "I realize there is something out of the ordinary here. I want to know exactly *what* is happening *as* it is happening, and do everything you can to see that this child is all right."

KATRINA: You had a strong feeling of caring that the child be all right?

ALEX: Oh, God yes! Absolutely! And I knew at that moment, "This kid is premature." I can quote statistics for you on prematurity. I know what happens. And I was aware "something may not be right."

KATRINA: Why mightn't you have *hoped* that it would die? It would have been—easier.

ALEX: The thought never entered my mind. Never entered my mind. And if the child had been born in a sickly situation, I would have turned that hospital upside-down to see that he had everything.

The thought never entered my mind. It was completely foreign to me. Anymore than if you were having a cat or a dog in your house, and there were complications, you would immediately wrap up the animals and take them to the vet. Uhm. How can I tell you how foreign to me it is? I was aware that there might be a problem, naturally, and I guessed that he'd have to go into an incubator: small size.

So, baby was born. They took him over to the little table. They told me it was a boy, I'm not quite sure just when. I didn't ask; they told me. And—they showed me the baby. And the only thing wrong with him was that he was underweight. That's all. Just the technical fact that he was born before an accepted time-factor. But I was assured when he left the delivery room that everything was in good order.

Place was busy as hell. One of the nurses took me out of the room and said, "Will you be all right if I leave you in this little vestibule?" She said, "We are having babies left and right." And I said, "How long?" She said, "Oh, just about five minutes. I'm going to move somebody in."

I was alone in the room. My little area—with a curtain. And I was aware that the child had been born. And I was tremendously aware that I was very calm. It was like I had done the job. Neatly. Safely. "Well done. Now you can relax."

It was over. I could have gone back to work the next day. The baby was in a premature section. He couldn't leave the hospital 'til he made the weight, which was something like two weeks. In the interim Miss Lander came to see me. She was a social worker for the hospital. It so happened that the social worker for the Judith Williams Adoption Agency was there also. She came and said, "When you get out, come to see me."

KATRINA: Did you see the baby at this time?

ALEX: Oh, sure! I saw the baby when he was born. And I saw him by walking down the hall. Jack came to visit me in the hospital, and we went to see him together. Including the significant fact that Jack said, "You know, I expect him to look like me." At one time, the question of what to do about the birth certificate— Jack said, "Use *my* name." I said, "No, that's, you know, a sliding way out." And on a birth certificate, you don't have to put down any father. I'm the mother. Who's the father? *Blank*. Don't fill it in. The child is born with your maiden name. Which is—the way I wanted it.

So— I got out. I started seeing the social worker. A psychiatric social worker at the Judith Williams Agency. We went into minute detail about the questions of telling my mother. My plans for his adoption. I think she wanted me to tell my mother. She said, "After all, she has a grandchild." I said, "Look, that may be great for you, but it's going to flap her far too much, and she'll raise hell with me." It ended that I did not tell my mother. And that the child was not adopted until November or December.

KATRINA: This was—he was born when?

ALEX: February 9, 1966.

He stayed in the hospital for two weeks. Then he went into the foster home arranged by the Judith Williams Agency. He was about a month premature. In every other respect, fine. No difficulties at all. I was very thorough about checking into this.

When I would go to the Williams Agency to see the social worker, he would, on several occasions, be there with his foster mother for his weekly check-up. So I saw him once or twice. Then. After he was born.

KATRINA: Was that done intentionally so that you could see him? Or was that a coincidence?

ALEX: I think that they took advantage of a coincidence. And Mrs. Burke asked me, "Would you like to see him?" And I said, "Yes." On one of those occasions Jack went with me and was there with us in our little conference room. And I was seeing her once or twice a week. We were also discussing the question of whether I should go into psychiatric treatment.

It developed that he was safely adopted in December. And of *course* he had to become a ward of the city. Technically he was, you know, on welfare. Because he had no parents, and he was placed in a foster home. I paid a small portion of the money that was going toward his support. The rest of it was paid from city tax-money.

KATRINA: Did you have any *desire* to keep him, or—?

ALEX: I had no desire to keep him. But I can tell you that the first time I went to see Mrs. Burke at the Williams Agency she said, "How do you feel?" And I said, "I feel fine." And she said, "How do you feel about the baby?" I said, "I can tell you that as soon as I can, I want to have a child of my own." I knew it *very* positively. No question about it. I gather this happens to a lot of people. And the feeling hasn't changed.

KATRINA: Why didn't—why didn't you change your mind?

ALEX: Then? And keep him?

KATRINA: Yes.

ALEX: Well, *what* would I do with him? By the time— Let's see, he was born in February. In June of '66 I got myself a very hot and heavy high-level job. Money was pretty good and destined to get much better—

KATRINA: Why didn't you keep him in April? In March? In May?

ALEX: I didn't want him. I had already made up my mind that he was to be placed for adoption.

Well, for one thing there was the obvious financial consideration. I might be able to keep him for a month or so. Although if you tell the Williams Agency that you're placing a child for adoption, they don't let you keep him in the intervening period.

KATRINA: No, no I don't mean, "Why didn't you keep him during that period?" Why— I'm wondering why you didn't

—have regrets. Because I feel that people might. Or that your answer, at least, would be interesting.

ALEX: I was sorry that I couldn't keep him. Sad, perhaps is the term. But I was tremendously well aware of the fact that I would not keep him. And I *know* why. Because I did not want that child to have any kind of life parallel to what I had!

What am I going to tell that kid when he starts growing up? "Tell me about my father." Tell him some cock-and-bull story? Maybe marry Jack, which would be all right. But how was Jack going to feel? And did I want to marry Jack? The whole thing sounded like it came out of a pulp magazine.

KATRINA: Did the fact that it *was* an echo of your own upbringing—?

ALEX: Oh, yes! "Here we go again." And I had read enough to know— I read an article shortly before he was born about "Illegitimate children tend to produce illegitimate children. It goes in a chain."

KATRINA: And was your mother's situation very definitely—?

ALEX: Oh, *definitely*.

KATRINA: I mean she had said that she was not married. But it wasn't that they were living together and being like husband and wife and hadn't bothered?

ALEX: No. They were not. They were—friends, lovers, but it was an out-of-wedlock conception. An out-of-wedlock pregnancy, an out-of-wedlock birth.

Subsequently, when I was a child, and so on, he would come back and want her to marry him. In fact, there must have been a time when I was a kid in high school that he really came back on her hot and heavy. This was of course after she had "remarried" and was settled down with my stepfather. But I do know—she subsequently told me—that at least at one point *before* she remarried, he did come to her and then wanted to get married and be a family. And with this eternal, goddam, fool pride of hers—'cause I think probably she loved him—she said no. And she was then *alone*. It's the Depression; she's got this kid; she's got an awful lot of flack and dirty looks from—

KATRINA: So your choice and your reasons for not reevaluating—

ALEX: Look, I had certain things that I could give to Alex. One was health, which I gave to him, and I was very much concerned about it.

KATRINA: You gave him that name?

ALEX: Yes. My grandfather's name is Alexander. And my name is Alexandra.

I gave him good health. I gave him a pretty decent heritage, coming from two healthy parents, two pretty bright parents. Basically decent folks. A little neurotic, okay.

I also could give him safety into a home that *wanted* him. And I mean [*hitting table*] *positively, intellectually, emotionally*, the whole bit. "We want him, we know we want him. We have gone through the hell of the question of infertility, and through the adoption situation. We're clear-headed." And when this kid spills his milk on the floor and you're about ready to slap his head, "That's all right, kid, I wanted you."

I didn't want him to have a mother looking at him, no matter how much money she had, no matter how much society has changed, looking at him and thinking, "Well, are *you* a mixed-up leftover from a mixed-up me."

Who may be by this time more mixed-up. I had very grave concerns about whether I could deal with the child emotionally. I didn't know what to do with him! Would I end up someday holding his head over the gas jet?

What would I do with him? The whole idea was completely— I—

KATRINA: Did you feel that was a possibility? That you might be a battering mother?

ALEX: An eeky small one. And I remembered that once, while I was married, one of my friends had had a baby. He was then old enough to walk. And he was a cute, nice kid. And he came around the coffee table. And I reached for him, to pick him up so he wouldn't fall down. And *at* the moment while I was picking him up, I had this horrendous urge to take that kid and bang him through the coffee table, which was glass. I was aware at the time what was happening.

I didn't do anything. I picked him up. You know. And Barbara was out in the kitchen doing something else. But I knew that at that moment I had wanted not only to kill, but to kill *violently*. The way that kids take cats and put them in paper bags. In fact, I thought of that: "My God, this is the kind of a thing that a child would do."

So— Alex was born and I saw him safely into what I felt was the best situation for him. Yes, he's going to have to deal with the mystery of "Who are my parents?" And Mrs. Burke and I talked about that long and heavy. But I think he stands a better chance of dealing and living with that mystery, if he's *got* parents, adoptive parents with him. And no matter how much he will scream at age thirteen, and no matter how many psychiatrists he *may* have to see, he still has the actuality of, "They wanted me, they came to get me, they kept me. I'm still here, and tomorrow they'll still be there." That he would have the kind of continuity and stability that I— I was very clear on this. Hard-headed. Absolutely hard-headed.

KATRINA: Do you still feel the same way?

ALEX: Oh sure.

KATRINA: I'd like to ask how you feel. But if it comes up later I can wait—

ALEX: It comes up later, because I subsequently had an abortion for the same reason. Exactly the same reason.

KATRINA: But you still, now—you do not feel regret?

ALEX: Oh, no! Absolutely. None. Because at this moment I do not feel that I have taken the action to put my life in order in such a way that I could take care of a child.

Now there are certain things you need in order to take care of a kid. One of them, obviously, is money. I think, in this time in history, and because of the way I feel, and having been to a headshrinker and so on—I think I could pretty well buck most of the people who would look down their noses. I think I have enough stability there.

But the one thing I feel I don't have, is a stable emotional relationship with a man. By that I don't mean marriage, and living in the suburbs, and so on. I mean a thing that is so good between us that we could say, "Let's have a child." Married or not married, whatever the case is. And take him to your aunts and uncles and all your friends and say, "This is mine and Joe Blow's kid." And it's known to me in my heart that Joe Blow and I have a good thing going.

So anyhow, I had this high-powered job. That was in June of '66 that I took that job. In November of '66 the relationship with Jack began to go to pot because a certain nurse from Sweden had come back from Sweden. And apparently they had had a thing going before. And goddam! it was going again. Uhm— In that late fall things were getting *very* bad. And I called Margo—the girl that I had originally gotten the name of a New Jersey doctor from. Because I knew that she had been to a headshrinker. And I said, "I think I need one." She gave me the name of the clinic that she went to. I was desperate. Oh God, I was desperate! I called them; they weren't able to give me an appointment until January of '67. I finally got to the doctor to whom they assigned me, whose name is D. And [*pause*] I was intellectually calm and cool. To the point of telling him the presenting problem and some of the back-up factors. I was also calm and cool about saying, "I think I am literally falling apart. Something has to be done."

I started to see him twice a week. He asked me to see him three times. I did. The classic case of psychiatric treatment. And upheaval all over the goddam place. And of course much of this was focused on Jack. He was a very convenient replay pattern for all my woes and griefs. I *would not believe* that the *absence* of a *father* could have *affected* me that much. Doctor D. was always saying to me, "It did, it did, it did!" And I was always saying, "No, no!" I was focusing everything on—on Jack. You know, "If he would do this, if he would do that."

KATRINA: The relationship with Jack was not all the way broken up?

ALEX: It was rough. It was involved with fighting, accusations, admissions, denials, detective-work. But it was still going on. Physically, emotionally and so on. I think he had a problem. [*laughs*] He didn't know which girl he wanted.

I started seeing the doctor in January of '67. A year later, in the spring of '68, the situation with Jack was really getting—

KATRINA: Can I ask you, how did February go?

ALEX: With the doctor?

KATRINA: No, February a year after the birth of your child. Any—?

ALEX: I was aware of it as an anniversary date. And thought pleasantly—not triumphantly, but satisfactorily— that I had *got* that *kid* through the difficulties of what could have been a medically problem-birth, and that he was [*hitting table*] *safe* and *sound*.

KATRINA: It was not a depressing memory?

ALEX: No, I wasn't depressed. 'Cause I have in my mind — It doesn't have to be depressing for me because I've got this good situation that I tried to set up for Alex. And I have the odious comparison of what he would have been involved in at any other time. "There but for the grace of God goes my kid." It's just like, in a way, saving your child from a fire, or drowning, or an automobile accident. You are aware that you're going to put that kid in a safe place. And having gotten him there, no matter how much you shake thereafter — And, you know, you always think, when you're going through Central Park and you see all the people: "Is that my child?" Yes, you do think of that. But it doesn't bother me. I can deal, I think, with that.

Spring of '68, my business had another big fat conference. I am about to go off to the conference, the evening session. I was talking on the phone with Jack and he tells me that the reason that he wasn't going to meet me at a certain place, was that Greta *was moving in* to his house.

Now you imagine *that* trauma. That was a Friday.

KATRINA: That sounds rather direct and clear, doesn't it?

ALEX: It should. But I didn't accept it as direct and clear. And Jack, although he wished, I'm sure, that I would accept it as direct and clear—he would have been back later. He came back often.

I called Doctor D. from the phone outside the conference room. He was very calm. And he always called me "Alexandra" when he was very calm. He said, "Now can you begin to think, Alexandra, about how we will deal with your life without him? It's done."

And I said, "Yes, I guess I'll have to." I don't know what other people may have told you, or what else you may know, about headshrinkers being supportive. He was supportive then.

I went into the conference la-de-goddam-da. Now this has bothered me many times: here we are passing pleasantries, and *my life is in pieces on the floor!*

I met this one fellow, who was very pleasant. A colleague introduced us. And this fellow said to me, "Have you ever thought of working in California? I might like to hire you away from your boss." Previously, I wouldn't have considered it. But at that moment I said, "All right. Let's talk money." And I gave him the figure, and he gulped. He said, "Are you open to negotiations?" I said, "Sure, we can dicker. Three hundred dollars." And he said, "A month?" I said, "No, a year."

But, you see, at that moment it was smacked to me: *"Yes, by God, maybe I would* go to California."

We went into dinner. And he came over to me when we had been seated. And he told me about this other fellow from another place. He said, "We have tickets for a concert tomorrow night. Would you like to go with us when we finish the meetings?" I said, "Great!" You bet I would! Take me to watch somebody play the piano, because, baby, I'm shattered!

The next morning—it was Saturday morning of the conference—I was reading *Vogue Magazine* and for the first time I learned what an excursion fare was on an airline. Previously I had been very careful about money. But I decided that I would go to California, just as a lark.

In the next two or three days, this other fellow took me out a couple of times. *He's married.* Very significant! Uhm —and I—I *knew* something was happening, I mean the electricity was *smashing.* At the end of that week, we were sitting in the Brasserie, and he said something about, "I think it's time for me to take you home." And I said, "Yes, with you." And he said, "You mean where I'm staying?" And I said, "Yes." And I went.

That was a big, smashing thing. He was here for another week. And we had a very nice time. He was tremendously troubled by it, 'cause it was the first time—

KATRINA: In other words, you seduced him?

ALEX: Yeah. I seduced him. But good. Though he wanted to be seduced.

He said something about, "Will I see you when you come to California?" 'Cause I'd mentioned that I was coming, you know, just to *go* someplace, to *spend* money, to be *away* from this *mess!*

KATRINA: You weren't going to California to accept his job?

ALEX: No! No! Had nothing to do with it. I was just going —the same way you'd go to Miami Beach. I wanted something pleasant—

KATRINA: But it was the same place where you were considering a job with him?

ALEX: I had stopped considering the job the moment the salary consideration had been settled. The job was out. And the only reason that I was on my way to California was that I knew I would have some time off. "I've got the money, I can afford to spend it, I need some pleasure. And the fact that you, my dear, are there, is a secondary coincidence."

KATRINA: Do you believe that?

ALEX: Yes, because I made the plan first. Before he ever asked me to go out with him *alone,* without his friend being along; before we ever got into bed.

I went to California, I was in the building and had seen some other people that I knew. I happened to go up the back stairway, because I don't take elevators. And there he was, in the stairway. We had a couple of lovely days in California. He was shocked by what he was doing. And yet for about a year he had been feeling in his own marriage, "Is this all?"

While I was in California, I ran out of pills. I called my office and said to Janice, "Get into my desk drawer, you'll find a package of some pills." She couldn't find them. "Oh hell!"

Now this other man, this friend that he had been with, was a doctor. I would have had no difficulty saying to him, "I've got to have some pills." Well, I didn't say a *damn* word! There we were in bed, time and again. And without the pills.

And so— I was pregnant again. Now the story gets very short.

I was back in New York. I went to my obstetrician and told him, "I think I'm pregnant," and he did the positive test. I was working with Doctor D. He said, "I cannot get you a legal two-psychiatrist abortion." He said, "For as nutty as you may think you are, you are *not now* that crazy." This is a girl who at one time he had thought of putting in the hospital. I said, "In other words that means across the river?" He said, "Yes."

KATRINA: This is in what year?

ALEX: The conception was early in April of '68, the abortion was in early June of '68.

I called the bank and said to Mr. Feldman, "I think I would like to borrow some money." "Oh, that's nice! What for?" "I think I'll go to Europe this summer."

Called Margo again and said, "Listen, tell me about that guy that you gave me the name of in New Jersey." She told me all about him and said, "He's a nice old-fashioned Jewish doctor, GP." I called him. I made the appointment. He was indeed a sort of old-fashioned Jewish family doctor GP, with a pretty well decorated office in a sort of rickety part of town. Not flashy, but comfortable. He took me in. Did a very classical D&C. Had a nice Irish nurse who held my hand throughout the procedure. Kept me informed, was supportive. She even made the remark at one point about, "He's a good doctor. You don't know how many people he has helped." Obviously a believer in what he was doing. He gave me a prescription on his own prescription blank for antibiotics which I—well, why shouldn't he? He's a licensed New Jersey physician. And he said something about, "That's one of the best D&Cs you'll ever have." And he told me at one point, "Now you're not pregnant anymore. But I just want to finish this up so everything is nice and neat." Well, I tell you, it was one of the best D&Cs that ever existed. No bleeding. No medical complications. No, I was not depressed. I came home. I went to sleep. Doctor D. called me about five o'clock and said, "Are you okay?" I said, "I'm fine." I went to work the next day.

And I would do it again. For the plain and simple reason that I think kids should be desired. Very strongly, that a child should be wanted and brought into an emotional climate—hang the money, and the food, and the so on— that can accept him and wants him.

Be a hippie if you want. Live in a commune. You know, do all these things—

KATRINA: Did you have this abortion for the same reason that you didn't keep the child?

ALEX: Yes.

KATRINA: Did you ever regret that you hadn't had an abortion the first time?

ALEX: Uh— Again, hindsight.

No, 'cause I got out of it pretty well. Uhm. And to the extent that the baby, Jack, and all these other factors got me to a psychiatrist—yes, goddamit, I am *glad!* Because I would have blown up without it.

KATRINA: Are you *glad* that you went through with it and *had* the baby and gave it up for adoption?

ALEX: Oh yes, definitely.

Because it led me to therapy. But also for the obvious reason: I am not afraid to have children; and now I want to. I would like to direct my life toward getting an emotional situation which *I* feel is stable enough for me that I will want to. I haven't got it yet.

Also, it wasn't my husband's child, and that in a way was very nice. I think if it had been, that would have really done great horrible things to me. In a way, it was sort of what I would call a "neutral child." I'd had no emotional involvement with the man. No, I'm not depressed. Yes, I would do it again. I have hellish regrets that abortions are necessary. I think it's *sad,* when you could solve the problem by public-health measures of contraception and education.

But if they are needed, have them safe, have them not expensive. Have them sufficiently anonymous that people don't get in all this hang-up. Because how long is it going to take before people can get rid of the inhibitions they have about an abortion? I don't go around broadcasting it. Last night the guy that I have now—when we were discussing the fact that I was coming here—he said, "Isn't it too personal? After all, it's a part of you." I said, "Yes. *But*—" And this is the same kind of thing I felt with Alex. Parts of it are tough. Parts of it I would rather not do. But you're playing the odds for what is more important. For *me*, I was willing to have *my* sweat so *he* could have a *decent life*. And now, although I have some regrets that these things need to be discussed—and some risk of publication—there are other people who *may* have life a little easier. All right, they're pregnant; but they don't have to get, you know [*making explanatory gesture of slicing off head*], like this.

KATRINA: May I ask you to correct your line, "some risk of publication" to "some risk *with* publication!" [*laughter*]

ALEX: Okay. [*laughing*] Publicity. The point is, you know, somebody may know. But I'm not that worried about it. And if someone comes to me and says, "Ah-hah! I read a book." Or, "I heard you on the radio." *So you may*. I have enough ego strength for *that*. I don't have enough ego strength to have a child without a father-figure. Hang the legal aspect. But a [*hitting table*] man in the *house* that looks at me and says, "I dig you, and isn't that a nice kid? And we wanted him, and we got him." That's all. The trappings don't matter. But that underneath *stability* I want for a child. So I would have to say that I would do it again, for the same reason.

I would do an abortion again. I would not do a pregnancy and give the child up again. Because I couldn't give the child up. I'll tell you that honestly. This time, I couldn't. I'm thirty-five years old. It might be my last chance. But I would have the abortion because I could not give up the child.

KATRINA: Do you think, by the way, that your husband was playing around?

ALEX: No. Absolutely not. *Absolutely not.* Not just because I trusted him, but we weren't the play-around kind. I tell you *now*—again, hindsight, and because of what I've learned—I believe that Rees loved me. It was not the way I wanted to be loved. But he did.

KATRINA: Do you feel this present relationship might be a stable one?

ALEX: No. I think the man in question is not the kind. I think he would like to be. But no, I don't think it will ever progress to a live-in arrangement. Um—and in all reality, I don't think I want to. But I am aware—shall I say, that I'm using him? In a way, yes. I'm using him to get used to somebody who really loves me. Which I need practice in.

KATRINA: Have you told your mother?

ALEX: Never! Never!
I have no contact with my mother now, except that she sends me occasional Christmas cards. And I would like to have lots of contact with her, *but*—she can't avoid recrimination for my divorce or anything else she may think I did that wasn't right. I truly don't want to have a surface relationship with her. I think I could have a mid-level relationship with her. I *miss* her. She's a fascinating woman. I'm not angry with her. *I have been in her position!* I *know* what kind of sweat she must have gone through to do what she did. How could I be angry?

And I'm not angry because she heaped a lot of her psychological trash on *me!*

KATRINA: Do you think she should have given *you* up for adoption?

ALEX: I have always felt that she should. And I could not understand *why* she didn't. Circumstances being what they were. It might have been easier for her. Did she keep me to punish herself? Did she keep me to punish my father, who would of course know that she had kept me? Did she keep me in the hope that he would come to her and want to get married? Probably not, because he did, and she didn't. Or maybe she wanted the ego satisfaction. Did she keep me because she really didn't know what else to do? Probably. That's why I kept Alex, or had him. I *could* have gotten an abortion. *She* could have had me adopted. People *wanted* to adopt me. My first foster home. And the second people that I lived with that are close to me—more close really than real parents—wanted to adopt me.

KATRINA: Why were you living in foster homes?

ALEX: Because it was in the 1930s and she was a maid in other people's houses. Cook, and so on. And had to keep me with another family. Until, in 1942, she [*hits table*] *married* and then had a home of her own. She was my mother, and she came to see me on Thursdays, and we did lots of things together, and I knew the grandparents and the aunts and the uncles. But I lived with other people. A matter of economic necessity. And first one family, and then another. Both of whom wanted to adopt me.

When the first one wanted to adopt me, she said no and took me therefrom; to home number two. Which is now where I go to visit, Christmas, Midwest. And what I consider close family. They also wanted to adopt me. They have two older sons who are adopted. And she said no. But they did not push the issue, and she left me there until such time— I think she knew then that she was going to be married. And in the spring of '42 she was married. Then established a home with my stepfather and took me there, where I've lived ever since.

Now I wasn't aware of the details of her situation until after I had made the decision for my divorce. In other words, Christmas '64. Christmas '64 she tells me. June '65 I got pregnant. I did not *think* about it until Alex was born. I really didn't give too much thought to—that I was repeating my mother's pattern. When I read that article, then I was tremendously aware of it: illegitimate children tend to create illegitimate children. "That's *me!*"

KATRINA: What was it that kept you from getting an abortion, do you think?

ALEX: I think it was because the whole idea was so foreign to me that I didn't really know enough about it. It was not something— In a way, it's like a kid who jumps from the top step to the sidewalk. When you stand up there to do it the first time, you think, "I never can."

KATRINA: Do you think if you'd had a best girlfriend who had had an abortion—?

ALEX: I would have very seriously considered it. If I had had somebody who not only *knew* about it, but was around to hold my psychological hand. But I didn't have very many friends. I had two in the Midwest, fairly close, who had had no abortions. But there was *me* and my *husband*. Rees was my best friend. He was the only person—you know, there we were, married to each other. We did not have that many friends. We worked awfully damn hard.

I think it's a question of education. If you could just get *information* about abortion. If you could walk into a hospital or a city clinic— You can get a TB X-ray, you can get a Wasserman, and a flocculation for VD. Why can't you go in and ask for a pregnancy test? And if it turns out positive, say, "Doctor or nurse, what is the next step?" In some places you can. In some of the hospitals now you are asked, "Do you wish to continue this pregnancy or do you wish to terminate it?" But to make it less of a hassle. Take a number, like at the barber shop. Make it *so* common that it is only a medical consideration: How do I cure this cough? How do I cure this growth within me? How do I deal with tuberculosis? What medical action do I take? Do I take it to insure the safe delivery of a healthy child? Or do I take it to insure the safe termination and the remainder of a healthy woman? Make it calm, and cool, undramatic, unhang-up. And then if you want to, maybe you could start teaching psychology in schools, so people will grow up with a knowledge of how they react to each other. Make it a part of your life so when you have a fight with your parents you can understand *why*. When you're growing up you can understand that all dating is not baby-marriage. Have a concept of yourself. Build some self-identity. Know who you are, and how you feel. Make it all so-o-o calm and cool.

Abortion in itself is not the answer. It's still a regrettable solution. Contraception is obviously the better solution. Education. Contraception. But people are going to go to bed with each other. They are going to do it outside the traditional confines of marital life. People are going to die of TB.

Abortion is certainly a better solution than going through with a pregnancy. Indeed yes. I was lucky. I had superb medical care. I had one guy who would let me hang onto him during the pregnancy. He was great while I needed him. When I didn't, when things got good, that's when it fell apart. But I was lucky. My child was lucky. Not every kid goes to the Judith Williams Agency. How many children are in the city's orphanages? How many kids whose eyes slant, or who have dark skin, are going to be there the rest of their lives? Absolutely. There are too many people walking around in the world right now. Not all kids can do what— My child was lucky. *Terribly* lucky. Part of it because I tried to tilt the odds for him. But not everybody can be that lucky. As it is, he was a premature kid and it took him ten months to be adopted. Yes, make abortions just as common as dirt. You'll phase yourself out of the business. You'll sell a lot of contraceptive medication, you'll have a lot of girls who at age four-teen know all gynecology. But you won't have unwanted children, and you won't have messed-up adults. It's called preventive medicine.

PATTI

Interviewed in June 1971

PATTI: Like when I found out I was pregnant, I went to the doctor's and he gave me—I don't know, an exam—where he puts the clamps in, and then puts his hand in. And like it was really freaky, 'cause he was talking to me the whole time, you know, askin' me all these questions about how I, you know, how I like school and everything, "Oh! I got your uterus in my hand!"

KATRINA: How did you know you were pregnant? You had missed your period?

PATTI: I had missed my period, yeah. I just—like—I don't know. We were drunk when we balled and I hadn't balled like since August. And I was late for my period, and I didn't, you know, I didn't even notice that I was late, and then all of a sudden I just thought, "I'm late." I just had a feeling that I was pregnant. I just knew I was pregnant about two weeks before I told Stig. And then, you know, he said, "Well, we'll take care of it, and everything." Like we weren't— weren't really even hangin' out together, really. We weren't goin' steady. And so then—I mean after that, we started seein' more of each other and then really got into it.

Like, I don't know, I was really scared. You know, after I went to the doctor he said like I was five or six weeks pregnant. And so then he gave me the number for *Clergy Counselors*. And I was really scared to call that—and I—like we didn't call for about three weeks.

And finally when we called, this—this guy was so fantastic—you know? Because he just said, you know, "Are you sure you want this?" You know, "You could have adoption. Or you could have this and that.

"But if you really want it, I'll tell you all about it. And I'll help you get there, and I'll do everything that I can for you. But like we just have this counseling in order to make sure that you know what's—what's real."

KATRINA: Did you really want it at that point?

PATTI: No, I didn't. I didn't want to have an abortion; no.

KATRINA: What did you want to do?

PATTI: Have the baby.

KATRINA: And do you feel this way now?

PATTI: Not now, not when I just saw a pan full of blood with this little blob in it; that's, that's all it was. But when it's inside of you, it's—it's so different—you know? It really is. But when you just see it floatin' around in blood, it's different.

KATRINA: Before you called the doctor, did you want to have the baby if you were pregnant?

PATTI: Yeah I did, but Stig didn't want to. Like he would have married me if I really, really wanted it. Or else I would have just gone to live with him and he still would have had the kid and would have taken care of me. But he said, "Lookit, you're just sixteen and I'm four years older than you. So when you're eighteen you just might look around and say, 'Here I am, eighteen, and my whole life's ahead of me, and here I am stuck with a kid.' " He says, "I don't want it to happen to you."

KATRINA: Do you feel he was wise? Or do you feel he coerced you? Or—?

PATTI: I don't know. I don't know. I really—I really wanted to have a baby, I really did. It was the first time I was ever pregnant. And I just didn't want to have an abortion. I told him if I had it somethin' would go wrong; I knew somethin' would go wrong. And it did. [laughs] But he said it was for my benefit. And now I'm kinda glad, 'cause I hated being pregnant. I was sick to my stomach all the time and I couldn't eat. We'd go out to eat— Like did you hear that chick talking in that other room? She'd order a big meal at a restaurant and she'd take two bites of it and couldn't eat the rest. And that's how I was. And everyone was gettin' down on him, you know, like, "How can you put up with that bitch?" "I wouldn't take that shit from her," and shit, you know?

KATRINA: So when you called the *Clergy Counselors*—

PATTI: I called them about three weeks after I went to the doctor. So like I was eight or nine weeks pregnant then.

And besides, we were tryin' to get bread together, because like I wanted to have a baby, but he didn't; and he said that I wouldn't want it. And he was trying to sell his motorcycle. And he still hasn't gotten his motorcycle sold. But that counseling is—it's really fantastic.

KATRINA: And you talked to the guy on the phone and he told you the alternatives?

PATTI: No; we talked to him and he said, you know, "Can you come down and see us?" So we went down to see him, and he was really nice.

But then he saw my doctor's note and he said that it was too late. Because, like when I went to the doctor's, I didn't know exactly when my period—my last period—was. I said, "About the beginning of the month, let's say the first." And the nurse wrote that down. But it did start March tenth, not the first.

So I had to go back to the doctor's and I took along my diary. You know, I never write in it, I just cross out when my period is. I just always have done that ever since I started my period, years ago. And I showed it to the nurse; and the doctor, you know, he changed it. She wrote up another doctor's note; and he came along and signed it and told me good luck.

So we took it back to the Reverend the next day. And the Reverend gave us the papers from the New York clinic— you know, like I showed you, what to expect and everything. And the telephone number, and directions how to get there, the whole shat. And he said to call as soon as possible; so we called Saturday, late Saturday afternoon.

We saw the Reverend last Thursday, and Saturday we called; and it was scheduled for Tuesday—yesterday. At eight-fifteen. But, I don't know. It was all really sudden, you know. Because I knew all along that I was going to New York to get an abortion. And all of a sudden I was on the plane coming here, and then I was in the clinic, and then it was all through. And that still hadn't penetrated me. And then when I was in the hospital last night, I didn't believe it: I'm here in New York, and all this has happened to me. It just—hasn't sunk in yet, you know? Now I know that I'm in New York. I've gotten that far. Okay now maybe I don't realize that I've had the abortion, yet, you know. Like it's— right now, it's just like I had a little operation, you know.

That's all it is. It's no big heartbreak; you know, like, "Oh! My baby!" But it was nothing; and—just nothing.

KATRINA: Are you Catholic?

PATTI: Yes.

KATRINA: How does that figure in?

PATTI: I went to a Catholic school for eight years, and I know a hell of a lot about the Catholic religion, and I think it's bullshit. What I do is my business, and what the Pope and the priest and the nuns do, that's their thing—you know? I'm not into it. It's not my bag, really.

KATRINA: Do you use—? Did you use birth control?

PATTI: No, I never have used that.

KATRINA: Why not?

PATTI: Like I wasn't planning on— You know, like I wasn't having like relations with any dude, for like a long time. Since last August.

Like last August I was engaged to this dude and we balled; a lot. You know? And then I broke up with him. 'Cause he was—he was spoiled around his mother. He didn't get attention, he pouted; and that was it, you know. He was no man at all really. So then, you know, I—I went with dudes but, you know, I didn't really get into any one dude. So like I wasn't—

KATRINA: So the time you got pregnant was—

PATTI: It was just one time. Just *one* time. It was the first time I had ever balled him, the first time I had balled since *last* August! And I got pregnant. I guess we're healthy; together, we're healthy. I don't believe it; you know, people try for years and years and years to conceive. And—one time.

KATRINA: And did you then learn you were pregnant, before the next time you had intercourse with him?

PATTI: Yeah. Yeah, I was late for my period and I told him. "Oh, well, we'll take care of that," you know. But then —you know, we really started hangin' out, and really got into each other.

KATRINA: He had no desire to have the child?

PATTI: I don't know. He said that he wasn't emotionally ready for a child—that, you know, in a couple of years that'll be fine, but not right away—you know. He had to get his shit together first—as he would put it.

KATRINA: Did you worry about getting pregnant?

PATTI: No, 'cause I had never used any contraceptive before and, you know, like never pulled out—withdrawal. And I have never gotten—you know, even been scared of getting pregnant. But I was late for my period, like it was due again in about a week and a half, and all of a sudden I just knew I was pregnant.

KATRINA: But you were not worried the other times?

PATTI: No, I was never worried. I wasn't worried; I just— All of a sudden it just hit me, I was pregnant. I just knew, I just had a feeling. And he said, "Oh come on," you know, "Go to the doctor's and find out."

I don't know. Like I said before, I really wanted to have a

baby. I—I even picked out a name if it was a girl. [*softly*] Laurinda.

KATRINA: Yet you say now that you don't regret it—?

PATTI: No. Because, I don't know, it's— What is it? Mother· hood? "The touch of mothers" or something, you know? To just want to hold a baby, I guess. But—now it's nothing. I don't know, we really weren't getting along that good. Because being pregnant's a hassle. I was sick to my stomach and I was really bitchy. And arguing all the time, you know?

KATRINA: Did you consider, at all, having the baby and giving it up?

PATTI: No. No. Not at all. If I couldn't have it, you know, *forever,* then just forget it right now.

One of the girls that he lives with—that lives in his house —she had a baby last April. And the guy wouldn't marry her. He just told her to fuck off. And he went and enlisted in the Army—in the Marines, for four years. So like she had the baby, and her parents weaseled her into putting it up for adoption, you know? They really talked her into it; they brainwashed her. And like, you know, she sees a little kid and she just—a little girl, about a year old, and she looks at it—and she just flips out, you know? Because like it just tore her apart, inside. And I—I've had one nervous breakdown, when my dad split—he split three years ago—and I don't think, mentally, I could handle—you know, cope with giv- ing away—

And that girl, she just *wishes* that she'd kept her baby. But she couldn't have kept it because she really couldn't have given it the care that—you know, a baby needs. And so that's why she did it. And like abortions weren't legal then, and otherwise she probably would have, you know. It's really the easy way out; it's a way of linking it, you know, because you don't have to go through all that mental pain afterward. 'Cause like she sees a little kid and she just, "Oh!" You know, she wonders, "Is that mine? That could possibly be mine. I'll never know." You know?

Like, she's twenty, you know. She—she could have done it but— She wanted the best for her baby—which is good. But still, you know, there's really an empty feeling; there's going to be an empty feeling for a while. That's—that's really a bummer. [*pause*]

KATRINA: Tell me what you were saying this morning about the problem of your age.

PATTI: Oh. Well the Reverend said that, you know, you have to be seventeen. "Take along something with your birth date."

Okay, I'm sixteen—

KATRINA: Did you tell the Reverend you were sixteen?

PATTI: No. No. I didn't. Like you were the first one I've told. I didn't even tell them there at the clinic. They were telling me, you know, to go get birth-control pills, and to lie and everything. But yet I didn't tell them I was sixteen. [*laughs*] Well, that's cool!

But I went through this— I worried— The only thing that was scarin' the hell out of me was they were gonna find out that my birth certificate was forged and call my mother. But they just took my word for it. They didn't really *want* to know that I wasn't seventeen. Because, like that chick was saying, they just want to help you and that's it. That's really a fantastic place.

KATRINA: What did you tell your mother when you left the house?

PATTI: I—I left the house Monday, at about one o'clock. She was— She works midnight shift; she works midnights and she sleeps during the day. And I didn't go to school, I just stayed home. And a friend of Stig's took me downtown to the city-county building, and I got my birth certificate and everything. And then we took it to where this chick works and she's got, you know, the size typewriter and everything, and she fixed the date on it. And it—it looks pretty good. Then we gave it the mud-puddle treatment and the wrinkle treatment. It looks like it's a million years old. And I—I was just so afraid that they would find out and they'd say no you couldn't do it.

So I was plannin' on goin' home and gettin' my things together before we left. 'Cause I didn't know what time we were gonna go. And all of a sudden he says we gotta get to the airport in a half hour. So I was at his house and I took a shower and I guess Tracy's suitcase. And a few other things that I didn't have with me, she threw in there—

KATRINA: Who is she?

PATTI: Tracy? It's one of Stig's house girls. He's got four of 'em. He lives with four girls now. And the rent went up when Mike and Rick moved out.

KATRINA: Did you say anything to your family? I mean, how was the actual departure from home?

PATTI: Well I—I didn't know that I was like going to the airport and everything, that I wasn't gonna go home. Like I — We left to go get my birth certificate, and then like I had to get a few things. Like they want us to douche and everything beforehand, and I had to go get all that equipment and everything. And then we just split.

KATRINA: Who was there at home? There's your mother—

PATTI: My mother was home, yeah.

KATRINA: And how many brothers and sisters?

PATTI: I have two brothers and three sisters, and I'm the second-eldest. One sister's thirteen, my older brother's seventeen, and there's one, he's going to be fifteen in July. And then I've got two little ones, five and six. [baby voice] And I got a dog named "Sweet-Poo."

KATRINA: Does anyone in your family know?

PATTI: No.

KATRINA: Any of your girl friends know?

PATTI: Yeah. Yeah, some of the people that he lives with. 'Cause like—I don't know, I feel different now, you know? 'Cause like we were having sex—big fucking deal—but, you know, some of them are just, you know, so righteous and holy and, you know, really holier-than-thou people. And, you know, I'm a slut and tramp to them. And like, my mother, you know: I walk in the house and I come home— you know, I've been gone for *two* hours—"Where were you? Out peddlin' your ass? Tramping, you little slut? You fucking bastard." That's my name, "fucking bastard."

KATRINA: And she uses that exact language?

PATTI: Fucking bastard.

KATRINA: And says, "out peddling your ass"?

PATTI: Yeah! I go, "I'm not a bastard, I know who my father is!" She doesn't like that. And then—and then in a little bit I'm "darling" "honey" "Would you do this?" "Sweetie, why don't you go clean your room?" Tryin' to weasel me into things, you know?

KATRINA: But, she did know you were going to be gone away for one night and one day.

PATTI: I— No, I really wasn't gonna—didn't tell her that. You know. Like I just don't know what to say—to some people.
But like, I've, you know, been gone for like two and three nights before.

KATRINA: *Without* telling anyone where you were?

PATTI: Without telling anyone where I was.

KATRINA: And what happens when you get home?

PATTI: Nothing.
One time she put out a Missing Persons Report, 'cause we went to Kennedy Park on that day and like I— We were havin' a big picnic, and I made ham sandwiches and took a jug of iced tea, and she thought I got kidnapped and raped and beat-up at Kennedy Park. 'Cause it's a really bug place, you know. But like what happened was, from bein' out in the fresh air all day, I fell asleep. And that's it, you know. I just didn't get it together to go home.

KATRINA: So it's possible that when you go home to-morrow—

PATTI: Nothing! She—she won't talk to me for a couple hours. She'll look at me, you know. But— And then she'll talk to me and we'll get on really good terms, you know?

KATRINA: Will she ask you where you've been?

PATTI: Yeah. I'll just say, "I never tell you where I've been. Why should I tell you now?" 'Cause I just say, "It's none of your business," or something.

KATRINA: I'd like to go back now: you got on the plane—

PATTI: Okay.

Okay, we got on the plane and I was—I was really excited 'cause that was my first plane ride, you know? And it —it was really neat. I mean it was far out. And then we landed; and I really felt, you know, bad. Like I felt sick to my stomach, and I had a fever. I always get a fever every night; almost every night I get a fever. And so then we were walkin' around the airport and got lost and finally we saw this thing about, you know, "You just push this button to call the hotel" and they'll "come and get you in their limousine." And the guy went past us three times without stopping. So finally we called back and this other man, this old man was there, and he was very upset 'cause they had passed him about twelve times.

So we got there and they weren't gonna give us a room.

KATRINA: Why?

PATTI: Probably because we walked in, in blue jeans. And we weren't very high-class looking, you know? "I'm sorry, we're all filled up." So I started— I don't know, I just said, "Why the hell aren't they gonna give us a room?" And the guy said, "Oh! Well! We just have one available." You know, "They just canceled the reservation." And probably because some other dude just came in, "Could I have a room for the night?" "Oh, yes, sir! Here we go!" And I heard that, and I didn't like that either. So they gave us a room. And it was a rip-off, twenty-five bucks—for one night.

And, like we got there about eleven-thirty. And then the restaurant was closed and I hadn't eaten anything all day but a bag of chips and a coke. And I was really hungry. So finally we found a candy-bar machine and we each had half a candy bar, and split a can of pop.

We didn't—like, we didn't have any money. Because he was tryin' to sell his cycle to get the money, you know. He still had his paycheck from last week and he borrowed the rest of the money; and it was like *just* enough. And we weren't counting on twenty-five dollars, and we weren't counting on staying over another *two* nights either! You know?

KATRINA: Right. But you had figured you'd have to spend a night in a hotel?

PATTI: Yeah, one night. Like we didn't really know what hotels were around here, or anything. They said at the agency that if, you know, we would have told 'em that we were going to be spending the night in a hotel, they could have given us the name of a cheap hotel, and, you know, made all the reservations for us. But like, you know, we didn't know that. It's Stig that called on the phone for me, because I'm really scared of . . . I was so scared, I couldn't even call the *Clergy Counselors'* number. And all it is, is a tape-recording! They give like to go see like Reverends, and all this stuff. You know, like "The North Side, go so and so; and the South Side, go so and so." So anyway, he called the place in New York on Saturday, and I didn't talk. But they could have done that for us.

So anyway I—I couldn't sleep, all Monday night. I was —I was just scared of the whole thing. I was scared that they were gonna tell me that my birth certificate was forged and— Or it was too late to do the oper—the abortion. And that's really what was scaring me. So like—

KATRINA: What about the abortion itself? Was that scaring you?

PATTI: I don't know. I was— Like I was kind of afraid of that. But I was—I was just so afraid that they were gonna say, "No, you can't have it; your birth cer—" [*shows her birth certificate*] Just lookin' at it, it doesn't look like it was right; there, you know, the four on it—and I was just so scared that they were gonna refuse me.

So we got a taxi to the clinic and I was shakin' like a leaf. And, you know, they—they were *all so pleasant* and *so nice* —you know? And like she told me to go up to the fourth floor, and she asked me like if I had my own sanitary pads and my belt and my doctor's note and the payment, you know, with me. And she told Stig where to go, to the waiting room, and that they'd call him in about three and a half hours. It was a long one for him; it wasn't three and a half hours.

So anyway, then I went up to the fourth floor. And I went to Room 402, I think. And there was like a screen, and this lady and this chick were behind the screen, and she took a blood sample from me and gave me this form to put my name on, and my number. And then she sent me up to the fifth floor. And when I got there they gave me these forms to fill out like, "How did you feel when you found out you were pregnant?" and, "How'd you get to this agency?" And then some things like, have I had any serious illnesses? And does diabetes run in my family? And so then the counselor came in. And her name was Lucy. She wears—she was kinda short, kind of on the fat side. She was a freak, which was cool. She was— Oh! She was bizarre, she really was. And they have this—she took me to this room, and they have like, this like diaphragm— No that's not a diaphragm, it's a —like a model of what your organs look like, you know. Like the ovaries and the vagina and the uterus, and the whole shat. I really didn't think it was supposed to be that *small*. Just really *small*.

And, I don't know, she was—she was really nice, you know. She really relaxed me, because she went into detail of exactly what they were gonna do. And one thing that she told me that really made a lot of sense, and that's: when the doctor is working on me, and like performing the operation, "Is it gonna hurt? Or does it feel funny or strange? There's a difference." Because some things—I never really thought of it that way before. You know, like when they put those— I don't know what they call them—"skepticles" or something; the clamps, the metal ones. Does that really hurt? Or does that just feel strange or funny? And, you know, lots of times, you know, I just, "Aw, that doesn't— That just feels weird, you know; that doesn't really hurt." And so that really helped me a lot. They tell the same bullshit to all the patients. That chick down the hall, she got the same thing, "You're a superb patient." "Oh, you're the *best* patient I've had in *years*." "You've really been good." And all this.

But like she had her hand on my knee the whole time. I don't know why. It was comforting. [*pause*]

Then I went in— Okay, before that she— 'Cause like this was the last day that they would accept me, was yesterday. Because they go three months, exactly three months after your last period. And so first the doctor gave me an internal examination. You know, like he just stuck his finger in there and pressed on my stomach. And if I was really big, you know, they would have known that my doctor's note was bullshit or something, you know. 'Cause a lot of people could do that, you know; they're not expecting that last examination. 'Cause I wasn't, you know. And then he said everything was cool, and that, you know, we could go ahead with it. But before that she told me, you know, to go to the bathroom. She said, "You got to crap? crap. I want your stomach to be as small as possible." That's exactly what she said. So I just went to the john. And, you know, she gave me a robe and everything. And he checked me and said everything was cool. So, I don't know, I think he split. And then she stayed with me.

The doctor came back like about ten minutes later, or

something. And then he started on it. Like they don't want you to see, you know, the blood and everything. 'Cause it— it flips a lot of people out. I wanted to see it. Because I'm— I'm glad that I did see it, you know? Because *that* is what my baby was. Right then; that's all it was—was just little— It was the biggest piece floating around. You know, there were like—like, you know, kind of mucous or something, you know, of blood.

KATRINA: Is that what it looked like?

PATTI: No, it was kind of—a dark red blob. That's all it was; and there was blood in there, too.

KATRINA: But it was *just* a blob? It didn't—

PATTI: It was just a blob.

KATRINA: It didn't *look* like anything else?

PATTI: No, it was just a dark blob.

KATRINA: And you looked because you asked? Or because you peeked?

PATTI: No, I looked— I peeked! [*laughter*]

KATRINA: And that whole procedure was over, you told me earlier, in three minutes.

PATTI: It just took three minutes, yeah.
   And then I went to the recovery room and they give you a coke if you want it, or any kind of soft drink. Then they come in and take your blood pressure. "Go and lie down for fifteen more minutes; your blood pressure is too high or too

low." So then I went back in fifteen minutes, "Go lie down for another ten minutes." And so finally, you know, I left.

Then we went out to the limousine driver. It's really a station wagon but they call it a "limousine service." We asked him when he leaves and everything. And the guy told Stig to take me out and get me something to eat, that I'd feel a lot better afterward.

KATRINA: Is this a limousine hired by the Clinic?

PATTI: Yeah. A guy that works there, he drives people to the airport. It's like eight dollars round-trip for one person, ten dollars altogether for another person. And like they start pickin' people up at eight-thirty in the morning and then ending at three o' clock in the afternoon. Just for—what is it called? La Guardia? Airport, they do that. And they tell you beforehand, you know, to try to go in, you know, to La Guardia, because they can pick you up there. And it's really —it's pretty good.

So anyway, we went out and it was lunch hour and all the restaurants were filled up. So we copped an apple, each, and we ate the apple, and we went back and we were sitting in the car. Stig was like asking me what happened and everything, was I really okay? Then I started—I don't know, I started feeling really funny; you know, I kept getting little pains, like I'd go "Ow," you know?

Then we split from there. And they were really gettin' harder, 'cause like, you know, I was going, "Oouw," you know, gritting my teeth and squeezing on his hand, you know. And I thought—they—they felt like cramps at the beginning, really intense ones that just came and went.

But by the time we got to the airport, like I was layin' on the seat with my head on his lap, you know? Oh, I was really on the suitcase, 'cause the suitcase was on his lap. And I really felt—you know, I had him roll down the window, 'cause I felt, I don't know, nauseous or whatever. Like—like I was startin' to sweat and I felt dizzy, and like I just wanted cold water, you know, and I was really shaky.

So we got out of the thing, and I ran into the bathroom and I thought—you know, like if I just went to the bathroom, like diarrhea or something. You know how you feel sometimes when you get diarrhea, you kind of feel, you know, sweaty and stuff?

But like nothing happened. And— You know, like it was really intense. And I was, you know, putting like cold water on my wrists and on my face, and everybody's comin' in and starin' at me. But nobody asked me what was wrong.

So finally I went out there, 'cause he was all flipped out, you know, and worried about me. And we sat in these chairs, and like that's—that's when it hurt the most, sitting out there. 'Cause I couldn't even stand up. And like, you know, he was pretty pissed off, you know, "Can't you maintain!" 'Cause like I was cryin'—'cause it hurt so bad. And I was breathin' really funny. I couldn't breathe—like there was something in the way. I was going "ehy, ehy, ehy"; like that. And so finally, you know, he kind of dragged me back to the john and said, "Go in there," you know. 'Cause people were looking at me. And he didn't—you know, he wasn't into that.

Then we went out and sat in these different chairs and I just—I just couldn't move, you know. And I was—I was really shaking, and he says, "Well, maybe I better call that place back, you know?" And I said, "No, it will go away." Like right after I had the abortion I had cramps, and they told me like to press on my stomach and push down, and that would make it go away. So I'd done that for maybe five minutes and I'd felt, you know, great after that. There were no cramps; no pain whatsoever.

But this time— And so finally, you know, I said, "Maybe you should call, maybe, you know. It won't go away, you know, even rubbing on my stomach." So like he went and he called. And he came back—you know, the guy was still on the phone—and he said that they wanted to talk to me. And I stood up, and I—I stood up like halfway, and I just had to sit down again. 'Cause I just—it was— You know, I just couldn't move, it hurt so bad, you know? And so he went back to the phone and said that, you know, I just couldn't even stand up. So they said, "Well, get a taxi, we'll pay for the taxi, just get—" You know, "Get her back here right away." So he went outside and got a taxi and put our bags in it. And then he came back in and kind of escorted me out, kind of draggin' me out to the taxi. And I got in the taxi and I kind of lay down on him again, 'cause it was— It's kind of hard to sit up when you're really in pain.

And so we got back to the Clinic, and then I could walk in and everything. But I was kind of like doubled over. And so we went back up to the fifth floor—and the one lady, Sally, that was in here—?

KATRINA: Yes.

PATTI: You know, when I saw her— You know, like when I wanted to leave, she was the one that kept tellin' me, "Go lie down for ten more minutes," you know? And she wasn't gonna leave me then.

And so she saw me. I said, "Well, I'm back again." She says, "I hear." And so then she told me to go to the john; you know, go see if I was bleeding heavily. And I wasn't. And so she took me into this examining room and put me up on the table and put me in a gown and everything.

And the doctor came in there. And put those dear old clamps back in me. And then like—oh that hurt like hell. But I don't know, I think— It did hurt, it really hurt a lot. But like if I wasn't *so* scared, I think I could have maintained, you know. But like I was really— I don't know—it just really hurt. And I was squeezin' on her hand and cryin'; and she's like—she was, you know, she *told* me *everything*.

She says, "Okay, now, they found some blood clots in you and he's gonna take 'em out. This may hurt." You know, "Hold onto my hand and everything," and she was really, really, *really* wonderful to me. They—they just couldn't do enough. Even before I came back, they still couldn't do enough for you. And that's why that place is really nice.

And so after that— I don't know, I think that it took about twenty minutes, you know? And they hid the blood and everything from me this time. They really hid it. And, but like he kept—he kept going in there—

KATRINA: And you didn't peek?

PATTI: I didn't even wanna look, 'cause I probably would have passed out. He just, you know, kept going in there and getting something and hitting it against the side of that tin pan. And I—I think I'll—I'll *never* forget the sound of that tin pan. For as *long* as I *live*.

So then she stayed in there with me and they brought an IV and everything. And this one lady doctor, she came in and pushed on my stomach, you know, to make me bleed. And I screamed. I must have scared the *hell* out of everybody. You shoulda heard me. I—I was—I was—I wasn't really that loud, but— And I was tryin' not to scare anybody, you know? 'Cause like that doesn't happen to everybody; that just happens once in a great while.

I think I triggered the whole thing because there's been *two more*. [*laughs*] Usually they say they have one every month, or every other month, one that has to go to the hospital. But [*laughs*] three in two days!

KATRINA: And then—? Did Sally stay with you?

PATTI: Yeah. Almost the whole time.

KATRINA: And you stayed there how long before they brought you over to the hospital?

PATTI: I was—about four hours I was on that examining —cold, hard examining table.

[*pause to change tape*]

PATTI: Right now, I've just got this feeling that in a while it will hit me that I'm doing an interview, you know? 'Cause it takes a while for things to sink in to me.

Because like—like I was starting to tell you: if I had read a book or something, that somebody said the thing takes *three minutes,* it's so *simple,* they sit down and *talk* to you and *relax* you and— You know, they're *all* so *casual,* and yet they take, you know, *fantastic* care of you. And, you know, when you're in the recovery room, they're in there every fifteen minutes to see how you are. You know, like if you've passed out or dropped dead or whatever. If I had known this. Like—like people say "abortions," and you think "ugh!" You know, right away that's what you think. But like, anybody—if they ever don't—if they ever get pregnant it's—it's the simplest way out, you know? Because, like it's *nothing.* It's—it's really nothing. That's why it's so neat, you know? Because I don't feel bad. I'm—you know, I'm *glad* that I did decide that. I don't know, it's really best.

Because, I don't know, I am kinda young, still at school. I'm really kinda young to have a baby. And be tied down the rest of my life.

KATRINA: How long have you been sixteen? Are you *just* sixteen? Or—?

PATTI: Since— No, since April.

I feel like—sometimes I feel like I'm a hundred years old, you know? [*faint laugh*] Doesn't everyone? But, I don't know.

I think—I think it was the wisest decision because like I really haven't been goin' with Stig that long. Like about maybe two—two months; really, you know, hangin' out to-gether all the time.

KATRINA: And that was only *after* you found out you were pregnant.

PATTI: Yeah. But like we used to see each other, you know, all the time; we were really good friends. And like, you know, he'd come over, "Oh, you're the only chick I can relate to. I got to see you for a while," you know? And we'd go out, or go to a show or something, and he'd have a good time. And yet, you know, he wasn't— He said, "I don't want to get hung up or anything now." And—and but—he changed his mind! [*laughs*]

KATRINA: He's been very helpful. I mean, that he came with you—

PATTI: Yeah.

KATRINA: Did it ever come up that he might not come with you?

PATTI: He wasn't gonna go with me in the first place.

KATRINA: He wasn't?

PATTI: No.

KATRINA: Whose idea was it?

PATTI: He just all of a sudden thought, "Wow, I really should go with you." Because that's when I started tellin' him that I have a feeling that somethin's gonna happen, somethin's gonna go wrong. I just had that feeling.

KATRINA: Did you feel bad that he wasn't going to go with you?

PATTI: I—I was scared. I get scared really easy, you know. Like I was even scared to call that counseling number. You know? It just scared me. Over nothing! Just calling a telephone number! I—I was afraid to do it. And—I don't know, he didn't decide—I didn't even know he was gonna go with me 'til we were talking to the Reverend and he was saying, "Fly to New York," and, "You get this and that." Stig says, you know, "Yeah, I'm gonna go with her." And I think, "Whoa! Far out!" you know. But I didn't say, "Oh, *before* you weren't gonna go with me." You know, 'cause he would have been pretty embarrassed. But he just decided to go with me, and I'm glad he did because now I have someone to lean on and I don't have to, you know, do all this by myself—you know?

Like if I had come by myself, I think I would have gotten on the airplane. It was he—he was the one that decided to call. He said, "I'm gonna call about you, because you're really sick and you're not supposed to be this way." And I think I would have gotten on the airplane. And they say I would have passed out on the airplane. In about a half hour, they said, I was gonna pass out. The guy from the clinic that Stig was talkin' to on the phone—that gave him a bed for last night—said that like if I hadn't of— You know, if I *had* passed out, I would have gotten clammy and everything, and they would have gotten an airport doctor to come, and he would have given me a shot, the wrong thing, and it would have counteracted or something or whatever. And it wouldn't have been right and it, you know, woulda screwed me up, really bad. And if I had gotten home, I would have been in a hospital for a couple weeks, you know? 'Cause alone I—I couldn't have—probably couldn't even walk to the telephone. Much less call! [*laughs*] Or had any change!

KATRINA: When you get home, do you think you will talk about your abortion?

PATTI: I—I don't know, I—I'd like to, because it's—it's such a good thing, you know? ' Cause I'd like to tell somebody that was—as afraid as I was. I would like to do something. I would. Maybe I could look it up, 'cause I really don't know what I could do. I'm—I'm—I'd like to help someone because—really—if I were to have a baby, I would have flipped out.

And, I don't know, I lost a lotta weight and yet I got fat. I couldn't eat when I was pregnant, and yet I got fat, right in the back, right here. And my stomach, my waist—I have no waist at all. And my stomach really got big, too. Give me three weeks, and I can get my hands around my waist. For sure.

LORNA

Interviewed in February 1971

LORNA: About six years ago, I had three children, was on the pill, and was having some complications. I was taken off the pill and was not careful, and I found myself pregnant.

KATRINA: How do you mean you were "not careful"?

LORNA: Well, I just was— I was trying to regulate my cycle and was not practicing any birth control. Which was a big mistake. I had always been on such a regular cycle that I thought that if I could just get back on it— But somewhere along the line I got pregnant; in a two-month period.

I was aware of it immediately. I called my gynecologist and I communicated to him that I was not interested in having another child. And I looked for an out. Like the doctor knew that I had a fibroid tumor and that this tumor ultimately had to be removed. So I was pressuring him—to the wall—to look for an excuse to make this be fibroid-tumor time. But he would not make any commitment.

Then I saw another doctor, who said the fibroid tumor was not anything, and I should go ahead with the pregnancy. When I communicated to him that I did not want to go ahead with the pregnancy and asked for names, addresses, I just got nowhere. Instead, he said I would have great trauma, emotional setbacks, and so forth. But I was determined not to have another child.

KATRINA: How old were your three children?

LORNA: Then, they would have been—let me see—four, I guess; eight—? Yes, four, eight, ten and a half. And my husband and I had really decided we didn't want any more children.

KATRINA: Had you and your husband talked about this before you discovered that you were pregnant?

LORNA: Oh yes. We really had decided that was it. We were delighted with our family. Although we had three boys, that was it. We weren't going to try for a girl. It was a definite decision on our part.

I tried to pursue any areas I could, in terms of information. And I reached a doctor I knew in Boston, who was an obstetrician, but was not practicing; he was here for further study of psychiatry. He came over and talked with us and reassured me that it was an absolute cinch to have an abortion, particularly at my stage of the game. He could see how apprehensive I was. He told me that if he had his instruments he would do it for me. He was a good friend. But he was completely not equipped for obstetrics here. Still, he kept reassuring me, and gave me a kind of confidence.

I didn't really have any strong feelings about the physical aspects. It was trying to arrange this thing. And then I remembered that we had spoken to some friends in New York during the course of the summer, who had, in conversation, told us about a gal they knew and her experience with abortion. This had been the typical phone call, five hundred dollars, meet the man at the brownstone in Brooklyn, have it done, walk out, no complications, and back to work two days later.

Well, this was just a fluke. So we called our friend, who was a radiologist in New York, and told him that we were looking for the same name. And he called us back, gave us the name. Then my husband made all the contacts—a series of phone calls—to set up an appointment.

Meanwhile, our friend gave us comfort. He also said that Puerto Rico—which we had talked about—was available, and to go ahead and pursue that, if nothing else should turn up. Also, he advised us to explore it with more of our friends; we know a lot of medical people. I did explore it with two or three friends, two of whom had names which were no longer in existence. They had to be current names. And these names were six months to nine months old at that time. You'd call and there'd be no one there, the phones would simply not answer. This was really, you know, very undercover. And these people move on, all the time. The names, interestingly enough, came from other psychiatrists. The psychiatrists had obviously gotten them from patients, therefore they couldn't check back; it had come out in patients' conversation. They could scarcely go back and ask their patients, "Now what was the name, and how do you reach him?" They're not in that position, you see. But nothing ever came of those names, although several did come up. So the best lead was from the radiologist in New York.

And we pursued it. I think the arrangements were completed within a week or ten-day period after we got the information. And it was very cut and dried. We were given an address, told to bring five hundred dollars in cash, not to say anything, to proceed with caution. . . . So we had an appointment, and we went down to New York. And it was like a grade-B movie: we got on the plane here, we landed at the airport, we hired a car to drive to the outskirts of Lido Beach, Long Island. In October—out of season—

which is like going to the hinterlands. We drove up to an obviously very middle-class—upper-middle-class—neighborhood. Split-level homes. And looked for the number. The houses were side by side. Drove in the driveway and rang the bell. Somebody peeked—like a speakeasy—peered through the door. And we gave our names and were acknowledged.

We walked into this house. No sign of anything. Asked to sit down in the living room. The doctor was probably seventy years old. Cigar-smoking, kind of distant, gruff, and asked me all the pertinent questions, like how late in my period, how many children I had. And after, he asked—I thought very interestingly enough—why I didn't want the pregnancy. And then he asked for the money. Which my husband proceeded to give him. Then the doctor asked for one hundred dollars more. Well, Roy said that this was all we had. This was what he had been told on the phone. And so the doctor accepted the five hundred dollars. He called a woman into the room and had her take care of me.

Then things sort of wheeled back and it was like a movie-set: there was this back room all set up for minor surgery!

The woman gave me a gown, shaved me; it was very medically correct. And she was warm and sympathetic—kindly—and it was a routine sort of thing for her, obviously. A very routine, around-the-clock experience. I was given penicillin and I was given sodium pentothal, and a local injection to numb me. And again, the doctor gave me the injections and then disappeared for awhile; and then, when she told him I was ready, he came in.

In the meantime he had sent my husband out of the house. Told him to go. Roy was extremely restless and apprehensive, and the doctor told him to go out and get coffee, or a sandwich, or something. Which Roy did. And he said he had an interesting experience in this little town, because he was driving around, looking for a delicatessen or someplace. And every time he was about to stop, he saw a police car.

Every street he drove down. He truly thought he was being trailed.

I'm sure he was much more nervous than I was. At this point I was completely calm; I knew this was what I wanted to do. The only thing that threw me was the doctor himself; he was gruff and mechanical. The woman was the saving factor. She was, I think, the equivalent of a European midwife, who kept talking to me, who was like a counselor in many ways. Who held my hand; who, when the abortion was over—the D&C was over—she did the cleaning up. The doctor disappeared. He just left. And this woman stayed with me and talked and proceeded to tell me the *number* of people he did, the *famous* people who came to him, the *fees* he extracted. I asked her why she did it. And she told me that she made extremely good money; she could put up with all his gruffness.

KATRINA: She dropped famous names without disguising them?

LORNA: She didn't drop names, but she told me "Hollywood," "New York," the locales of the people. So she was quite discreet. Quite discreet. She was a very warm human being. And she explained to me that she was bringing up her sister's child. She might even have been a German war refugee; she was from that part of Europe. Also, she told me that some of these things were done at night; and she was always on call. He scheduled so many per day, or per night; whenever it was convenient. She said that this was strictly, for her, the best paying money she could possibly make in this country.

KATRINA: Did she say what other fees he extracted?

LORNA: Oh yes. She told me some people pay one thousand dollars, fifteen hundred dollars. I asked her about the young, unmarried girls who came. And he got even more money from them because they were more intent on doing it; they didn't have the kind of situation— They would somehow get this money up. Many of them could afford it. He certainly wasn't getting the young school kid with only two hundred dollars, who didn't have parental support or—

KATRINA: He wasn't getting her at all? Or he wasn't extracting huge fees from her?

LORNA: I don't think he was interested in her. Or that girl wasn't getting to him. But he was evidently well known.

Oh, the other thing she told me was that he was a—disbarred. Is that the word, for a medical man? He'd been doing this for years and years and had been caught at it probably once or twice, or three times. But she said that he was so experienced, and so good, that he had been in business all these years. And he moved his front constantly. Constantly. Because this was the same man who had done the gal my friends knew, in Brooklyn, in the brownstone, you see. This was only four or five months later. And he was now in Lido Beach.

She also told me that many people came back more than once. That, since she had been there—she'd been there a few years—she had seen some of the same people two and three times. And this really threw me. I couldn't understand how anybody— But it was a simple thing. They had the money, and it was a simple way for them to take care of it.

I had planned to come back home the same day. We were flying home, and the doctor had suggested, before we started, that we change our plans and stay over in a motel. But we said this was impossible. We had kids at home; we had already made arrangements for the day. And then he said okay; we could stay here in the house until we were really ready to go. But this was, again, rather reassuring in that he had wanted us to stay over. This sounded to me as though, in case there were complications, he would be available. He didn't verbalize this, but it was sort of unsaid. And he gave me medication when I left. Or rather she did. He had all these things ready. And I think we must have stayed three hours or so, afterward.

KATRINA: Did your husband come back by then?

LORNA: Oh, yes, he was back long before that and was greatly relieved. By then, the doctor had left and the woman was alone with me, and she welcomed him into the room. She told him I just had to get this wooziness over with, and then we could leave.

And I felt tremendously relieved, tremendously. I had no apprehension. I didn't have any feeling that I was going to have any complications or any remorse. Two of my friends knew that I was going for this, and they came over to my house the next day. And the only complication I had was that I was silly enough to have something to drink—tea—before I got on the plane. And I upchucked that on the plane. But that was my only complication. I got home that evening, and my kids were in bed. I sort of took it easy the following day because I had these friends around who were catering to me. And by the next day or so I was up and around.

And I was aware that to me it was a very positive experience. *I* was tremendously relieved. My *husband* was tremendously relieved. And from then on in, I let it be known around that I knew of a name of someone I felt was good; and I told my professional friends. And I think two or three times that same name was called. I didn't follow up to see if they had ever reached him. But when, more recently, a friend's son was looking for somebody, they couldn't reach this man. They did reach the New York contact for the first consultation; so I guess the old man must have passed away. And this was two or three years ago.

So that was my only feeling about it afterward. You know. It was not at all a weird, unusual, horrible experience. I never had any complications. I never had any misgivings.

I had told my gynecologist that I was not going to go through with this pregnancy, and I went back to him for a check-up three or four weeks later. It was like unsaid, you know, that I had had an abortion, a D&C. He must have put it in the record somewhere but he never discussed it. I just said I was coming in for a check-up, I was no longer pregnant, and we proceeded from there. He had never delivered any of my babies; he was not the obstetrician. I had decided I was through with obstetricians and all I wanted was a gynecologist to check me once a year, and this was a top man in Boston. I've had a past history of complications of minor surgery, of ovarian cysts, and polyps, and now this fibroid thing—which I since had operated on.

KATRINA: Do you think this past history affected your choice not to have more children?

LORNA: Oh no. No. My choice not to have more children was: we felt our family was complete. We were old enough to decide this. And our family was set; we really didn't want anymore children. And there was no question in our minds that we should produce anymore kids. My husband and I were one hundred percent agreed on this. And this is the feeling that I've had so strongly about abortion . . . about unwanted pregnancies: I was in a good position. I could come up with the five hundred dollars. I had a husband who would not *allow* me to go down to that place alone, who was in *full* support. What of the numbers of thousands of people that don't have this? And who have to go through the same kind of thing, only worse? And who don't have professional friends who can put them in touch? Who are the unknown people? I feel very strongly about this.

My husband's reaction— Mine was, it was over and done

with. My husband's reaction was—the *indignity*. For the first time in his life he felt like he was doing something criminal. And he knew it wasn't criminal. But the whole subterfuge has always bothered him. The whole intent, and the whole feeling, was that he was doing something illegal. It was not a question of morality. We had no question of this is immoral, or we were killing a fetus, or any of this mythology. But the feeling of "we've got to work like it's under the table"—this goes against his whole grain. I just wanted it done and over with. His feeling was, he wanted it done and over with, but he always resented the fact that society makes it—this kind of a situation. After all, you know, it is a person's own right to do what they want. And this does not come within the bounds of a state's legality to arbitrate. My husband feels very strongly about this. I do too. But I, you know, my reaction was much more personal. I just wanted it over with. Though, you know, abortion reform serves the man, as well as the woman. For the *man's* protection as well. He was put in this position, and it's not a fair position to be in. You know, it's, "I'm doing something illegal." What's illegal about it? It's a crazy kind of system and it has to be changed.

KATRINA: Were you confident all along that you were going to get your abortion?

LORNA: First of all, I had plenty of time. I was very early. Probably by the time I had it, I was seven and a half weeks. So there was the security of thinking, well, I'm not going to run into problems. Besides, I knew that if we couldn't get a name in New York, we would go to Puerto Rico. I mean, there was no question in my mind. And that if we had to go to Mexico, we would go to Mexico. So the kind of assurance which I had, that we could swing this, made me perfectly— But, you know, it's not the same for everyone. I'm working . . . I've been working here for six months, and the whole thing is incredible. The barriers that are put up to people, are incredible.

KATRINA: How old were you?

LORNA: Six years ago I was thirty-nine, which is not, I feel, a time to bear more children. My husband was forty-two. So this had something to do with our feeling about "our family's complete, and we don't want to start raising new babies."

KATRINA: Did you have a feeling of the risk to you at thirty-nine—?

LORNA: In terms of a pregnancy?

KATRINA: Yes, and giving birth.

LORNA: No. No, because I *knew* I wasn't going to. I'm not going to produce this child.
   The only thing . . . I'm not bitter; I've never had any bitterness about the doctor, although he was sort of offhand. And I was delighted with this woman. My real chagrin and debate comes when I think of the two top-notch gynecologists in Boston who knew I was thirty-nine, who knew I had all my faculties, who knew that I was probably going to do something, and who wouldn't give me an out when I thought there was a good out.
   They never even suggested to me that I go through the psychiatrist thing; they never suggested anything. It was *I* who suggested to *them*, "What do I do to get rid of this?" I went to them with this perfectly good out, with a fibroid tumor, which was sizable, and I had the abortion, and then I did have to have that fibroid tumor removed three years later. It's major surgery; but, you see, that would have taken care of everything. I knew it was going to have to be done anyway. So I had to go through the abortion and then the

operation. My feeling was that they could have pushed it. Now their feeling is, you see, they're both connected with big teaching hospitals and they're not going to put me on the table and have medical students question what's going on.

I just felt I had a legitimate thing going, and they wouldn't capitalize on it the way I wanted them to.

KATRINA: And you feel they definitely knew that you were going to have an illegal abortion if they let you down?

LORNA: Oh yes! I made it very clear to them when I left both places. I made it very clear to them that I was not going to have this baby. I asked them, I said, "What do you know about Puerto Rico?" And one of them said, "Oh, Puerto Rico is tightening up now. It's possible though." "Well," I said. "Do you know about any other place?"

The second one said, "Make an appointment with my secretary for a maternity check-up a month from now." I said, "I'm not making an appointment, I'm not going to have this embryo in me a month from now, I will seek out somebody to do it." And they just— It was like they had their hands tied; they were so involved in *not* saying anything, and *not* giving me any information. I just felt, right along, they could have given me information and encouragement.

Since then, by the way, both these men have become very active, locally, on the abortion scene.

KATRINA: Supporting?

LORNA: Absolutely. Very involved! Very actively trying to get a clinic located here in Boston. Now I think this is a difference in timing. Again, I was not bitter about them or upset about them, because I really knew that—according to their ethics—this is the way they had to do it.

KATRINA: But it wasn't according to their personal ethics —because they're now personally involved.

LORNA: Right.

KATRINA: So their ethics were dishonest to themselves.

LORNA: As so many things are in the profession! There's a lot of facing up— But I feel that there has been growth with these guys. They've probably seen enough women like me, and a lot more unfortunate ones, to have grown a little bit with the situation. And of course the whole timing is different. I give them credit for at least moving with the times.

KATRINA: Did you have any remorse afterward?

LORNA: None.

KATRINA: Do you think of the date the baby would have been born?

LORNA: You know, I can't even recall the time sequence now. My greatest remorse, I think, would have been if I had produced another child and had not been able to give it the time or the . . . . Because my family was very demanding at that time, anyway. And I had things of my own that I wanted to do. And my husband didn't need the additional burden, the pressure of another child. There were many factors. I never, you know . . . I recollect in terms of the trip, how it took place. But I certainly don't go into an annual depression nine months from the time that—the time I might have delivered. Because I never figured out when the delivery date would be. I never got a future date; I never cared.

To me it was a simple medical procedure, and that's all. It was just more complicated in terms of appointment and traveling and getting there and coming up with the money, and subterfuge—which my husband resented more than I. My intent was so great that I really didn't get involved in what I had to go through to do this. But, in retrospect, it's always —not as a personal matter, but in terms of the whole big scene— I feel so strongly about the girls that I see, and the kinds of things that they have had to go through to get an abortion. It's much simpler now, with New York. But before that, it was just an unfair situation; the barriers put in front of people are tremendous—in, supposedly, our free society!

And I found that as time went on, and as the subject came up, I spoke very freely about it. Well, I would scarcely have told my mother. I did tell my sisters. As the occasion came up, and I saw them, I told them. And at that point it was very interesting, because my older sister said to me, "You know, as we were growing up, I'm sure our mother had several abortions. I can remember Mother going to a doctor, coming home, Aunt Letty going with her, and kind of a whole big thing. As I think about it now, I think Mother went and had abortions now and then; and I think her friends did the same."

Now I keep hearing this more and more from girls that I've talked to whose mothers were women of my mother's generation. They were without birth control, you see, and were constantly pregnant. They were not aware of when they were fertile and when they were not. They just really didn't know, and they wouldn't face up to any kind of discussion about sex or their bodies or fertility. So, in thinking about it, it would have been an interesting study to do in terms of how many women of that generation went to the doctor, went into his office, he aborted them, they came home, they stained, and they carried on. They had a relationship with a family doctor, and that same family doctor delivered the babies in those days. I think that lots of women were getting doctors'-office abortions in their day, because otherwise these women would have produced a lot more children.

Now this is not the sort of thing that was ever discussed, of course. My mother was still alive when I had this done, and I would never have discussed it with her. But she would not have disapproved. Not in any way. The fact that I didn't want another child, she would not have disapproved of. But she would not have liked to think of me going through any kind of . . . having a tooth pulled would upset her because it was "her child" suffering something. But the idea of an unwanted pregnancy, I think she would have been extremely sympathetic with. In fact she was very upset with my sister —who is a trained nurse—who has produced six children. She always said that, "a trained nurse should know better." You see, Mother was already saying that this generation, with their knowledge and knowhow, should know better than to be pregnant and deliver six children. So she was very, I think, forward-looking.

Someone else said something to me— We were talking, and this gal said that when she was at college she had a conversation with her mother . . . her mother calling her for some other reason, but mentioning to her that "the well-known-name Doctor who performed abortions in Boston"— this must have been twenty years ago—"had died that day. Therefore tell all your college friends to be careful." Now this is certainly an interesting thing to have brought out.

One other thing I've always felt about the abortion was the number of women who have had it without any kind of shot or anesthesia or . . . I mean, I'm always upset about this. Now I'm sure that this is the way my mother would have had it, the way women in those days must have had it. And there are *still* girls having abortions without any kind of medication. Again, I feel this isn't right. They shouldn't have to be subjected to this. Because I think with that much . . . with that kind of pain, there's going to be more trauma. The immediate situation is painful, and then there's the trauma, afterward, of thinking about it— I mean, it's going to be much more lasting. Also, I think that in terms of bearing children, they're going to be more apprehensive. They're going to have a different feeling going into it than they might have . . . if they hadn't had this kind of situation, if they had been numbed, somewhat. So, again, that's an unfair kind of situation.

There are so many discrepancies. And it's not just the young unwed girl who suffers. There's also the *married* woman who doesn't have this kind of security with her husband, who doesn't have the kind of relationship that affords her this kind of ease and freedom. Which is unfortunate, but it does happen. And she shouldn't be penalized for not having this kind of relationship. But she is, constantly. It's just not . . . it's barbaric. Some people say abortions are barbaric; the kind of situations that women have to go through are barbaric. It's the least civilized thing I can think of, really. The penalties of not-adhering-to-the-line or of simply the-misfortunes-of-nature-at-that-point, or of any other thing —it is just not fair. And can be remedied. But we move so slowly.

My experience here, as an abortion counselor, has been somewhat frustrating in that I feel that the great need is for this kind of understanding in the social-service field. The whole picture of family planning, and birth control, and abortion counseling, has been a neglected field. Social service stays away from it. They shunt it away as the medical profession has shunted it. And my own frustrations in this have sent me back to applying to graduate school. In fact, I've just been accepted for the fall semester.

I simply feel that this field is wide open, with not enough people understanding it, working in it; and that it hasn't been financially provided for. United Fund is not interested in promoting this kind of information; and they should be. United Fund funds all these family service agencies. I've talked to enough social workers—who call me at home now —asking for information for their individual clients. They call and ask me for specific information about birth control —which they haven't really gotten clearly from Planned Parenthood; or they have, but they need some qualifications.

KATRINA: Does that mean that their own agency hasn't given them enough information?

LORNA: Their own agencies, in some cases, want to, but their own agencies are ruled by boards of trustees, or directors— Planned Parenthood is working, and the forces are there, but the resistance is still great.

Now an individual social worker can do a hell of a lot of good, if she's got the information. And what I would like to do, after I get this little piece of paper that says I have a degree, is to work with these people. Also, I think that two years from now, the timing will be much better in terms of acceptance. The people who work in agencies want to help their clients, but they can't without the information—which they're not getting in school. I can see the enlarged service they will be offering to the client in two years. Now I may not end up in this field at all, in two years, but I do project.

KATRINA: Do you think, if you'd not had an abortion, that you would have gotten into this?

LORNA: I think I feel much more strongly about it because I've had an abortion. I think that the field itself, I probably might have gotten into. Though I might have been working, instead, for the Civil Liberties Union. The time has arrived that my youngest child is old enough so that I can do something with my free time. So whether I would have been directed this way, I'm not sure; because my heart is with the ACLU also. You know, it's a combination. You really have to make your decisions as you go along. And it's a matter of exposure. I've seen the need for family counseling from my volunteer work as a counselor here. That's a direct thing. I may have been aware of the need, but now I'm sure of it.

But I can tell you that they're not looking for women my age in social service. And I think it's a big mistake! I've had to *bludgeon* my way into school.

LYNN

Interviewed in December 1971

LYNN: Start with a question. That's easier for me.

KATRINA: I'm interested in—particularly—the first story.

LYNN: Oh, that's all I thought you *were* interested in.

KATRINA: Well, you said you also had an abortion—

LYNN: My dear, I've had *two* abortions since then.

KATRINA: So where does the story—?

LYNN: The story begins, probably, with the reason for having gotten married. Which was—I *think,* not having been through thousands of years of analysis—a kind of loneliness, more than anything else. And tremendous respect for someone who seemed to have only one goal in life which was "his work." And I was a rather minor part of his life.

I had left home—at what? Seventeen, I guess. He had been through a rather similar experience. We were not in love. I mean it wasn't anything like *love.* It was companionship. It was two sort of lonely, lost kids.

KATRINA: Did you know that at the time?

LYNN: A little, yes. We also knew, when we got married that the chances of—you know, we talked about divorce immediately. It was really—it really was living together, but in those days you got *married*.

Anyway, we got married, and I discovered to my horror that this guy—who, seemingly, was very talented, very ambitious, very one-directional; rather, to me, awe-inspiring— was very, very weak. The whole thing was a kind of awful façade. He also—though I've never known for sure— No, he must be, because he certainly has proven it—was an alcoholic. Our whole relationship prior to our getting married was parties and stuff, and we both drank a great deal. But it wasn't until we were married and living a life, that I became aware that his drinking was not just a sort of party thing.

And we were married two months, I guess, when I discovered I was pregnant. I was literally about to leave. I had *literally* begun to pack, when I discovered this.

I was very young. Twenty. I had no family. Or, I should say, I had a mother out in Michigan who was nuts, and a father who had remarried and had thereby acquired a new family of four kids. And not only that, but he and I didn't like each other. And it was a sort of ghastly moment in my life. And the thing is, what I can't do right now is summon up—the emotional—kind of thing I went through when I first found it out.

Um— I didn't know I could get pregnant. I seem to have a screwed-up, upside-down or whatever, ovary. And I had had a gynecologist actually tell me that the chances of my conceiving were very slim.

KATRINA: Were you using contraception?

LYNN: Yes, but it doesn't work for me. *Nothing* works. [*laughs*] Nothing. Except, probably, a condom. But that's a little much to—

Also, I must have gotten pregnant literally the night we got married. And the other problem I have is that I get a "sort of" period. Sometimes for two months. So I didn't even know I was pregnant until I was in about my second month, or a little over. I just had a strange period and I thought it was because I was married and having a regular sex life. But things were happening to me physically, like—you know— big bosoms, and morning sickness, and I began to realize "I must be!"

There was absolutely no money. This is all in New York, by the way. I only came out here two years ago. We were living in other people's apartments, under *incredible* circumstances. Like, at one point, we were staying with an ancient derelict friend of ours in a loft that happened to have a little el in which this old guy's bed was. He would sit there all day typing out his memoirs, but at night he would get screaming terrors in his sleep and cry for his mother and vomit in the wastebasket. That was pretty incredible.

Um— Anyway, we went through, you know, horrible moments of, "Yes I am," "What are we going to do?" "Get an abortion." So we started shopping around, trying to find an abortionist. Which—well, until it became legal, it was messy anyway. But it was really messy because we were—if we could dig up a hundred dollars we would be lucky.

I'm just wondering about windows. I don't know how loudly I'm talking.

KATRINA: Very softly, actually.

LYNN: You can hear everything in this place.

KATRINA: Do you want the windows closed?

LYNN: Yes, I think I'd better. [*crosses to window*]
It's so top-of-the-head, Katrina! It's weird. [*closes window and returns to sofa*]

Discovered I was pregnant. He was not working. I was. I was selling at a store and I was making thirty-five dollars a week. My take-home pay was twenty-nine, right? There was also a tiny bit of money which was a part of the settlement that my parents, who had just gotten a divorce, had arranged. It literally was not enough to pay rent. Oh no, wait a minute; they'd already gotten a divorce when I was seventeen. Eighteen? No. No, what happened was, they got a divorce when I was seventeen. Mother got the money for a long time. And then, arrangements were made so that it would be sent directly to me, because I never got it from Mother. And it was—was fifty dollars a month. It was not — You know, you couldn't live on it. And, uh . . . anyway . . . I think something I— God, it's *beginning* to come back! I mean I don't think this is valid unless I feel it. And I'm not feeling it yet.

KATRINA: I know what you mean, but it isn't— If you don't have the internal approach, then the intellectual . . .

LYNN: Yes, but I've been turning this off for a long time, baby, I really have!

KATRINA: Why you didn't get an abortion is . . .

LYNN: [*intensely*] Because the abortionist was the most filthy little woman you have ever seen in your life!
I went to— I guess she was the local Barnard abortionist, Columbia University. She was on 115th Street. She was middle-European, I believe. She had a waiting room that was *so* dirty, I mean just *awful*. With *masses* of people in it; women, all women, no men. Of all ages, all a wreck. Obviously there was nothing else she was doing, but giving abortions. And I left my umbrella. I'll never forget it. I left my umbrella. [*softly*] It was black and it had a silver handle.

Um— It was finally my turn. I waited maybe two hours, as all these awful people— They went in and they went out another door, by the way. And I went in. And lay down on the [*pause*] table. And she had long stringy black hair. Which in those days—I mean nobody had long hair. A sort of gypsy look. A white off-the-shoulder peasant blouse. And *enormous* breasts. Small woman, but huge. And she bent over me and everything sort of fell like this—Oomph— In the middle of it was a gold cross! And there was something so ironic about it—as she is telling me how one arranges a hundred-dollar abortion!

It has to be done in my place. I will need a bottle of liquor because there is no anesthesia. And I need at least two men, to hold me down.

And so I told her "I would call her." [*laughter*]

And I sat in the 110th Street subway station; Seventh Avenue. For another two hours. Thinking about what I want to do with my life. Like throw myself in front of the subway.

Finally went home. To face, of course, an irate husband. Irate—ooh—that's not the word for it. Who—who was furious because I had not solved our problem.

KATRINA: You went for a consultation? You didn't go to have it done then and there?

LYNN: No, not to have it done then and there. To be examined, to get the final. . . . What I did, was get a positive rabbit test, and then she did the final examination and said, "Yes, you're two months pregnant, a little over two months." Which gets a bit dangerous, even legally. And she was dirty. I mean she had spots on this white blouse, and things like that.

I went home. We were still living in a loft with old men and vomit and stuff. And it's very funny: I can't even remember that night. I just remember Stephen was—was absolutely furious. And scared shitless. I mean, suddenly he was presented with someone who was not. . . . You know, I just refused to go through this. I decided then and there that I was going to go ahead with the pregnancy. We could not afford a fairly safe abortion, and I would not do this. I decided. I would not have this—you know, be *made* to do this, for his sake.

KATRINA: Were you afraid for your life?

LYNN: No, not my life, because I—I got very close to [*pause*] killing myself—that night. Closer than I've ever been, really. I was afraid of—the hour or two before I died. One is not afraid of dying. One is afraid of pain.

And it sounded ghastly. I was disgusted at the idea of her filth; that she didn't even wash her hands, by the way. As I was leaving, she had not washed her hands—that was something I was terribly aware of. At just this long, *greasy* black hair that was sort of swinging in front of her face, and then she, you know, put her hand up you. The dirt of the place; the—the *pathetic* people in the waiting room, some of whom were really young kids. I mean, I was young, but they were younger. And mothers with young daughters. There was one woman with a young—sort of lower-middle-class lady with her *kid*. I mean who was maybe fourteen or fifteen years old. And from all indications, this woman was not a normal gynecologist. I mean it was just a mill, it looked like.

Um. . . . Went home, we had the mess. And this is what —this is funny: I remember how upset and angry he was. And scared. And then my just putting my life— Also I'd asked him to come with me, and he wouldn't. Also, he was drunk by the time I got home. Anyway, I literally sort of—I guess it was anger at that point—just put my foot down. I said, "I'm going to have this child, whatever, I don't care. We'll solve that later."

And uh— Then we just had absolutely ghastly months of

— The next two months I got very sick, morning sickness, and fainting and things.

KATRINA: Were you checked by a doctor?

LYNN: Oh, I went through the clinic at Manhatten Municipal, dear! They don't tell you a thing, they just sort of— You know, all the interns come by and you're stand—you're lying there with your legs apart, and they all go "Oh."

And this is where, Katrina—where it's all such a—so sort of weird, because I really don't remember that period. I remember what happened to *us*. But I don't really remember the real details in terms of when, in the pregnancy, decisions were made.

Uh— Very shortly after that, we moved. Found an apartment, a sublet on the Lower East Side, for fifty dollars, which I could afford. He was still not making any money; he was not working. He was doing little sort of funny verses, and stuff like that. He was a poet. And he was doing things like writing other people's captions. Anyway, we took an apartment. He decided that, all right—and this is where I can't remember at what point he decided this—that he would try to support me until the birth of the child. But he would *not* have anything to do with that baby. Under *no* circumstances would he be financially responsible; *anything* like that. And I still sort of hadn't decided what to do. I had not— You know, I was thinking "adoption" but I didn't know how you went about it or anything.

KATRINA: Were you thinking at all of—?

LYNN: I was just thinking, "How the hell do I get through the next seven months of my life?" Particularly when I started getting sick, and couldn't even support myself anymore; I got fired. I was sick so much that I would have to lie down. They were not very nice about pregnant ladies in those days. Horrible. I think, now, it's illegal—but at the time, I was fired because I was pregnant. And of course I couldn't collect unemployment. It was very messy.

KATRINA: So you don't remember too much what your thoughts were, about after the baby would be born? Or did you really know adoption was—?

LYNN: No. Sort of as time went by— Particularly when Stephen really, you know, *said* that he would have *nothing* to do with it. He never wanted to see it. He wouldn't support it. The minute it was . . . that was it. There was nothing else that could be done, except put it up for adoption. My mother was nuts, absolutely out of her mind, which is why I had left home. My father—as I say—I never got along with anyway; and certainly there was no reason to think that he would in any way help, either financially or in any other way. And my prospects were, at that point, a possible salary, afterward, of thirty-five or forty dollars a week. I had no, you know—I couldn't do anything; I couldn't even type at that point.

Oh, what I did do, in the very early stages, was start checking foster homes. To see if I could continue working and keep the child in a home until I could— Like, eventually, I figured I'd make *fifty* dollars a week. And it was just incredible. It was impossible: fifteen dollars a week for a foster home, at that point. And my take-home pay was twenty-nine. It just became, you know, absolutely impossible. And because of my own upbringing, I didn't really approve of bringing a child up under these circumstances anyway.

And then my sister and her husband, who lived in Baltimore, mentioned the fact that some people they knew there were dying to adopt a child. And, very briefly, there was a little communication. I actually wrote these people a letter. Sylvia and Paul had told this couple about me. Paul, my sister's husband, was an adopted child by the way. And the couple got desperately interested. It was really sort of horrific. They wanted to take over, pay my expenses, all that jazz. And the more I thought of it, the more dangerous I thought it was. Because it would be people I knew. If I had any kind of change of heart later, I could go scream and yell on their doorstep. And, again, I did not think this was fair to a child. I mean I was pretty convinced I wouldn't, but you just don't know yourself that well. So I finally, after maybe a month of this going back and forth with them, decided no. If I was going to do this—which was the only solution at that point—it would have to be put up for adoption through normal channels, so that I had absolutely no way of changing my mind later and *ruining* this kid's life.

Also, I felt that if that child were in a foster home, and I were spending fifteen dollars a week on it, and going out to, maybe, Queens, wherever—you know, weird, out-of-the-way places—I would resent it terribly. I'd hate that child for what it was. . . . I was afraid—I was afraid I would resent it tremendously. Even though intellectually I could avoid this. Still I'd *have* to. Because, one, I was young; two, I wanted this marriage to be over. As of the minute this episode was finished, I was going to be out of that. I wanted to not have my life stop, all that jazz. But also, because I was afraid I would remarry as fast as possible for "it." And make a tremendous mistake in doing so. I mean marry the first sort of, you know, stable, stockbroker type. And I wasn't sure at that point in my life, as screwed up as I was, that I'd make, you know, the right decision. So when I finally decided to put it up for adoption, it was a very clear concise thing in my head.

And Stephen just sort of— He did one thing, and I have to admit— It took years to do it, but I now respect him for it tremendously: he finally got a job, and he made a hundred dollars a week. In a factory. He was a kid, he was about twenty-two. I must confess that on payday he would come back with about ten dollars, and lots of booze, and lots of books and records. He'd come back at ten o'clock, having spent it all. But he *tried,* he really tried—for him. And I hated him for it, I mean he'd come in the house—I lived on spaghetti, my dear, and baked potatoes—and I *hated* him for it. It wasn't until, you know, years later, that I realized that that was the *best* he could do. That he *did* commit himself to at least supporting me until it was over.

And this way the months went by, and it was pretty ghastly. We were impoverished under those circumstances. God, did we have a book collection though! And records. And a fantastic hi-fi set! In those days hi-fi sets, you know, nobody had.

And terrible fights and what-have-you. And I sort of slowly went through the Judith Williams Adoption thing of going to see them. And then going through the Manhattan Municipal bit, which is just awful. And yet in a funny way it was sort of good for me, because as sorry as I felt for myself, the kids that I went there with were in such worse shape. Oh, there was one little girl— We'd all go, you know, like once a month to start with and then once every two weeks or whatever toward the end. There was a whole slew of people I went at the same time as. And there was one little girl, sort of a side-street girl, who was about seventeen or eighteen; very pretty, not very bright; who had married a sailor. And her parents hated him for some reason; he wasn't good enough for her or something like that. And they annulled the marriage. Legally, she had been married to him; and they annulled it, at which point she discovered she was pregnant. And they were *so ashamed,* that she was put into this place for unwed mothers. And she was not going to be *allowed* back into their *house* until she'd gotten rid of that child. And things like that made me, you know, feel not quite so put upon.

And the rest of it was sort of, you know, waiting, just— just waiting *forever.* Because I really felt that my life had sort of stopped until, you know, whenever it was going to be.

We lived in this little two-room apartment, a tiny little apartment that was painted emerald green. It had two beds in it that were red felt, absolutely bright, crimsony red felt. And I lived in that little house, and Stephen would be away all day and all night, drinking. And I spent a lot of time there because I had nothing else to do, and no money. I would lie on one of the red felt beds and read. And my eyes would fuzz because of the red next to the green, just so close, all the time. And I would sort of come up trying to see again.

KATRINA: You didn't try to get another job, because you felt so awful?

LYNN: I couldn't, I couldn't. How could—? I was beginning to show, for one thing. You can't get a menial kind of job, pregnant. I tried to do a couple of odd things, like take care of children in the neighborhood. But it just never came about. I think at that point I ran about two ads in a local newspaper 'cause I thought that was a possibility. But nothing ever—

I lived literally— I paid the rent and we lived and ate— although he wasn't home that much—on maybe forty dollars a month. And as I say, I lived on spaghetti. Anything to fill up on.

KATRINA: How was the Judith Williams Adoption Agency? You went several times I would imagine.

LYNN: As I recall, it was cool. Concerned, but very cool to start with. I don't think they believe you in the beginning. You know, because the final things are not until later.

Oh, wait a minute, I did that through Manhattan Municipal. I didn't go to Judith Williams on my own. I think when I first started going to Manhattan Municipal—which would have been maybe when I was three months pregnant—just for, you know, a check-up and kind of, "What do I do?" That's right, it was—it was at Manhattan Municipal. In the very beginning, in one of those first interviews. Yes, I do remember now— And I told them I wanted to put the child up for adoption, and they questioned me quite thoroughly about it. And wanted to know why, you know, particularly since I was married. And then they set up—I think the whole thing went through Manhattan Municipal until the very end; until, you know, it was actually a thing, a baby. I dealt with a psychiatric social worker, I think, as I vaguely recall. Or a social worker. Yes, a woman. And I am absolutely blank— I mean this is—I—this is all blocked out. [*pause*] I don't know if I could ever pull that back. Uh—but it was a woman. And it was that cool but concerned. . . . That's all I can say. It was sort of a very distant kind of thing. There was no "Poor thing." Which is just as well! And also disbelief at the— They kept saying "You can't tell until—later."

However, two things came out of that: one, fairly early on you make the decision as to, you know, you do not see the child if you're putting it up for adoption. And I did not want that. I wanted to see this child. I thought it would be very unrealistic not to. I was warned about it and "It's too hard" and "You get attached and you cry a lot." And I just thought that was absurd. So I made arrangements, fairly early on, to spend the time in the hospital with the baby. Not breast-feed it, but, you know, just be there for those—what? eight or ten days, I think it was at that point. And they still are not convinced you're going to go ahead with this, at all. It really is all very last minute; they come and see you after you've had the child. That may have changed by now.

KATRINA: Was it hard on you that they weren't convinced?

LYNN: No. No, because I—at that point, I really knew why I was doing this. I think I was quite honest with myself in knowing what *my* feelings would be like if I tried to keep her—*it*. I had grown up in a family where my sister was an unexpected child, and I knew how my mother felt about her. And I did not want this to happen to a child of mine. You know, spend the rest of my life thinking, "You've ruined my life, you little bitch." And I think that, in a curious way, something happens to you in dire straits. I think you think very clearly. I think some of my decisions were, in a funny way, less emotional than many I've made since. Because I had a long time to think about it, and a long time to really decide what was best for me and for the child.

KATRINA: You were certain in this period that you were going to go through with the adoption?

LYNN: I had to. There was absolutely no—at that point, no out.

KATRINA: And did this make you sad for yourself? Or were you . . . ?

LYNN: No. I was afraid I would be afterward. No, there was a kind of, as I say, crisis in my life. There was no reason to be sad; I was in a mess; this was the only solution. It really was at that point.

Now, remember, my father and I hardly spoke to each other. And he did cause problems later. I mean horrendous problems. Because—well anyway.

KATRINA: In this?

LYNN: Later, oh yes, horrendous *emotional* problems for me. Um. [*pause*] Everybody did. I mean, up until then nobody else really cared, except that Sylvia and Paul had talked about it with some people. They were the only people who kind of—friends who offered any kind of help. Meanwhile one of the things that kept me sane was an ex-beau who would still take me out. [*laughs*] My stomach out to here! And I kept thinking, "He has to love me for *me*."

KATRINA: Did you hope to be "saved" by the ex-beau?

LYNN: Oh no—no, we'd had it. I just thought it was terribly nice for him to *care* enough that he would take me to a movie occasionally. Because it was—you know, I had no money and Stephen was in his cups all the time.

By the way, the marriage was absolutely ghastly; which did not help. If you believe in prenatal influences, that's a pretty screwed-up kid. Plus, no vitamins. My entire life was —because, as I say, we had no money—was cooking a dinner. Maybe Stephen came home. If he came home he was so drunk it was not to be believed. And then he would bait me all night; and I couldn't have fights. I can now but I couldn't then. And I would sit there, night after night, while he, you know, "explained" myself to me. And told me how I was ruining his life, and he couldn't work anymore, and he was doing this only for me, and all this crap. And he had no responsibility for this; he had nothing to do with it. It was almost as though he was not—in fact, a couple times he did sort of suggest that maybe it was, you know, somebody else's child. Which it couldn't have been.

And there was the night he raped me; which wasn't too pleasant since I was rather pregnant, very pregnant. And I cracked his elbow.

Um— And then finally it all came about. And, oh, you know, all those sort of funny little things that happen, like you can't laugh because you pee, and you can't lie on your stomach anymore. And just the terrible inconveniences of it all; except with none of the pleasures of . . . whatever; you know, the future.

Except I had this *incredible* need for freedom. And freedom to me was the day I went to the hospital. And I think it was a physical freedom, too. I think there was a sense of a tremendous physical burden. Plus the thing of—of starting my life again.

And anyway, it came the night. And *that* was fantastic. The whole thing was beautiful. It really was, it was marvelous.

KATRINA: You mean the giving birth?

LYNN: Oh, it was just incredible, yes. It's—*That* really is very vivid. Still.

One, I thought I'd be out. You know, you have no preparation at all; there's no breathing exercises or anything like that. I thought I was going to be drugged, and then I wasn't. And there were funny things like breaking the bag of water at home and thinking, "Gee, I should go to the hospital"; and nothing happened. And then finally trying to get a cab at like four in the morning and no taxis. So we walked the thirty-odd blocks to Manhattan Municipal. [*laughs*] Me, you know— And then the endless waits while they do all those things. They shave you, and you sit around and you wait, and you're starving to death and you can't eat. And *still* just an occasional little "oop," you know. And then finally being put in the labor room.

And I happened to be in a labor room with a woman who later died; who had some sort of terrible messy delivery, I gather, and she'd come in so late that there was nothing they could do about it. I mean I don't even know if I was in pain, because it was so ghastly being with her. There were two beds in this one tiny room, and I was with this woman who must have been in excruciating pain, and who screamed, not — I mean, you heard other screams there, but this was like —absolutely ghastly. And they finally dragged her off, and as it turned out she did die later. I never found out too much about it.

KATRINA: Did this frighten you or just preoccupy you?

LYNN: It preoccupied me, I think, more than— And it was *horrifying*. And it was that weird thing of, if somebody is in worse straits than yourself— Which was the remarkable part about this whole experience: that there was always someone whose situation was so much worse than my own. It always made me feel that, "Honey, it's just not that bad. Whatever's happening to you, there's somebody who's going through something so much more ghastly."

Anyway, finally one went into the delivery room. I got a shot of glucose; it was natural childbirth. And I was awake for the whole thing. It was fabulous. It was just incredible.

And they said it was a girl. And they went through all the things of holding it up and, you know, slapping it.

KATRINA: How did you feel?

LYNN: I was very tired at that point. I lost thirty-five pounds in something like half-an-hour. I had gained fifty pounds; I weighed a hundred and eighty-five pounds when I went into the hospital. No one told me not to. They just came along and stuck their finger up you and said, "Okay. Come back in a month." Absolutely nothing; that's what was so appalling about that. And I didn't know anyone who was having children. I didn't have friends who were—you know, who knew about cocoa butter on the belly and things like that. And as I say, part of it was I couldn't have afforded to do much about it anyway.

And then came sort of the nitty-gritty oh— Um— Oh, funny thing— Oh, I'll have to. . . .

KATRINA: You may jump around . . .

LYNN: All right, I'll jump around because—

This is something that in this day and age is a horrific idea: but having a baby to me, at that point in my life, when

I was a very strong, independent, whatever—ambitious, I think, though I had no real direction—female; I had terrible problems with men. This is pre-Women's Lib, remember. And I went through that thing of, "My God, I've produced a child. I never have to prove myself as a creative person again. This is it, baby; anything from here on in, is gravy." [*laughs*] Of just—the pressure of not being a serious painter, not being an I-don't-know-what, a musician, or a, you know, writing the great American novel. Which with the people I knew, was sort of what one had to be. And in a funny way it was a tremendous release. "I've done one thing that I am very good at. And *that's it.*" It was very much a freeing thing—from all the pressures. Because of the kind of people I knew and was friends of; and even my husband who was, you know, a creator. That I just didn't have to write the Great American Novel now. I could just be me. That was very nice.

KATRINA: That lasted?

LYNN: Oh, tremendously, yes. I mean now it sort of doesn't matter anymore. But for a long time. . . . Because of the two areas of my life that were tremendous problems. Which is coming from a family where the father was a nothing; and the—the mother was this creative brilliant genius, who produced these great works of art. And at the same time having the problem of being a rather strong and individual female—of, you know, having men tell me I was a ball-breaker. So I was sort of, you know, in between these two. Which were rather common problems in this day and age. And feeling guilt at wanting more than just being a wife and just producing a child. And so there was a funny kind of "Oh, it's all right, it really is *good* for you. It's—it's a creative act. That's what you're here for, in terms of your just being an animal. And you've gotten it over with, baby; you don't have to worry about it anymore. Nor do you have to prove yourself in other areas. You've *always* got this to fall back on. *You can have a baby."*

KATRINA: Could that have been, in any way, an incentive for turning down the abortion? And going through with—?

LYNN: Oh—oh no. I didn't even *think* about it. Absolutely not. No, I was— Katrina, *that* was a *crisis.* I mean it was like, you know, a knife in my tummy. I had to *do* something. I had to *save* my life. No, I was in a situation where something had to be done and I had to do it; and I had no choice. No, that really, for me, was the only alternative to a situation that had to be solved.

This feeling was something that didn't even really happen until sort of I was in the hospital with the baby. It wasn't even an immediate thing. It was not— I mean, like I got out of the delivery room and I sat up in the bed and it's like eight o'clock in the morning and everybody's having breakfast, and I said, "I want breakfast." And, "But—but, you can't—" *"I want breakfast."* [*laughter*]

KATRINA: Did you get it?

LYNN: I got breakfast, and my first visitor arrived. [*laughs*]
And then about—like two hours maybe— I don't know what time it was, but there was some point that was the next feeding, and the babies arrived. By the way the Manhattan Municipal maternity ward—and it's probably worse now— was incredible. Oh! Everybody's in a bed; there are like eighty beds in one area, just on top of each other. You have one sort of either stool or chair, usually partially broken, next to your bed. And we were on a porch because there was not room. We were on one of those things where, as you're driving up, you can see these sort of lovely, open, glass sec-

tions. That's where we were. It was where you're supposed to sit when you're an invalid, you know. Very chilly.

And it was May. [*very soft voice*] It was beautiful; it was. It was sort of that first spring— It was very nice. And then I went through the whole thing of seeing "it" and holding "it" and, you know, just sort of preparing myself for [*pause*] whatever I thought I would go through afterward [*voice soft and distant—very slowly*] Of being ready if it happened, you know, that—the guilt, the desire for it, the wanting in some way to—get it back. All of that.

And— I was there for ten days 'cause they screwed the whole thing up. I think I was supposed to be there for five. And I had to stay three extra days because I had kept it, which was—was unusual. And it was very cute and it did all the—those things, you know, like babies do. And uh— [*pause—distantly*] Parts I can't remember.

KATRINA: Was that hard and trying at the time?

LYNN: No, oh no, that was marvelous. It was sort of, "I've made my decision." I knew that I was going to be faced with emotional problems afterward. But in a funny way I think I enjoyed that whole time, tremendously. And I really—made the decision. I'm tremendously sensualistic or whatever that word is; and I'm very good at enjoying things while I've got them. And it was— That whole thing was just fabulous. And also, you know, more so probably because this was it.

And then the emotional problems sort of arose. Like my mother arrived from Michigan, having heard that I was in the hospital. She knew I was pregnant. And the story was that the child had died. And then trying to get the hospital to keep her away and out of the ward—was just a mess. But that finally worked out. I didn't see her, and she sort of went wandering off on her own.

Then I heard from my father. He knew about the adoption. He'd known what my plans were all along; he'd known the whole thing. And, out of the blue, he said, "We will take the child."

And I then went through that incredible— I mean like in two days I had to make the decision: *"Suddenly* there's something I can do with that child."

KATRINA: Take it in a fostering situation? Or take it to adopt it?

LYNN: They would take the child not for adoption, but they would keep it until I could— There was no plan or anything, but they would take the child.

And then Stephen appeared one day, my husband. And —started crying. And [*very softly*] said he would help to— that he—if I wanted to keep it, he would try to help. [*pause*] Having already said, you know—

And—all this made it very difficult. Because suddenly there were alternatives. Which I had not had. *Ever.* It was ghastly.

KATRINA: Did you feel resentment that these alternatives came up?

LYNN: No; I just felt as though I were being *attacked.* By people who I think in a funny way were more immature than I was. I mean there was a kind of funny realization, "Kids, where were you when I needed you? This is nine—seven months of my life I have been planning to do something because there was *no way out.* And now, *suddenly* there are things I need another month to think about."

And I just decided, "No, it's not going to work, I don't like my father, I don't approve of him. I'm going to— If I'm not there I'm going to hate what he's doing, I'm going to disapprove; I don't like his own kids, they're the dumb-dumbs of the world."

I couldn't trust Stephen. I mean he might mean well but —forget it. And so I went ahead with it.

KATRINA: And do you feel you made that decision completely out of the good sense you mention now? Or out of any pay-them-back? Or anything like that?

LYNN: No, no. No, Stephen was not paying back. Again I sort of thought, you know, "He *means* well." Like his ten dollars a week. But he just— You can't trust him.

And my father, I was very resentful of him for finally making this decision at the last minute. And I kind of suspected that he must have known I couldn't do it. It was just too last-minute.

But it was a horrendous couple of days. It was really just ghastly. And I had to go over— I had to go over seven months of decisions which I had thought I could live with. And come to the same decisions. And *justify* them.

I may have been very wrong. I mean maybe Stephen *could* have somehow or other earned a living. Maybe my father— I don't know, I—I just doubt it.

No, I think I was right.

But anyway.

Well, under the circumstances, in a funny way I began to realize that even—even though I seemed to have alternatives, I didn't. I was right back where I started. I just didn't see that these possibilities were really possibilities. And I, again, did not think it was fair to her, to go— I mean just— just a kid. You know, my parents were I guess in their fifties then. Daddy was late fifties, his wife was younger. She had four children. The youngest child was like about ten or eleven. And just thinking of—"All right, let—let them bring the child up until I can somehow or other. . . ." That's not a life for anybody! You know, with older people. I would be somewhere else, I couldn't earn a living there; I certainly couldn't go *live* with them and live *off* them, you know. The minute I began to think of the practical aspects of it, it was —it just couldn't work. And again, the child would have surrogate parents and then have me. It would go through that ghastly thing of, you know, maybe at six I could afford to take my child and bring it up. Maybe I would be married and maybe I wouldn't, I didn't know. I went through that whole thing of "What I'm going to do is marry somebody as wealthy as possible who can support me and it." Some idiot.

But it was—it was not a good time, I'm afraid.

So I went ahead with it. And I got out of the hospital. And Stephen picked me up, and we got in a taxi, and we went to the Judith Williams Adoption Agency. Straight from the hospital with the baby in my arms. In Manhattan Municipal's little blankets. And by the way, I was a charity patient; they decided I couldn't afford to have a baby [*laughs*] under the circumstances. I never got a bill. And that was sort of embarrassing in a funny way. In spite of everything. I don't come from a family that "accepts charity." You know, they don't even know what it is, I don't think.

And little ladies arrived and they took it, and it cried. And then it had to go off and be examined by a doctor. And [*very softly*] we waited. Because I guess they would have refused it if it wasn't okay. You know, there I'd have been, with a—I don't know, child with some terrible problem. And uh— [*pause*]

Anyway, it was examined by a doctor and we sat for quite a long time. And then they came back and said yes, the child was okay. "Do you want to see it again?"

And it was another decision.

And I couldn't. That *had* to be it.

Said no. And that was that. And I went home. And Stephen left the next day. And I bought several gallons of white paint and I painted the apartment white.

[*long pause*]

And—Uh—

[*long pause*]

And— [*pause*] Oh, wow! [*voice cracks*] Sorry; it's getting me.

KATRINA: Do you want—do you want to jump ahead a couple of weeks or years?

LYNN: [*body shakes with sobs*] No; it's just that every once in a while I do this.

KATRINA: I'm sorry, Lynn. [*pause*]
  I feel very apologetic.

LYNN: No; it can— It just happens occasionally. Next thing I was going to say is [*fully weeping*] that every once in a while I break down.

KATRINA: I'm— I feel deeply sorry.

LYNN: And there's another thing, which is sort of scary, which is—I think, I'm not sure of this—that when she is twenty-one, she can find out who her—who her mother is.

KATRINA: No, I don't believe this is true. I don't—

LYNN: Paul did! [*Lynn waits, alert, crying stopped*]

KATRINA: I can only say that, because someone else I've talked to—who was adopted—went back at the age of twenty-one to the agency. And they said, "We can tell you everything we know, except your mother's name."

LYNN: You're kidding! I have *dreaded* this!

KATRINA: No, I don't think they can give the name.

LYNN: Then how did—?

KATRINA: They can give whatever information—

LYNN: Maybe—maybe with Paul, because it wasn't a legal one.

KATRINA: How do you mean?

LYNN: It was sort of an arrangement via friends.

KATRINA: I guess those can be risky—

LYNN: Do you know that all these years I've felt that it's going to come a day when the doorbell rings, and I have to *confront*— Because most adopted children have this terrible myth about their—their real parents. I suppose I should look into it. I suppose I've been afraid to.

KATRINA: I—I do really strongly believe that they cannot tell the real name.

LYNN: [*gently*] "Baby Evans."

KATRINA: They can describe her parents, what their interests were. But definitely not the mother's name. That's what this girl said she—

LYNN: Well, you see, as an adopted child, your person wanted to look into her past the way I thought this thing would want to look into its.

KATRINA: Yes. But she did not want the confrontation—

LYNN: I don't know. I've known some adopted kids who have just this *search;* they are—they're *born* almost, with a search for parents. No matter how well-brought-up they have been—I don't mean well-brought-up; I mean no matter how loving and secure and all that jazz, the family they've come from—the minute they know they're adopted, there is this idea that "somewhere are these mythical parents." And the idea of *being* that myth. And being *confronted* with—you know, whatever this dream was. Just horrifying. I mean, just awful.

KATRINA: Now one thing your child will be told, if in fact she does go to the agency, is that her parents were *married*.

LYNN: Katrina, that *does* matter! My aunt, my mother's sister, just discovered— She wanted to go to Italy; she's never been out of the country, and she tried to get her birth certificate. And she was "Baby, her-mother's-maiden-name." Her parents didn't get married until after.

Well, she almost died. And she got pulmonary pneumonia and emphysema in about three days. It was such a shock. [*laughter*] We just died when we heard, it was so funny. This terribly straight-laced, proper family lady. She's the only one in the family who, you know, digs up things like famous people in our ancestry— [*laughs*]

Do you have any questions? Because it's—it's sort of hard to think of it broadly and still tell a story which is a very personal one.

KATRINA: Right. I was wondering what year this was.

LYNN: Nineteen-fifty-one. Fifty-one? Two? One, I think it was. I don't really remember.

KATRINA: I'd like to ask you how you felt about it in the years afterward. At the same time, I don't want to— I don't want to make you miserable.

LYNN: No, no, that was all right. It just happened. It's all right. It's quite—actually, it's quite all right. It's just that I haven't talked about it for a long time. This happened every once in a while early on; and less and less as time went by.

I have *absolutely* no regrets about it. I can't believe, knowing how adoption agencies function, that this family, wherever she went, could have been *any worse* than the situation she would have been in had I kept her, under *any* of these possibilities. At least there were *two parents*. And I have a *thing* about growing up without a father, which is my own hang-up. They could be neurotic as hell. But I still think two neurotic parents is better than one neurotic parent. [*laughs*] Plus tremendous financial problems; plus, you know, being shifted about and all that sort of thing.

So that whenever I've had— As I say, it happened much more often in the first couple of years. You know, tremendous *guilt*. God, every once in a while I'd feel so guilty about it. And then when I'm rational and I think it out again: I know it was the *best possible* thing I could have done. I really would have hated her, I know that; I would have resented her tremendously. I was too young, I had a whole sort of crazy, mad life I wanted to lead. I would not have wanted to stop going out. If I had been *saddled* with a child who had cost me *financially* and *deprived* me to that extent, I'd have loathed her. I know that. And she at least was wanted by whomever adopted her. Whatever the reasons—they could have been very neurotic—but she was *wanted*.

KATRINA: Did you look at children of the age—?

LYNN: No, no.

No, as a matter of fact, I turned off kids. To a great extent. *Now,* yes, I'm sort of developing funny rela— I've always gotten *along* with them and I sort of had *friends* who were kids. But—

I—I also never wanted children again. I mean for numerous reasons; not just that. But I just was never in a situation where I wanted children. And I just, you know—

KATRINA: Do you think that's at all because of—?

LYNN: Very possibly; yes.

But I also think it's because having *had* a child, I don't *need* a child. Do you know what I mean? There's not that female thing. See I'm—in a funny way I'm very, very lucky: I've been married and I've had a child. And I don't ever have to do— They are *not* all-enveloping drives, and they haven't ever been since. So that other people I know, who are, oh, even in their early thirties—Why, people that are twenty-five are getting desperate because they're not married. I was *freed* of that. Which was marvelous.

KATRINA: Looking at it with hindsight, if you were. . . .

LYNN: Doing it all over?

KATRINA: Twenty today.

LYNN: Yes?

KATRINA: But with what you know now. . . .

LYNN: All right, if I were twenty today, my dear, I'd have gotten an abortion. Absolutely.

KATRINA: And with the hindsight of the good things that have happened, the pressure off about having babies, you know, the good things that have happened to you as a result of having had a child— With *that* knowledge, and you were twenty today, would you still have an abortion or would you go through with it?

LYNN: No, I would have had the abortion.

KATRINA: Why?

LYNN: [*slowly*] Because those months were very destructive to *me*. Very destructive. I haven't really ever thought about this—clearly, but uh— [*pause*] That was the end of my trust in people. Really, to a great extent. When I saw that both my husband and my father came through at the *last* minute, when it was *safest* to do it—that was it. I have never really trusted anyone ever since. I've been a sort of funny, "Okay, I'm on my own. There is *nobody*—that you can ever depend on." And I think *that* did it. More than anything else in my life.

Yes, I would have had the abortion. Though in the same — It is also possible, on the other hand, that twenty years later— I mean there are whole other situations. On the basis of the kind of person I was then, I might have been living in a commune now. I might—it might have been quite a different thing. I might conceivably have had a way of having a child. One, the whole thing about *living* with someone is so different. Ways of earning livings are so different. The social pressures are very different. And possibly— It's very—I— I really can't judge.

KATRINA: Should we whip through your abortions?

LYNN: Well, I guess they're pretty messy, I suppose. As it turned out—I didn't know it till later—I am very impregnable. Supposedly I'm not; but I am. And because I am so physically screwed-up I cannot wear a diaphragm safely. It just doesn't work. I mean it does most of the time, but it doesn't always. And it turns out that the pill doesn't work either, because I tend to— I have one leg that swells up, so doctors don't— It isn't safe.

Very simply, the second pregnancy: the abortionist was a very nice guy in Brooklyn. The whole thing was very fast. I was very early; it was painless; he was a real doctor who, I think, was a pretty altruistic guy. He was very nice, very understanding. And it was not that dangerous. I was probably a month and a half. I was more alert to the possibility of it, because of the first time. I had one of those kooky little periods and I thought, "oh-oh," and the breasts were going and stuff.

KATRINA: Was your first thought "abortion"? Or—?

LYNN: Absolutely; that was it. Also I had a friend who had just been through it about three months earlier, with the same doctor. Everything was fine with her. There was no fear. He was one of those, you know, *doctor*-doctors, who just was very straightforward. Yes, you were pregnant; made an appointment, went back, it was very fast. Plus I was *out* for it. The next time I wasn't; I was awake for it. But that first abortion was just very simple and very uncomplicated and no complications afterward.

The next one was a *mess*. Again, I did not know I was pregnant because I had two almost normal periods. And I also had amoebic dysentery at the same time. This child should have been aborted, whatever. I was going through arsenic treatment. And I was so sick anyway that I didn't know the difference. I was already about two-and-a-half months pregnant; and it was awful, it was really awful. My first doctor had disappeared. The person I was involved with dug up the abortionist. And a friend of his had been—she was okay, no problems—four hundred dollars.

I called this doctor up, and he was leaving for Florida the next morning and I had to go that day. And it was not four hundred dollars, it was five. Actually I got out there and was examined, when he told me it was five hundred. And he was horrible. It was also in Brooklyn, but a ghastly place right off some main highway. As he examined me he said he was leaving tomorrow morning, and it had to be tonight, and I had to have another hundred dollars. I screamed and yelled about the hundred, "I can't get it." He said, "Well, what about this man? The father? Hasn't he any money?" And I said,

"No. He gave me everything he could." He'd dug up two hundred. I believe in equal responsibility by the way. And he was a nice guy; I liked him and he liked me.

And then this doctor said, "Well, the *next* time, don't sleep around—*unless he's rich.*"

And just the whole thing was so sick-making.

So I had to come back into New York and run all over the city trying to dig up another hundred dollars. Which is not easy if your friends are not rich and you can't tell them why you need the money. [*laughs*] I went back out there around five o'clock, with my poor roommate who had dug up twenty-five of it herself. The man was a doctor and had a normal little office, unlike the first lady. But as I say, he was a sort of leery horrible man. And I scared the shit out of him, because I almost died.

I really did. He was terrified. I was supposed to be able to get up in about an hour afterward and go home. Well, it started about five. And he packed me, and I kept bleeding, and I kept bleeding, and he got scared. He had a gas mask which he finally just attached to my wrists. There was this incredible thing of the hand—I could *feel* it move. And I'd slowly come to, and then try to lift, you know, this heavy thing— I would try to get it back to my face as fast as possible so I'd be out again. And this kept on, and he obviously was getting more and more scared. You could *tell;* he was getting terribly nervous.

KATRINA: Were *you?*

LYNN: I didn't know. I was half out at that point. I knew something was the matter. I knew that I was supposed to leave in an hour. He *finally,* at about eleven o'clock, packed me— He kept unpacking me and then packing me up again. And the sheets were all— It was a mess. And the funny thing was that since I was not married, there was the whole social thing of my poor family: What if—what if I died? [*laughs*]

Finally around eleven he gave my roommate back five dollars—we had no money—and he said, "Take a taxi home." She had to go out without me to find a cab. She came back to get me and walked me one block away to the waiting taxi. He didn't want me on his doorstep!

And I went home. And I went to bed thinking I was not going to wake up. You know, if *he* was that nervous about the whole thing, and if I'd been bleeding that badly, I really thought— But I didn't really care what happened at that point. I was just sort of conscious of the embarrassment it could be since I wasn't married anymore. It could be embarrassing to my daddy out in Texas [*laughs*] if this hit the newspaper, you know, "carved-up body" and all.

I woke up the next day; I was *exhausted*. I had this sense of being incredibly drained. I don't think I've ever looked quite so ill in my life, but again I was pretty ill anyway. Then I went to the doctor who was treating me for amoebic dysentery, and he shot me full of pencillin for about a week. I had asked him, before I went for the abortion, if he would see me the next day. And he said, "Yes; but don't tell me who he is. I don't want to know anything about him. I *can't*." But, legally, he *could* treat a patient *afterward*. So he gave me incredible doses of penicillin and then said I was okay. And the whole thing worked out because it was one of those funny situations where it didn't affect my job. It was right around Christmas and there were enough long weekends and stuff so I—you know, I didn't get fired and they didn't get suspicious.

KATRINA: What form of contraception were you using at the time of the two abortions?

LYNN: The first one, diaphragm. Second one, diaphragm. Knowing, you know, that it didn't always work.

KATRINA: So they were diaphragm failures?

LYNN: Yes, but in my case— And I guess it's not *that* uncommon. I've even had one gynecologist say, "Oh, come on, you're crazy. It doesn't fall out." And he put it in one night, and I went back the next day and *he* removed it. And it was out of place.

KATRINA: But you definitely were wearing it?

LYNN: Yes, oh yes.

KATRINA: Both times?

LYNN: Oh, I always wear it. [*laughs*] Just in case it'll work!

I thought the pill would solve everything. Well!

I've asked my gynecologist—whom I've had ever since I've been out here, he's a most marvelous man—to give me an operation. He says it's major surgery and he won't do it. I've thought of going somewhere else; though I sort of think he's right. But I don't *want* children now. I'm too *old*. It's getting more and more dangerous. And if I got married I certainly wouldn't want to have a child for a couple of years anyway. And it's just—you know, it's getting *silly* now. So I was really sort of upset, having made that decision, to have him say "No!"

I must say, Katrina, that in this day and age to still have problems about getting pregnant—seems absurd. You know? Really. I mean what if you live in Chicago? What if I lived someplace where the abortion laws—? *Now* I don't feel the tremendous *fear* that I used to. I'd just go up the hill to Seattle Women's. [*laughter*] You know, it's very simple. Not pleasant. By the way, legal abortions are not that pleasant; they really aren't.

KATRINA: Is there anything in particular, in the years since you gave the child up for adoption, that you feel would be informative, or helpful, to other people who have also done it?

LYNN: There is a very difficult moment when you start leading a comfortable life, yes. When I began to make enough money so that I could conceivably have supported somebody. I have to admit she would have been in a foster home for ten years by then. But I would say that when she was about nine or ten I could have had a child, could have managed to support a child. But the minute I would go through the sort of guilt of that, I would think: *"But"*—going back to my original set of reasons—*"I do not approve of a neurotic single lady trying to bring up a child."* And you cannot be a single female without having a lot of the problems of being single.

KATRINA: I can't think of any other questions.

LYNN: Oh, there is another one.

KATRINA: There is another?

LYNN: That, because of the business I'm in, I'm constantly confronted, or, you know, dealing with young kids of about that age. The age she would be. Now. And every once in a while I see, or, you know, meet, or have some kind of contact with a kid [*pause*] who could be—my child.
And *that* is *unnerving*. But that's only happened recently. It never—I never went through the thing of, you know, the child age one or two, "Could it be mine?" It's only recently that I think that "God, that could be my kid!"

KATRINA: How do you cope with it?

LYNN: I think we'd get along well if we ever did meet. 'Cause I like that age-range and they seem to like me.

KATRINA: Now I don't want to *press* you, you know, because I don't want to upset you.

LYNN: Oh, no, you— No, I have no— Don't worry. Really. As I say, it's very rare, and I was surprised it happened.

KATRINA: And the confrontation is your biggest worry? Or not? Or has been in the past? Or—?

LYNN: Yes. I—it terrified me for years.

I almost think, on the basis of what you've told me, I should look into it. Because if it's not—if it can't happen, it's almost as though a huge kind of *thing* has been lifted. I was convinced that someday my phone would ring, or there would be a knock on my door. [*pause*] And I would have to *explain* myself.

And I never could. Because I've known enough adopted kids to *know* that there is *no* explanation. They would never understand. They couldn't. They might intellectually, but not emotionally. You have in some way failed them *so* horrifically. And someday I thought I would [*pause*] have to face that. Not right away. Because at first it was, you know, so far in the distance.

KATRINA: Have you ever talked to other people who have given up children?

LYNN: No; unh-unh, no. I've talked to kids who've *been* adopted, and discussed it with them because I'm sort of fascinated by what it must be to discover this. But I've never known anyone who— Ever. No. But I think even if—if I did know someone who'd given up a child, who was *not* married, I think the reasons would be quite different and the pressures would be so much greater.

KATRINA: It might be helpful to you. You know, you might feel better.

LYNN: I don't—Katrina, I *don't not* feel good about it. I know that I did the right thing. I don't have to convince myself. There are just little moments of guilt.

I think the *scare*, as I got older and she got older, was that —that it was something *she* would never understand. Unless, you know, maybe years later. But if I *ever sat in a room* with that *child* and *tried* to explain—Because I think she would want an explanation: "Why, Mommy?" Or just that terrible cold thing of *"You're*—??" You know, it's—it's just an *awful* idea, it really is. And a complete *stranger*.

And also if—if one ever did "meet" shall we say—the trying to be— I mean a—a feeling that one had to *be* something awfully special to someone. Because you would be. Whether you liked it or not, you'd have to be. That's rather demanding. And I thought that demand would be made someday. And I think I'm going to look into this further. It's silly to think about, if it's not possible. I just always assumed, on the basis of Paul's experience, that at twenty-one you could go check the records. You say you can't.

KATRINA: I say you can check the records, but they're— As this girl said, "I can tell you everything I know—"

LYNN: *"Except."*

KATRINA: "Except your mother's name."

LYNN: I think I'd better look into it; I really do.
[*pause*]
Katrina, if it happens, it's going to happen next year. I will be forty-two, she will be twenty-one.

KATRINA: I think— I think you'll be all right.

JEAN

Interviewed in April 1971

JEAN: Last year I had an IUD put in, around January, in the belief that I really—having had two children—didn't feel like having any more. At least not for a while. And it worked pretty well for a couple of months, or anyway I thought it was working pretty well.

But in the beginning of June, I hadn't had my period for a while. I'm usually very irregular as it is, and I didn't think too much of it, but I began to feel rather woozy and dizzy and logy and I just had a sense that I was pregnant. So I went to see the doctor who had put in the coil. He examined me and he said, "You're not pregnant. Not a chance that you're pregnant. The coil is in place; everything's fine. Go away for the summer. Don't worry about it."

KATRINA: How did he explain your having missed your period?

JEAN: Oh, well, I'm *very* irregular and sometimes I don't have a period for six or eight weeks. Also with the insertion of the coil, often your period gets irregular, and you have some bleeding, and everything's very mixed up. But, to give him credit, I will say he said, "Oh, it's *possible* you're a week pregnant." He said, "I can never say 'never.' But don't worry about it."

And I left his office feeling pretty relaxed. Although I had a sneaking suspicion in the back of my mind that women always know better than their doctors about things like that. [*laughter*]

So we went away to our summer house. And by the end of June, I was feeling very, very sick and very nauseous in the morning. I had all kinds of pregnancy symptoms, but I just assumed that . . . I didn't want to believe I was pregnant. So I just kept on going and I—I altered my diet; I thought perhaps I had hepatitis, which I've had before, and I stopped eating fats and I stopped drinking alcohol. And I felt a little better.

And then in the very beginning of July, I got what I believed was my period. So I thought, "Oh, it's all over. There's nothing wrong with me; I've got my period and everything is fine." And I continued to feel sick, nauseous, and just all kinds of symptoms. Plus bleeding for a week, which is the usual time; and then more afterward. But that had happened before with the coil, so I really didn't think much of it.

By the second week in July, I was so sick that I felt I just must go to the doctor. But I didn't want to go to the gynecologist; I'd already *been* to *him*. [*laughs*] So I went to my internist. I had to wait a week for an appointment with him, as usual. He examined me and took blood and he checked my liver and my blood-pressure and everything, and he said, "You know, it seems to me that you're pregnant." I said, "Oh, no, I couldn't possibly be!" He said, "Well, I want you to go and have the pregnancy test." So I did, and the next day I called up and sure enough I was pregnant. Which made me feel much better, because then I realized I wasn't dying of stomach tumors or hepatitis or [*laughing*] anything really horrible.

So I immediately called my gynecologist who had put in

the coil, and I said, "My internist says I'm pregnant. I've had a test." This was a Friday. Well he was going away for the weekend. And he wanted to *stall* me. So he said he didn't believe in that pregnancy test and I should take another one, at *his* hospital. He didn't want to be bothered seeing me Friday; he didn't want to deal with me 'til Monday, anyway. Meanwhile I'm bleeding and feeling *absolutely* miserable, and also thinking, "I do want to have an abortion, since I am pregnant. I really have, you know, made it clear that I don't want to have another baby, by getting this coil."

So Monday morning—he makes an appointment for Monday—so Monday morning I *pack* my *bag!* [*laughter*] Because I'm convinced I'm going to go to him and he's going to put me in the hospital and remove the coil, thereby causing an abortion, and thereby getting the whole thing over with.

I pack my toothbrush in my pocketbook, and my husband and I go down to his office, which is in the hospital. And he examines me, and he can't believe it. He just can't believe it. [*laughs*] That I could be pregnant. I'm one of the first people he's ever inserted a coil in, and he had looked at me and the coil was in place in the beginning of June and he just— he just can't believe it.

So we sit in his office, my husband and I, and he says that —Well, I said, "I've been bleeding a lot and I really would like to have abortion. I feel something is wrong anyway; even if I didn't want to have an abortion. I really feel that something is wrong because I've been having so much bleeding, I've been having pains, I've been so sick I can hardly get out of bed—" And he says, "No, you can have a perfectly normal pregnancy with the coil in. It doesn't make any difference."

And then he proceeds to give my husband and me a lecture. About how the third child is really great, and how it's wonderful to have a third child. How people brought up as we had been— How he knew how we'd been brought up, I don't know, since he'd only known me for about six months —people brought up as we had been would regret it all our lives if we had an abortion. And on and on, and that he— he'd "never done one," he said. Which of course is ridiculous because he must have done a D&C at some time or other in his gynecological career. And he assured me that it would be a perfectly normal birth. He drew a picture about where the coil was during all this time and how it couldn't interfere with the baby. I had visions of the baby being born with the coil in its head, in its stomach. And he gave me some pills for the nausea and he said I'd be fine and we would deliver the baby next—nine months from then, and don't worry about it.

Oh, and then he said, "And another thing I want you to realize: the hospital is very full right now, the schedule is very bad, and I probably couldn't get you *in* for an abortion before the fifth or sixth month. In which case we'd have to do 'salting out.' " Well, I was just horrified. Because I had no intention of having an abortion that late. And just the idea that he would—sort of *threaten* me. But, at the same time, I was very persuaded, and I felt very bad. And I left— Oh, my husband was great; he stood up for me and he just sort of looked at the doctor and said, "It's fine for you to say. But *she*'s the one who has to put off any sort of career plans or school plans, or any sort of plans, and stay home and take care of a third baby. And it's easy for me; I just come home at night and it's another one to run up to me and kiss me. But it's not the same for her."

Well, I left the office feeling, "Maybe I shouldn't do this. Maybe he's right." I was in such an emotional state anyway. [*laughing*] You know, when you're pregnant you do kind of feel—you cry very easily. And I was sort of persuaded; and I started thinking, "What if it's a boy?" because I already have two girls. And I thought, "Well, he assured me nothing would happen; I'll just be sick for another month." And for about an hour I entertained the whole idea of being pregnant and having another baby.

And I had—in my previous two pregnancies I had enjoyed them very much. I really had; I'd liked the feeling. I've always been the kind of person who feels that I must *do* something, I must accomplish something, I must achieve something; and I've been quite driven in many ways. And being pregnant kind of took all this off my shoulders. The two times I was pregnant, I just really relaxed and pampered my body and [*laughs*] enjoyed myself. I had natural childbirth. I had wonderful births and everything was great. So I left his office and I went through this idyll, "Well I'll have the baby, and nothing—Everything'll be fine."

And I went home and I felt *so* sick. And I was having pain. So I decided— I really did want to have an abortion by that time. But I just—this doctor had me so *intimidated*. I—I just felt I couldn't call him up and say I wanted one. From him. So I called my internist, and he recommended that I get "an opinion" from another doctor. And at that point I thought, "If I can only get an opinion of someone who says, 'Yes, you'll have a deformed baby if you go through pregnancy with the coil in there,' that will take the onus off my shoulders. And it will be very easy to make the decision because then it won't be *me* deciding to have an abortion, it will be a *necessity,* a medical necessity." Because really underneath, all the time, I just didn't want to have another child.

KATRINA: Was the idea of killing a fetus and murdering—?

JEAN: No, that really didn't—Well, I didn't really think of it in those terms. But I did think of it in terms of— I usually think of these things in terms of: "This is something natural that happened to me and I shouldn't fight nature. I should go along with it and not fight it and accept it." But all the time

I felt a little bit like it wasn't *quite* natural, because that plastic thing was in there. [*laughter*]

So I went to see this other gynecologist and he—he unfortunately wouldn't tell me what I wanted to hear. He said, "Yes, you can have a perfectly normal baby with the coil in and don't worry about it." But *he* was very nice about it. He said he'd seen enough women arrive chopped-up at Bellevue to know that when a woman decides she wants an abortion she's going to get it. And so if I asked him to give me one, he would certainly give it to me.

KATRINA: By women "chopped-up," he meant illegal?

JEAN: Yes, illegal abortions, or people trying to do it themselves.

So I went home from him, also, going through this idyll of, "Well, I'll have another baby; I'll live through the first three months somehow, and then everything will be all right; and I'll have another one. And he says nothing can happen, and I really shouldn't do it."

KATRINA: But he had said he would perform the abortion.

JEAN: He had said he would do it. But I was so *ambivalent* by that time, and I—I—I just—Inside, I really didn't want to have another baby, but I really didn't have enough courage to make the decision. I—I felt I needed some outside force and obviously these doctors weren't going to give it to me. And my husband—I think rightly so—said it was *completely* up to me and he would go along with whatever decision I made. [*laughs*] Which didn't really help. [*laughs*] Because I wanted him to say, you know, "Do one thing or the other."

KATRINA: What did he feel?

JEAN: Well, I—I honestly think he—I think he felt that it would have been nice to have another baby. But I don't think he felt it strongly enough to, you know, try to influence me in that way. And also he did see how miserable I—I was. And how our life had completely deteriorated since this whole thing had come about. And he wasn't anxious to, you know, prolong this for me if— Part of the problem was that the *decision* was the hard thing; I mean I wasn't really suffering physically that much. But I was just agonizing, because I *knew* I didn't want to have a baby but I was just *afraid* to make the decision to have an abortion.

I went home that night from the second gynecologist, and I had what I felt was a hemorrhage. It wasn't, [*laughs*] but it seemed to be; and I went through the whole night simply having labor pains. I woke up in the morning and I thought, "This just can't go on." And I called up this second gynecologist and I said, "I want an abortion." So he said, "Fine. All right." And he got me into the hospital that day at twelve— twelve noon. He happens to be the head of gynecology and obstetrics, [*giggles*] so it was easy for him to get me a room. Which is not always the case.

And I got to the hospital and then I was scared. Oh, I was so scared! I'd never had an operation. I was scared of the anesthesia. I was just a wreck by that time. [*laughs*]

But I really was glad that I had—that I had made the decision. So I went through the whole thing, and it was really very very simple. Do you want to hear about that?

KATRINA: Yes. I'm interested.

JEAN: It was—it was very, very simple; but all the time I kept thinking, "I would never have the courage to have an illegal abortion. Here I am in one of the best hospitals in New York, and they're taking my blood and they're testing all my reflexes, and they're doing *absolutely* everything," [*laughs*] "and I'm *still* scared to death. I can't imagine what it'd be like, you know, in an illegal situation."

When I got down there for the operation I saw it listed on the board as "Impending Abortion." By that time everybody pretty much agreed that I might be miscarrying. Then I was knocked out completely, and the doctor did a D&C. By that time I was at least ten, if not eleven weeks pregnant. From all this time of not knowing whether I was pregnant, and then, you know, going from one doctor to the other, it was pretty far along.

So an hour after the operation the doctor turns up in my room; he puts his hand in his pocket, holds out this coil, and he says, "Here it is; it was imbedded in the placenta, and you would have miscarried in the fourth or fifth month, anyway." Which really got me angry because I realized that all these doctors were going to let me go on, here, there, and then have a *late* abortion, a late miscarriage—which is more serious and more dangerous. But none of them were able to predict this, or didn't want to predict this.

KATRINA: Do you think they knew? Or not?

JEAN: Well, I—I think they should have listened to me when I was telling them something. I was *telling* them that this was not right, that I felt this was wrong. Just the way I'd been telling the first doctor I was pregnant, very early on, and he didn't accept it. And particularly when I had all the bleeding. But none of the doctors ever said, "Maybe the reason you're so sick is that you're going to miscarry later." And my guess is that this is a possibility that did exist all along and they knew it. But they never said a word. Because they don't want to do it. Well, the second doctor said something to me which I think was fair on his part and very real. He said, "I don't like to do abortions. To do an abortion is abhorrent to a gynecologist who has spent all his life trying to save the fetus. *But,* I will do it." Because, as I said before, he'd seen too many people—who wanted them and got them illegally—get butchered.

But I think that, you know, they—none of them laid the possibilities squarely on the table. And none of them could really tell me why I was bleeding so much, or why I was having pains. I mean if I would have miscarried in another month or two months, they must have had some inkling. They could have mentioned it was maybe possible. And I think it would have made my decision much easier, if they had just simply said that. Because then I would have felt, "Well, it's a fifty-fifty chance."

But in a way—You know, I'm the kind of person who likes to do everything the hard way! And in a sense, afterward I thought, "Well, it's good; I was forced to make this decision, and I made it. And that's *character*-building." [*laughs*] You know, despite the trauma.

I think it's also the way doctors practice now; they just don't do anything about anything, they just let nature take its course. And I was a little resentful of that, since— I suppose I couldn't rightly be. I mean I suppose they did the right thing. They couldn't tell me: "Have an abortion." It had to be my decision. Luckily this was all a month after the law came into effect. So there were no—no problems. And Blue Cross paid for the hospital. The doctor charged two hundred and fifty dollars for twenty minutes, [*giggles*] which was the time the operation took. And that was the end of it, and I've never had any— You know, I left the hospital the next morning. I had it at noon on a Friday; I left the hospital Saturday morning by *myself;* my husband took the kids to the beach. And I went home and I stayed in bed for the day. And I was fine and I have never regretted it or felt bad about it.

I am—well, I'm nearing thirty this year and I, I feel this great identity crisis coming on. Both my children will be in school half the day next year. And I'm just so *thrilled* that, you know, those early years with the children are over. Not that I didn't enjoy them, but they're very trying. I—I love my children, and I enjoy them; but it's very trying when they're one and three, and I'm glad those days are over. And I'm beginning to feel like a person again. I feel like my head's coming out from under the water. And I can start to think about possibilities for my life as an independent person again.

And so I don't feel bad at all. And maybe—maybe five years from now I'll decide, you know, "Maybe I want another baby." Although I don't think I will, because the population people have really gotten to me. And I feel very strongly about population control. I just can't see people having more than two children. Also, I know personally, for myself, that emotionally and psychologically it's better for me not to have more than two children. I—I can give just so much. I feel I've reached my limit.

And I had decided not to have more when I had the coil put in. Some friends of mine had had the coil and found it very satisfactory. And it was great while it lasted. But obviously, as the doctor said to me, it just had *never* worked for me. It wasn't that it had worked for four months. I simply hadn't conceived in four months. Probably. That's probably what happened.

KATRINA: What were you using before the coil?

JEAN: Well, before the coil, I'd used the diaphragm.
And the funny thing is: I had been on the foam for a year and a half before my first child. And I had used the foam for another two years, in between my first and second child. And never got pregnant.

KATRINA: Just foam?

JEAN: Just foam!

KATRINA: That's not supposed to be enough.

JEAN: [*laughs*] It's not supposed to be good at all. But it worked for me. For almost three years.

But the coil just didn't work. Usually the problem with the coil is that it becomes dislodged; though it didn't become dislodged in me. It was in place when I was already at least four weeks pregnant—in June, when I first saw the doctor and *told* him I was pregnant. What happens is, after you get pregnant the coil is sucked up into the uterus. So that the coil was no longer in place by the middle of August. There was some speculation as to whether it had been sucked up or whether it had just come out. But I knew it hadn't come out. It's a big thing! [*laughs*] It's an inch and a half long! I don't really see how people could lose it and not know about it.

One amusing thing—if you want to call it amusing—was that I went to my regular obstetrician when I first decided I wanted a coil. I went to my regular obstetrician who delivered my first two babies. And he said no, he wouldn't give me the coil. He just didn't believe in it and he didn't think it was a good idea. But this is a man who really believes that women should have babies all the time. I mean he—he used to tell me how I had "a halo of pregnancy" around my head. This doctor doesn't give pills either. He just really doesn't see any need for contraception at *all,* as far as I can gather. So it wasn't my regular gynecologist-obstetrician who had given me the coil. I had gone to somebody else.

KATRINA: Was this the same doctor who gave you the foam originally?

JEAN: Yes. This was the same doctor who gave me the foam! [*laughs*]

So really his birth-control advice was pretty bad. I mean he really had *no* birth-control advice, I don't think. But I love him, I must say, because he delivered my two *babies* and he was so *nice* to me. . . .

So now I'm waiting for— Well, we discussed sterilization for my husband, and we decided not to do it, not yet. My husband's perfectly willing to do it. But it bothers me a little bit. I don't know, I'm not quite sure why. I feel that we're still young. I still have a few child-bearing years. And if, you know, our life were to change drastically, or we were to move to the country, or inherit a lot of money, or something — [laughs] if I were to go through psychoanalysis—things might change and we might want another child.

But I must say, to the credit of my final gynecologist, he was great. I find most doctors are so conservative and so backward about these kinds of things. But he said, "Look, by the time you're thirty-four, thirty-five, you should know. And at that point, stop fooling around with all these devices and hormones and come let me tie your tubes, or send in your husband and let me tie him."

KATRINA: Does the fact that you kind of got intrigued with the idea of a third child—even though it was brief—?

JEAN: Well, I was intrigued with the idea *mainly* because I had had such *beautiful* experiences with pregnancy and child-birth. I mean I really dug the whole thing; I don't know how else to put it. The first time was glorious, I loved being pregnant, it was wonderful; I felt a little sick the first three months. The second time was a little harder because I had the first child; and I felt a little *sicker* the first three months, with the second child. But both times the births were exceedingly easy, my husband was there, I was a total princess for a week after. *Then* I got home. [laughs] *That's* when the bad things started. So that it was easy for me to fantasize into a lovely, you know, six months of feeling great, and round, and full, and—And also I must say that I'm a kind of tense, you know, nervous person. And when I was pregnant both times I felt great; really relaxed. I mean it just changed my whole metabolism. So, you know, it wasn't such a horrible prospect. The pregnancy and the birth weren't a horrible prospect at all. It—it was just that I knew by that time what it meant, taking care of someone; and how rattled I get.

KATRINA: And did this brief interest, or the happy recollections, influence you toward any sort of regret?

JEAN: No, no, I really have no regrets. I would think— I —I think I would do it again. I would have another abortion now if I got pregnant again. That's the way I feel; you know, this year. Maybe things'll change. But I've really just never had any bit of regret. From the moment it was over, I was *so* happy. The *instant* I awoke. No, the instant I awoke, I threw up. [*laughs*] About ten minutes later. By ten minutes later, I was just thrilled. And this has never changed. I've never felt bad about it at all.

KATRINA: Do you think about the *date* the child would have been born?

JEAN: No! I don't think about the date the child would have been born.

It never occurred to me to ask if it had been a boy or a girl; I just never— It occurred to me *since,* you know. But at the time, it just didn't occur to me at all.

I wonder now, you know— The one thing I do question is: if I get pregnant again and there's not a coil, you know, *maybe* it wouldn't be quite so easy for me to do it again. I don't know why; somehow the coil was my excuse. You know, that something was wrong. Maybe if I got pregnant again, and I *felt good,* and I didn't have any bleeding, and everything was going well, it might not be so easy for me to just go and have an abortion.

But, for that particular abortion, I was up for it.

CATHERINE

Interviewed in February 1971

CATHERINE: I'm just trying to think of my story, I'm trying to think back. It's a long time ago—1948. I was twenty-two years old. Twenty-two years ago, I was twenty-two years old, yes, right; I'll be forty-five next month.

But I think my story is essentially the common one of my generation, which is now known as "the middle-aged group." I also think it's a common one, an exceptionally common one, for today's generation; in other words, for girls who are also, today, twenty-two years old. I had been going along assuming, these last twenty years, that my generation, having learned all sorts of things—human physiology, and birth control, and being generally better educated—were imparting this information to the next generation. And what I've been doing the last two years has convinced me that they're not.

KATRINA: You mean that really there's been no progress?

CATHERINE: That's right. There's been a little progress, but I am startled today to find out that girls who are twenty-two years old, as I was; who are in college, as I was, are as ignorant in many ways as I was—about human physiology, how you get pregnant, what you do to prevent conception, and literally what an abortion is all about.

Which is why I'm talking to you: because I don't think that things have changed that nicely in twenty years.

KATRINA: Do you think that's an educational fault? Or do you think there's anything psychological about—?

CATHERINE: Well, no, I don't think it's psychological at all. I think that my generation was not as educated as I thought they were in this area. In other words, my mother told me nothing because my mother knew little; my generation, in theory, knew a great deal more. Now I know a great deal. But I have assumed, erroneously, that all of my peers knew a great deal, too. And now I find that my peers really don't know basic physiology. The bulk of the counselors at this institution do not know basic physiology. Which is one of the things that horrified me when I first came here. A lot of the ladies here do not understand their own bodies. And if you don't understand your own body you cannot understand birth control, or anything else.

KATRINA: Don't they cover that in their training to be a counselor?

CATHERINE: Well, yes, they do, but I think it's got great gaps in it.

Anyway, my story is essentially that I was a twenty-two-year-old girl, I was educated by nuns, Dominican nuns, in convent schools until I was eighteen—when I managed to escape, with great loud shouts and noises, and insisted on going to the University of Chicago. Which in those days was considered a very radical, a very communistic, shocking kind of institution. My insistence on going there was not just intellectual; it happened also to be two blocks from where I lived, and I was terribly poor and I had to go to a school that I could walk to, and that I could work at, so I could help support my siblings. So it wasn't all "I'm off to a liberal institution." Part of it was just plain stark reality: this was the best place for me to go.

So anyway, I grew up in this marvelous world, knowing nothing. I went off to the University of Chicago and discovered that there were all sorts of splendid things in the world, like cigarettes, and boys, and blacks, and Jews, and just all sorts of things that I'd never heard of. I should tell you that my parents were immigrants from England. Essentially they really had lived in a very small world; there were the English and "those other strange people out there, whoever they are." Imposed on that was the fact that they were terribly proud about being English Catholics. Which, as you know, gives you a certain status in certain worlds, since you can trace your lineage to holding up the faith when—

Anyway, so there I was. I went off to the University of Chicago, and among other things I discovered boys; and therefore I discovered sex. And without the foggiest idea at all, literally, like most young girls, of what it was all about. Quite literally, not any real understanding. But it was just absolutely smashing. I enjoyed it thoroughly—thought it was great.

When I got to the University of Chicago, I had credits from a high school that taught me biology and sociology. And when I got to the University of Chicago I discovered that in biology one is supposed to learn about the reproductive system. However, in my biology courses in high school, we did not touch on the reproductive system, including the reproductive system of the frog! Although we had dissected the frogs, we had just never mentioned how new little frogs came into being!

KATRINA: Where *did* babies come from?

CATHERINE: Well, we just never discussed that. I mean it simply was a very taboo subject.

I knew a certain amount about pregnancy. I knew that there was a baby growing inside my mother and all of the ladies that looked pregnant; and that at the appropriate time this baby came forth from the general area of the vagina; yes, I knew that. But I didn't have a very good notion of how the baby got there.

All this—you know—marvelous, confused, kind of noninformation—along with some realistic information. For instance, I knew that one of my younger brothers was delivered breech birth. Which is a very sophisticated concept for a kid as little as I was. And I knew what that meant, in the sense that I knew how the baby came out.

KATRINA: But you didn't know that intercourse led to, could lead to pregnancy?

CATHERINE: I knew that intercourse led to pregnancy. I just didn't know how intercourse was really done. In that sense of ignorance, I had no concept about intercourse itself. I was like most girls, including the girls of today. You can sit in on interviews upstairs and still be startled with the idea that most girls have it in their heads that intercourse is one activity, and pregnancy is another. And "one just doesn't get pregnant." A lot of gals have this magic thing in their heads that "Pregnancy is at a time." You know, "You get pregnant when you get married," "You get pregnancy part of your life when you're of a certain age." This is a very common belief with girls. Whether they articulate it or not.

So that it just never occurred to me that I would get pregnant. I'm sure that the connection between intercourse and pregnancy was there in my head. But it just didn't occur to me I would get pregnant. Because obviously I was not *ready* to get pregnant yet. In the sense that we weren't married and I— So I was fine.

You must understand that in my family . . . my grand-mother, for instance—who would allow no discussion of anything of this nature—would happily say, when one of my aunts became pregnant, "Kathleen is in a family way." At which point we knew that Kathleen was going to have a baby. But we did not discuss that until, nine months later, my grandmother said, "Kathleen has had a boy." And in be-tween, there was no mention. This was the general tone.

I did not have an enormous sex life; in other words, I didn't go from boy to boy, and boy to boy. It seems to me, yes, I think the condom must have been used: this is my guess, but it's a long time ago. I would think so. It was something that didn't involve me, anyway. Needless to say, I had no concept whatsoever of venereal disease.

KATRINA: Did you feel that you were "sinning," or any-thing like that? You were still a good Catholic girl?

CATHERINE: No. No, no, I wasn't a good Catholic girl. No, I made an enormous and very vocal break with the Church at sixteen and was kept in a kind of confinement, kept in the Catholic school, because I was considered an exceptionally bright, vocal, nattering, yapping kid—which I was—and I was very active in the labor movement early on. So it was thought that I would be a very good person, as a young Catholic person, doing great things for the future of the Church's position. Unfortunately, I could not see their posi-tion on so many issues; and finally there had been this one great row—so that intellectually I was long out of the Church.

My "sinning" was being a radical. I was very well aware that I was stomping hard on much of society's conventions by my political and social attitudes. Sexual attitudes were not, you know, involved. In some ways that makes sense, I think, psychologically. Because I poured an enormous amount of energy—I presume sexual energy—very early on,

fifteen, sixteen, seventeen, eighteen, and nineteen years old
—into the causes, the political . . . the important issues of
the day. Which were primarily, for me, black and white relationships in our society. So that I think an enormous amount
of energy and thought went in this direction, rather than into
worrying about my sexual being. Maybe I was repressing it,
who knows? But this was not an important aspect of my life,
you know, whether or not I was an attractive-darling-teen-
ager-type, were-boys-going-to-love-me? It never occurred to
me that they wouldn't. When I got around to it.

I didn't really have a lot of sexual activity until I was
nineteen years old. I did not become pregnant until I was
twenty-two. So I'm presuming that the condom must have
been working, because I know I'm fertile. In my happy way,
of course, I had three years of substantial evidence—so to
speak—that of course pregnancy was not anything you gave
any consideration to.

KATRINA: And then?

CATHERINE: And then I got pregnant.

KATRINA: Did you know right away?

CATHERINE: No.

KATRINA: You missed a period, and what did you think?

CATHERINE: I didn't think anything at all about missing
periods at that point in my life. As I try to explain to many
young women, the two ends of your life are fairly normal
times for missing periods: the end of the menses and the
onset of the menses; and all through adolescence as well.
There's an enormous variation. And I went through life perfectly happy, thinking, "Well, there's a period every month,"
and if there wasn't one that month it didn't particularly un-

nerve me one way or the other; the period always came. It always does, sooner or later.

So, I had missed a period, which had given me no thought at all. The one thing that gave me a clue that I was pregnant, was that fortunately I was involved with a young man who knew a great deal about human physiology, and my problem was I began to swell; my ankles were swelling. I had a certain amount of edema, and I mentioned this to him. And off I went to the doctor to find out about the edema. I think I was now into my second period in terms of all this mad counting, which in those days by the way I didn't do. There was no concept of counting, and knowing whether you're twenty-eight days. It came once a month, you know, that was it.

But Pete felt that there would be a very definite reason for retaining this water, and pregnancy could be one of them. And since we had an active sex life this was a reasonable assumption.

KATRINA: So it's lucky he was bright on this subject.

CATHERINE: Yes, right; right, otherwise I would have gone happily on, probably for another two months. So off I went to the doctor and I was pregnant. And there was no question in my mind; I certainly was not going to have a child. That —was impossible. By now, I knew a little more about physiology, needless to say, and I certainly knew that it was possible to abort people. I said flat out, "I must have an abortion; that's it." And he agreed, and—

KATRINA: How did you take it, when you discovered you were pregnant? Just "I won't have it"? Or was there anything else? Horror? Or disbelief?

CATHERINE: No, by this time I knew that it was perfectly possible to become pregnant. I must have accepted that much of the reality of the world. My immediate response was, "No, I cannot have it. This is not the appropriate time."

KATRINA: Why didn't you consider marriage with the young man?

CATHERINE: Oh, because I hadn't the slightest intention of getting married that young! I had much too much to do! Well, I started early on in life realizing that if you married—you must undertand that I came from a family of six children—that if you married, you married; you did very specific things, you stayed in the home, you took care of the children; and that's what you did. And I had no intention of doing that until a later point in my life.

KATRINA: Did the alternative of having the baby and giving it up—?

CATHERINE: No, I don't approve of that! Not at all. I have very strong feelings about that. I think you have no right to do that to another human being.

I don't think you have any right at all to create a human being and *give it away*. That is not your job in life. Just because it makes *you* feel a little better. No, you have no right to do that to the child. And you have no right to do that to society.

KATRINA: And, I suspect, to the person herself . . .

CATHERINE: Well, there's a certain amount of theory that some people need to do this, otherwise they will be very damaged emotionally; that they need to bear this child and then they'll— I think this is a lot of *claptrap*, myself. I think you should get to their heads and handle it a different way. Because I just don't think you have the right to do this to human beings. And most babies that are "given away" are not put into darling little homes. Most babies that are "given away" are institutionalized.

KATRINA: Is that still——?

CATHERINE: This is true around the world. You know, when I think about human beings, I think internationally as well as nationally. In our country we are all patting ourselves on the head, saying, "My goodness, we are reducing the number of children up for adoption!" We're talking about, of course, Caucasian children only—preferably with blonde hair and blue eyes—as opposed to black hair and brown eyes.

And, of course, children who are healthy, extremely healthy; bright; and all sorts of other things. Well I don't think we have reached, in our society, a situation where we *don't* have babies for adoption: primarily because of that operative word, "babies." It's very hard to get kids out of institutions after they're six or seven years old. Nobody takes them.

KATRINA: So the other route open to you was to have the baby and keep it?

CATHERINE: No, absolutely ridiculous! I was already supporting five kids! You're out of your bloody mind! I was working full time and going to school and conducting my political life; I slept four hours a night, sometimes three. I would never have considered bearing a child and keeping it. First of all, my commitment at that point to rearing children was already there and had been there since I was twelve years old. I had young brothers and sisters who had to be fed and housed and educated. No question about there being children to take care of. Commitment was already there; and they existed. I didn't have any fantasies about "Wouldn't it be nice to have a baby?" I had had an involvement with babies for a long time.

KATRINA: Why did you have so much responsibility?

CATHERINE: Which I shared with my mother.

KATRINA: Your father was—?

CATHERINE: My father was—my parents were separated not too long after my youngest sister's birth; and this was, you know, a shared adventure.

KATRINA: Your mother didn't receive any financial assistance?

CATHERINE: No, none.

KATRINA: Except from you.

CATHERINE: Right, right. And she also worked. She worked one shift, which we managed very neatly, in that she would come home and I would shoot out the door.

KATRINA: So—you said to the doctor—

CATHERINE: So there I was, yes, and it was agreed— We agreed that this was the only feasible thing to do. The only sensible thing to do. Fortunately he had his head in the right place. And in those days, of course, this was not an easy thing to do. But fortunately he knew a very fine OB man who did a few of these in his own office. This very fine OB man was not in the abortion business, he was in a regular gynecological practice. But, on occasion—for special people, I presume—he did it.

And so I dropped in to his office. I should tell you, of

course, that it did not occur to the physician I was talking to that I really didn't understand what an abortion was. Because, like most young women, I had a lovely, lovely veneer of sophistication; and in many areas I *was* sophisticated. Which is one of the things that I'd like to get through to everybody in this particular kind of work here: that they should *not* be taken in by this veneer of sophistication. When they say, "Do you know?" people answer, "Mm-hm"; and then the conversation goes on. Because a lot of people who pretend sophistication, who are sophisticated in many areas, carry it through to other areas where they know nothing at all.

So I hadn't the foggiest clue what in hell an abortion really was, in the strictest sense of the word. Here I was— you know, this person who knew so many other kinds of things—not having a bloody clue in terms of— Even though, at this point, I had done some better physiology and biology, I still really wasn't sure in my own head what was going to happen to me and my body when I did this.

So I went to the OB's office and I had an abortion. That was it, and I left. And again, nobody bothered to—

KATRINA: Was it—?

CATHERINE: Uncomfortable? Yes.

KATRINA: Yes, was it painful?

CATHERINE: Oh yes! Of course!

KATRINA: And were you forewarned at all by the doctor at the time?

CATHERINE: No, no, no.

KATRINA: So "something very strange" was done to you; and "that's what an abortion must be."

CATHERINE: That was what an abortion was, right. An abortion was this painful process. But I'm also aware, both now and then, that I had a fair threshold for pain, so I couldn't say I was going to die; I mean I didn't have any great drama attached to this. But it is a painful process without any anesthesia at all.

KATRINA: About how far along do you think you might have been?

CATHERINE: I probably—Well, I'm sure that he would not have done this— I can't remember, but since I was already having signs of edema—which is what really drove me to all this—I must have been eight weeks pregnant, in all likelihood.

But I had no clear-cut idea of what this was all about. I felt very strongly that obviously this was now some sort of a disgrace. In the sense that I could not possibly tell anyone I was going to have an abortion. Aside from knowing the full legal implications of what I was into; that much I was very aware of.

KATRINA: Did that upset you, then, as a political young lady? Or not?

CATHERINE: Yes. First of all I realized that my major responsibility was to the OB. And it made me very angry, in the sense of knowing that not only was there a problem in terms of what would happen to him as a doctor, but since he was a black doctor, he'd really have had it! So I was very annoyed with this, without question.

I insisted on going alone, I mean this was my responsibility; and the reason I insisted on going alone was this *enormous* sense of having to protect both the OB and the referring physician. Of course, I had this incredible amount of independence; I don't have to tell you that. But I felt, you know, that I just had to protect these two guys.

So off I trotted and had this procedure. I think probably it was not as traumatic to me as it might have been to a number of other girls, because I had already had a lot of physical procedures. I had already been in hospital; I'd already had surgery. In other words I was not having the human body assaulted for the first time in *that* sense; you know, it didn't spook me. I already had had a lot of association with physicians and hospitals and that kind of thing. So it didn't have *that* kind of fear attached to it, as I think it might for girls who are going for this procedure and have had no prior medical—real medical experience.

I had set it up: obviously I could not trot home after this. So what I did was to check in to a hotel; and Pete came pounding over, and there we sat. Actually he sat, and I was lying down. Because the one thing that everybody had forgotten to tell me was that I would need a Kotex with me! So of course I didn't think of this, since I still was not associating, in my thick head, abortions with menses and the whole total thing. And so of course I had no sanitary napkins with me, which was absolutely unbelievable. And this is one of the reasons why I urge the counselors to write it down, on the referrals here, "Take a sanitary napkin with you." Otherwise this connection is not made. And I know this because I've had, since then, a lot of experience with this particular activity over the many years, and it is something that women do not connect.

KATRINA: And the doctor who performed the operation didn't think of telling you much about it?

CATHERINE: Well, abortions in those days were not discussed. This is, I think, something that most people are not aware of. There just wasn't the concept. Probably because of the social pressures; probably because the whole thing was so terribly illegal, so fraught with fear. In others words, what everyone was trying to do was to keep the contact minimal. Unlike today, where we're sitting and nattering for an hour or two hours with the girl. And then the doctor is also going to sit and natter with her for two hours. In those days, contact was to be minimal. There were abortions done over the years, in that city and others that I have been involved in, where the girl very often didn't even know the doctor's name. In order to protect him, you see. So—no, he didn't get into any discussion.

He certainly greeted you in a pleasant manner and proceeded to tell you what *you* were to do. This is, as a matter of fact, the way most physicians handle their patients, for all sorts of procedures. You go in, they say, "Take off your clothes," and then, "Lie down," and they thump you on the back. They don't tell you why they're doing it or what they're doing. I mean, it's a standard medical way of behaving. So I don't think it's so terribly strange, when you think about it.

So we went to the hotel and I did a good bit of thrashing around during the night, because of course it was an uncomfortable situation. Fortunately, I had been a poverty-stricken child and knew perfectly well how to make sanitary napkins out of towels. As a matter of fact, in the earlier menses I wore them, as there wasn't enough money to buy regular ones. So this was no great crisis for me; I think it would have been a terrible shock to somebody else, you know, coming from a different kind of background.

KATRINA: Were you having any emotional distress at this time, of "what had you done" or whatever—?

CATHERINE: No, no, no, you're not— And I would like to point out—not only out of my own experience, but out of the experiences of a lot of other gals that I have gone through this with from day one to day three—you don't feel

awfully good if you've had an abortion without any anesthesia. If you have a lot of cramping afterward, what you're
really concerned with is not your emotional state at all; you
are physically uncomfortable. And I think most people do
not get into their emotional discomforts until after they finish
with the physical ones. I just don't think they're going
through high trauma—psychic trauma—at that point. They
are physically uncomfortable, they're concerned about their
own body, they're not concerned about what they've done.
It's not until the physical aspects of the abortion are disap-
pearing that they can give their energies to other aspects of
it.

KATRINA: And what happened to you?

CATHERINE: Well, what happened to me, physically, was
of course that the whole thing was over physically in a couple of days. I felt perfectly fine. Needless to say we both had
the problem of coming up with the money, which was a
great source of anguish and aggravation. It was—uh, let's see
—we managed to pull together five hundred and fifty— That
was very high in those days. But I was able to borrow some
money, and Pete was able to borrow some money.

KATRINA: Did you resent the fee? Or did you feel you got
what you wanted and—?

CATHERINE: I think we— I think probably you did not resent the fee in those days. Because there was no concept that
it could be done cheaper. And you did not really relate the
fee to the procedure; you related the fee to the illegality of it.
    You must understand that, if you have any consciousness
at all in the city of Chicago, you're well aware that there is
an enormous amount of protection money and gangsterism
and other kinds of pay-offs done in that city for all sorts of
things. I was well aware, for instance, that one had to have a

jukebox, even with a live band, because that's the way it was. So that both of us were much more inclined to think of the fee as something with which to pay off various people who had to be paid off. Rather than the doctor making a lot of money for himself. Which he may have been doing, by the way. But our thinking was that of course he had to split this money with other people. We just never thought of it any other way. We were paying, because this was an illegal activity. And that always raises the cost of what's going on.

No, I don't think we resented the money; we certainly didn't resent the man. In other words, I had no sense of "this bastard is—" you know, "has got me over a barrel." On the contrary, I felt that this was a very good fine human being who would walk out on a limb for me. Which is what he was doing, no matter which way you cut it. So I had very positive feelings about him.

KATRINA: Did emotional thoughts set in? Or were you soon busy with your other activities? Or did you have some sort of postabortion depression?

CATHERINE: Well, frankly, I wasn't sophisticated enough in those days to know what a depression was, so that if I did— I may have. I certainly was concerned in later years that if I'd had the child, it would now be of X age.

KATRINA: You did have that?

CATHERINE: Oh sure, I think everybody does.

KATRINA: To a large degree? I mean, how—?

CATHERINE: To a crippling degree? A very upsetting degree? No, I don't think so. No, I don't think so. I think that this is a fairly normal thought that goes through the mind of any woman that is aborted. And it may have nothing to do with the abortion at all. It may have to do with lots of other emotional things that are going on.

KATRINA: In other words, it's not grounds against using abortion as a means of solving an unwanted pregnancy?

CATHERINE: Oh no!
And not only do I think that's true in terms of my own psychic process, but I think the statistics bear us out.

KATRINA: How do you mean, "the statistics?"

CATHERINE: Well, many women have more than one abortion. Many women. And if they had enormous emotional hang-ups, if their grief over this particular, quote, "child," was such, they wouldn't do it the second time. I mean, if it *really* was a hang-up, they wouldn't be able to do it. And it's pretty apparent that this is a very ambivalent kind of a thing; in other words, "This is a child, but it's not a child."

KATRINA: Even though you had rebelled against the Church, were you influenced—torn in any way—as a result of your earlier background with the Church? I'm thinking particularly of the idea that "you've killed a human being."

CATHERINE: No. No, I think the reason that there were not enormous feelings of guilt, that I had "murdered a baby" as far as the Catholic Church's teachings are concerned, is that I had spent a lot of time, and enormous effort, in working through the teachings of the Catholic Church. To the extent even of going very heavily into other faiths and their theology. I spent a lot of time with Aquinas, and many other kinds of things. So that *that* wasn't a reality for me; it wasn't even left subconsciously; there was no conflict. I had already thought through the theology of the Church very carefully. I had read all the Papal Encyclicals, for instance. I had spent a lot of time worrying about this, thinking it through, and discussing it with people who were capable of discussing Church doctrine. So that I was not "an ordinary Catholic little girl going off to have an abortion." I had already thought through, not just the question of when and where the soul is, when and where one is human, but I'd also thought through euthanasia and lots of other things that are involved with, quote, "human life." So I think that's probably the reason there was no big hang-up about it.

KATRINA: Do you have anything to say, now, to a Catholic girl who is troubled by this question of it being murder? Have you any advice, as someone well-versed in Catholic—?

CATHERINE: Well, I think generally—at least what I *have* done—whether it's good or bad I don't know— Generally, with Catholic girls who are troubled by the concept that they have "a baby that they are now going to murder" (and, of course, a fair percentage of the problems ladies have with abortion would be eliminated tomorrow, if we would all stop referring to this as a "baby")— Where we conjure up this little thing that you're holding in your arms with its blue eyes and its little face.— This is *not* what you're dealing with, when you're talking about an eight-week pregnancy. But in talking to gals about that, I talk a great deal about the physical development of this creature. Very vividly, in terms of where it is, week after week after week.

If they are prepared to *think* about the position of the Church and the position of all the people within the Church —which has great variation, as you know—then I'm perfectly happy to sit and talk about this a great deal; because I can. And I think generally for Catholic girls, if they haven't ever been exposed to the notion that there is more to Catholic dogma than just what they've heard from their local parish priest, it is a very liberating thing for them—to know that there are great and famous priests, great and famous

Catholic doctors, who give serious thought to this question; to know that it isn't just as simple as Father Jones, around the corner, says: that the moment, bong, you become pregnant, you have within you another human being. And most girls are quite prepared to talk about this.

KATRINA: And are there great Catholic thinkers and great Catholic doctors who are really *good* practicing Catholics—?

CATHERINE: Oh indeed! This is one of the big arguments within the Catholic Church at the moment: "What are we talking about when we talk about human development?" The question of when-the-soul-arises will never be settled, by the bare nature of what-is-a-soul. However, whether or not you're talking about a viable human being is an enormous argument in the Catholic Church right now.

KATRINA: And you feel there are definitely ways a Catholic woman can still feel a good Catholic and stay a good Catholic—?

CATHERINE: Yes. Yes, yes.

Unless she is totally hung up on believing that the Pope has the final word. Now there are many Catholic theologians —they're in public print—who are saying, flat out, that it is unfortunate of the present Pope, that he will not rescind his most recent Encyclical. Because of course his successor is going to; there's no question about this.

There's no question about it. This will happen. And it is tragic that that man felt compelled to speak in the form he did, because we *know* what's going to happen.

Most Catholics are very relieved when they learn that there is a discussion within their Church. And there are so many marvelous little examples of how the Church changes; you can use them in talking to almost any age, grade. Most all people alive today can recall when it was really a terrible thing to eat meat on Friday! Most people can remember when it was a shocking thought to have mass at anything other than before twelve noon of the day. They can remember these small changes. And if there can be small changes, there can be large changes!

Anyway, the point is that you can talk to Catholic women. I spend a lot of time talking to Catholic women. I think that in many ways I can be more helpful to them than I can to people who have other kinds of hang-ups. I know the faith very well; where it stands, over time, on this issue.

KATRINA: To get back to your abortion—

CATHERINE: Back to my abortion: Where am I? Yes, well, I'm in the hotel room now, and I finally got over the various pains and aches that are associated with this. Which was very uncomfortable; I slept off and on during the night. I think probably the abortion, in some ways, was harder on Pete than it was on me, in the sense that he sat up all night worrying. I, of course, went to sleep, when I wasn't being too cramped; I just dozed off and slept. So the next morning I was in much better shape than he was. I hadn't eaten anything, having had operative experiences in the past. I had not eaten before I went for the abortion out of my own knowledge, rather than anything that was said to me. So the next morning I woke up ravenous. And the greatest treat, I should tell you—and I sometimes wonder if I should say this to young men—was that Pete said I could have anything I wanted for breakfast sent up to this hotel room. Which of course was also a new experience to me; I hadn't been in many hotels before; any, as a matter of fact. And I had this big thing for what was, for me, the world's most expensive fantastic thing—which was lamb chops. So I had lamb chops for breakfast. And it was, you know, a very pleasant, happy experience. We ate this enormous breakfast, served to us in this elegant fashion, which impressed me out of my mind. And then we packed up and paid the bill and off I went.

And then I went back to the original physician. There were no complications, no infections. Needless to say, he then suggested I be fitted with a diaphragm. Which is when I first heard about other kinds of birth control; and I was fitted with the diaphragm.

KATRINA: Did you have any regrets? Do you ever have any regrets?

CATHERINE: About having an abortion? No.

KATRINA: And about that child never being born? Any kind of regrets around the whole thing?

CATHERINE: Well, you must understand— My regrets were not so much around the abortion. I went through a period in my life where I regretted not having children, because I do not have any. And in the course of that regret, which is tied up into a lot of other things, in other words *why* I do not have the children—

[*At this point the tape ran out. In the several minutes which followed, Catherine spoke, among other things, of motherhood in general, marriage, an ectopic pregnancy that occurred while married, and finally her feelings about her childlessness. It was only as she was finishing these remarks that I discovered we were no longer recording. We were both pressed for time, and I was not able to learn, then, how much of the conversation had been lost. We began the next tape, presuming, erroneously, that less than a minute had gone unrecorded, and trying to pick up from the last few sentences of our conversation.*]

CATHERINE: What we were saying, at the end of that other tape, was that I have no doubt at all, that the feelings I have had, and the feelings I've worked through on not having children at all—are completely unrelated to the first pregnancy. Because they have nothing to do with it. I regret it as would any other person of my age who's never had children. Whether or not she's had an abortion. And probably for some of the same reasons, although I think they're generally individual reasons.

I don't say it's not *possible* that a woman who has had an abortion and then subsequently, for whatever reasons, has not ever reproduced, might not get hung up on the first pregnancy. But that is— You know, I could just as easily get hung up on the ectopic pregnancy which I had at another point. And those are not the reasons that I did not reproduce. So that I think the abortion essentially is not involved; for me anyway.

KATRINA: I want to ask you about the work you're doing now. You're doing work in this field, right?

CATHERINE: Well, no, I don't like to sell myself as "doing work in this field," because it's not essentially true. I'm going to be very involved in working out methods of disseminating family planning—birth control, conception control—whatever ridiculous euphemisms people are going to use to discuss these things.

And I am also here at PCS at least one day a week, sometimes two. I am concerned not so much with what this organization does in terms of abortion referral, which I think is its main activity at the moment. I'd like to see them into true pregnancy counseling. Pregnancy counseling involves a lot more than just finding out where to get an abortion. I mean, one of the reasons a fair percentage of these ladies are getting abortions is that they don't know how to *prevent conception*. And this is the thing that this organization should be very heavily into. Disseminating birth-control information. Pregnancy counseling is sex education to begin with; and that's known as "human physiology" as far as I'm concerned, not "sex education" which is a stupid word. And human physiology then leads you to conception control. And the failure of conception control leads you to abortion. That's a very simple route; and all three are part of pregnancy counseling. Which is what I think this organization technically was set up to do, but isn't doing; it's doing abortion referrals, a very separate thing.

Then, of course, in our state, as you understand, we have some rather strange attitudes. And this state is in desperate need—which is why I feel strongly about pregnancy counseling—really desperate need of as many resources as it can lay its hands on, to disseminate all three pieces of information. And as far as this organization is concerned, they are certainly well aware of my attitudes! I'm not saying anything that they haven't heard me tell them many times! And I never ever, ever, counsel a client without finding out what she knows about contraception. Because "abortion referral" itself is a waste of time. You'll have them back in nine months. Six months. If you are going to have intercourse you must prevent conception, if that's what you want to do.

KATRINA: What about the girls who "get themselves pregnant"?

CATHERINE: Well, we will always have a fair proportion of that; sure.

KATRINA: It came up, talking with someone else, the concept of "If I put on a diaphragm, I'm preparing for a seduction, which is wicked, so I won't." I mean, this is screwed-up thinking, but it will continue to exist.

CATHERINE: Sure; right.

KATRINA: I asked her what she would suggest as an improvement for other people in this situation. She felt that the pill was a potential solution: if you took the pill, you were less preparing yourself for the—

CATHERINE: Well, one of the interesting things about the pill, in terms of what it has done and is doing to people's heads, is that today young women are galloping in to doctors and saying, "I"ve got to go on the pill." At which point they are put on the pill. Unfortunately, what everyone is forgetting to ask is a rather obvious question: "Why do you need the pill?" There are girls who are on this pill for a number of months before they ever have a sexual encounter.

KATRINA: Do you think this is all that bad?

CATHERINE: Well, if you start going on the pill when you're sixteen years old, you're going to have to come off the pill when you're nineteen in all likelihood, maybe twenty.

KATRINA: Because of the side-effects of the pill?

CATHERINE: That's right, that's right. And you may need that pill when you're nineteen or twenty much more than you needed it when you were sixteen.

The reason they're asking for the pill is because that's all they've heard of. Our responsibility is to say, "If you're maybe going to bed in seven months, you could use *this* for the one time. If you're going to establish a permanent relationship with seventeen people—I don't mean permanent in the sense of one man, I mean a permanent sexual activity—then you consider the pill." But for people who are hopping into bed once every eight months, the pill is a bit ludicrous, you know.

KATRINA: Well, I see your point. But you're expecting a lot of complex thought— This is not only intelligent and educated—which is what you're working for—but it's also "not screwed-up" thinking—

CATHERINE: I think the resolution to the problem—the problem of pregnancy, abortion, and population generally —is *unscrewing* the thinking!

Yes. Pretty soon we'll tell people in the grade schools about physiology, and then we'll tell them about conception. Either we'll do that, or we'll have it done by law. Which I would prefer not to do; you know, make laws which will start penalizing the people who bear.

KATRINA: Oh! That's a terror to me.

CATHERINE: Is it? Well, it's coming.

KATRINA: That's why I feel—why I personally feel that birth control must be accomplished now, before we get a law saying, "You're allowed X number of children."

CATHERINE: That's right. And that's coming.

KATRINA: Because I think that's inhuman.

CATHERINE: That's coming.

KATRINA: But does it not offend you?
[*pause*]
Not the way it offends me, I guess.

CATHERINE: As you probably notice, I'm a highly rational human being.

Yes, it offends me. I like people to have freedom of total choice. I don't know that we will do it *first* quite that radically. I think probably what we'll do *first,* is we'll start using the penalty system. You see, this country, which is very pronatalist, is now penalizing the unmarried, or the people who do not have children, according to our tax laws. We are encouraging people to bear by giving them deductions on their income tax. I expect we will reverse that. And you'll be given rewards for *not* reproducing. I think this will come before—at least I would *hope* it would come before a law which says, "Here's a chit and you may have a child." Because that's the way it'll be worked out: you'll have the legal regulations.

I think it would be better to interfere with the thinking of people. We live in a society where it is almost *indecent,* and it is certainly fraught with social pressures, not to reproduce. There is something "wrong, wrong," with people who do not get married; there's something "strange" and "sick" and "ugly" about them. Right? There's something "wrong" with people who choose not to have children. There are enormous social pressures on them. I know a couple who have made a conscious decision, and who are under enormous pressures. I don't think they go out anywhere without somebody, you know, giving them a just-who-do-you-think-you-are kind of attitude. Until we change the pronatalist attitude of people, we have little hope for population control. And we will go to these—what I consider very rigid and unpleasant laws.

I think we need to get education so that we understand two things: One, the process of conception and controlling it. And, simultaneously, we need to change the attitudes about the usefulness of reproducing. In other words, so that we understand that there is nothing *evil* about people who do not reproduce, nothing *evil* about "old maids" or "bachelors." You know, any man in our society today who's forty years old and hasn't gotten married is either a "weird" man or "one of those other terrible things" known as homosexuals. Until society is prepared to move in other directions—I think some of the kids are doing this. This is an aspect of what the whole thing about not-getting-married is all about. It's a psychological delay, in many ways, of the imposition of society's attitude that "the only good thing you can do in life is to marry and have children." I think the rejection of marriage is coming first. Those who are marrying are delaying their children, many of them. So these attitudes are changing slowly. But you know as well as I, that a woman who is married for one year and still shows no sign of being pregnant will already be having a number of comments about it. "What is wrong with you?" the question always is. The immediate assumption is, of course, that you are sick in the physical sense; there is something *wrong* with *you,* the woman. It's always the woman, by the way, it's never the man; in all societies, as you probably know. And this is a heavy burden. I think this is one of the reasons why girls get pregnant. And why single girls get pregnant.

KATRINA: In order to prove that there's nothing the matter?

CATHERINE: To prove their womanhood, to prove that they have a reason for existing, to prove their status. It isn't all bound up in their overwhelming desires to be maternal. It's also bound up in their image of themselves as a human being. Society says—all societies say, "A woman, and her greatest function is—"And if that's the way you define women, if that's the way you define her function, I think there's a fair percentage of young women who want to be defined as women. If we had a social climate where women were human beings who could pursue a number of careers, including motherhood, but that was not the *only* definition — In other words, your status doesn't come from being a mother; it comes from being a human being, who, as it happens, is a mother—this is a very different thought. I think it would remove a lot of the incentives for women to become pregnant. One of the incentives to become pregnant in very young girls is obviously the desire to get out of the home; you know, to leave. It's one of the ways of becoming an adult, one of the ways of getting out from under Mum or Dad or whoever it is you're getting out from under. Those things are all operating. And until we face some of the attitudes, we're always going to have this problem.

KATRINA: But you feel it will be decreased with this education?

CATHERINE: Hopefully, hopefully; and if some of our more marvelous mechanisms of conception control work out. If implantation works out. Probably we'll get desperate enough in our society, I think, to use implantation as a social rule rather than as a matter of choice. That would be my guess.

KATRINA: What's that?

CATHERINE: Well, I think we will get desperate enough in a population situation so that we'll implant. And in order to have the implant removed you will have to have official permission.

KATRINA: You mean women will be forced to go and have a "thing" put in?

CATHERINE: Yes. You will have a small implantation which will change the hormonal balance of your system, so that will change the ovulation.

KATRINA: I think it's absolutely horrible!

CATHERINE: Yes, I don't like it myself. But I think these things are quite possible in terms of looking at the whole problem.

Now if you want to stop that kind of activity, the first thing you do is sex education—conception control—*now*. Preferably yesterday. In other words, have it done as a voluntary kind of thing. Because if it isn't voluntary, eventually it'll be compulsory. There'll be nothing for it.

KATRINA: You speak about this as "not just an American problem"; you talk about the "international situation," and you obviously know something of the larger—

CATHERINE: Well, as you probably know, there are many people who think America has no problems at all, because America's birthrate is not, quote, "getting out of hand."

KATRINA: Yes: "Let's just worry about India and only help them."

CATHERINE: Right, that's the position they've taken. They're wrong. But, you know, you can play statistics lots of different ways—!
  Anyway, the international situation is bizarre, to say the very least. In Latin America and South America, where they have an incredibly high abortion rate—

KATRINA: Because of low conception control?

CATHERINE: There is *no* conception control, legally, at all. In some of the countries there's an absolute ban on importing the items into the country.

KATRINA: Does that make for more illegal abortions?

CATHERINE: You know, there's a really ugly thing that I say to people, and it scares them right out of their bloody wits when I say it:
  All societies, when they are desperate to control the population, reach out to the most extreme methods they can find —including infanticide. Most people don't realize that, but it's true. When you must control your population and you

don't know how to do it, what do you do? You kill the babies that are born. That's the only logical thing to do. And that is still being done in this world. And it's always been done.

KATRINA: Do you think that, here, we could——?

CATHERINE: I don't think America will go to that unless they go the route of eugenics control. Which they may do.

KATRINA: You're talking not about a public infanticide, but rather a private, quiet, personal——?

CATHERINE: Well, the whole society knows about it! I mean it's not a secret!

KATRINA: Can you be more specific?

CATHERINE: Well, the whole tribe knows what you do. In other words, all the babies born on a Wednesday, die. China, for years, used all the girls—a percentage of the girls—died. That's the way it is. How are you going to keep the population down otherwise, if you don't know any other way?

KATRINA: So you mean a sort of happily accepted thing?

CATHERINE: Of course. Americans look at me with this look on their faces as if I have just, you know, said the most hideous thing in the world—because I'm prepared to realize that people murder other human beings, *which they must do. All human beings survive,* and they think of ways of surviving. If there's not enough food, *they do not encourage more mouths.* And they find ways to stop this. The Eskimos have a splendid system. They have limited resources; and what do they do with limited resources? There are X number of people they can feed; therefore they must take care of the old, to eliminate *them*. They let them die. Take them out on the ice and they die. That's what they're supposed to do. At a certain point in your life where you can no longer be part of a productive society, you're very old, you're useless, you're taken out on the ice and you're supposed to lie down quietly and die. And this is a culturally accepted mode of behavior. This is done. In some ways I think it's kinder than the American style of locking them up. The same is true of babies. A percentage of babies *must* die. And a percentage of babies *do* die. They're born, and then they are left to die.

KATRINA: Where?

CATHERINE: Well, in their particular culture they don't have a bush, so they leave them on the ice. If you live in an ice culture, that's where you leave them. If you live in the bush, you leave them in the bush. This is done informally in some cultures, and it's done formally in other cultures.

KATRINA: But you don't feel it's done here?

CATHERINE: In America? I think in America it's not done; as you know we have rigid laws about this. I think, generally, in America it's not practiced. I think people who are very upset about reproducing themselves find other ways of killing their children. I think this is probably one of the reasons why we have, now, units in hospitals for battered babies. It's all part of the same thing.

KATRINA: Can you give me another example like the Eskimos? Specific like that?

CATHERINE: Oh, there are many. There's a splendid tribe in New Zealand that does this, still.

KATRINA: Might the rebuttal to your remarks be, "Well, they're less civilized than we are"? Or is that irrelevant?

CATHERINE: We happen to be in a country where we have enormous resources for food production. So we don't have to take a public position of killing off the old or the very young in order to keep the food in the mouths of the bulk of our society. However, in a society where we have this fantastic production of food, we kill a segment of our population every year. Through starvation.

I don't know what civilized means. If civilized is the way the middle-class American views his particular suburb, sure, I don't think that there are people out in Newton deliberately killing off their babies because they're starving; because they're not. And I don't think society is doing that to them. But I do know that in Mississippi our society is deliberately, by omission if not direct commission—I think by commission, but let us say omission—killing off a percentage of the society, both the very young and the very old, by starving them to death. Which I don't think is any different from what the "more primitive"—as we like to think of them—people are doing.

This is . . . part of the real-world horrors.

LOUISE

Interviewed in September 1972

LOUISE: My husband and I were not *planning* on having another child; not right away. And we were using contraceptives. But obviously something went wrong. And—I found myself pregnant. I knew I was. I made arrangements to have a check-up to see. My husband took care of the test for me, and I was indeed pregnant.

KATRINA: What kind of contraception were you using?

LOUISE: Well, my husband—my— A prophylactic! I had a bad experience with birth-control pills, and I had to go off those—completely, forever. So we've had to turn to other methods—which just aren't as reliable.

My husband and I talked about this. There were several things to be concerned about. The primary factor was the fact that our child is an asthmatic and had been in and out of hospital numerous times. With serious attacks, in which she almost died.

KATRINA: How old is your child?

LOUISE: She was a year then, just over twelve months. This was about two-and-a-half months ago.

We had been told by the doctors that, because of family history on both sides, we couldn't expect ever to have a non-asthmatic child.

KATRINA: Were you told this before you had *her?*

LOUISE: No, because we didn't even know about it at the time. Nor think to inquire about it! We had no idea that we had the asthma problem, it's not in the immediate family. Neither of us is asthmatic, there are just allergies on both sides of the family. Later, they did find that back in my husband's side of the family there is some asthma. But it's very remote. Of course [*voice shakes*] if you have two children and they're both asthmatic—a mother could quietly go insane.

Also, with two children, I just wouldn't be able to divide my time properly between the children. I would always be being unfair to one, if one were in the hospital. I had seen —when I had been in the hospital with our child—mothers who also had children at home, and who could not be with their child in the hospital because of their responsibilities at home. And it was very sad to see what would happen to these other children who had to stay in the hospital day in and day out, not always seeing their mothers. I felt it was really important for me to be there *with* my daughter. I mean when she's ill she needs a lot of attention and love and care and holding. She needs reassurance that Mommy's there. And I want to give that *to* her. And especially because of—you know—everything they were doing to her. I, you know, I don't want to— I didn't want to jeopardize *her* well-being—

KATRINA: Is she likely to continue with these problems?

LOUISE: Well, she has to be constantly on medication. And frequently on—uhm—even stronger—you know, steroid-type things, which are very dangerous. She's—a *very* severe case. And we have to wait awhile, to see if this is going to clear up. Sometimes it's just a couple of years and it clears up. Other times it seems that when they go through puberty it clears up. And sometimes it doesn't clear up at all. The doctors say there's a fifty-fifty chance. They don't know.

So it's been, you know, a very trying period. She would be up and down all night long. So I was up and down with her. She would go into these attacks and we'd have to rush her off to the hospital as fast as possible. An attack, I should explain, is tremendous wheezing. It's audible across several rooms. It's the child not being able to breathe. And she just kind of lays—you know, she can't get enough breath to even have—for any activity at all. We'd rush her to the hospital and she'd have to be—They'd have to put her in Intensive Care, and she'd have to be intubated and put on a respirator—

KATRINA: Intubated?

LOUISE: That means that they immobilize her completely. They give her a nerve-block; she's totally immobilized. And they put her on the respirator. All this is terribly fright—frightening to see. And to go through.

And she had to have numerous cut downs—where they have to actually, you know, cut down into—to get the vein. Then of course this leaves scars. They just become a pinhole for blood-samples and blood-work. Because you have to test the blood gases and everything. And of course when a child is on the critical list it's like—you just sit in *agony*. Because, you know, this is your *child,* and you *love* it so; and—there it *lays*. And you just don't *know* what's going to happen to it. It's a terrible, terrible thing to go through. And I just wouldn't wish it on anyone. And when this happens *repeatedly;* not, you know, not just *once*. But you turn around and the very next month you're in again, and *again*. It's a horrible thing.

And it's a strain, a terrible strain on your *marriage*. You have to—to really have a good, stable marriage, and really *love* each other, to be able to pull through this kind of a crisis. Because you're under such emotional pressure that any little thing and you just explode. And you have to have, you know, have someone *understand*—understanding, with you. Or else it could be— You know, I could see where it could completely *ruin* a marriage. Even though, of course, *both* parents are terribly concerned about the child. It's just the pressure that you're under. And this is what— After going through this, we just, you know, we just realized we could *not* take the chance of having *two* children going through this. It would just be unbearable. Just unbearable. I know I —I— My husband felt that I couldn't stand the strain. And I probably couldn't. Because I was so upset with—with her. You know, *really,* I think you could have a nervous breakdown. From being under this kind of— Especially if you had *two* children like this.

You know, there's the constant medication; and the constant listening, during the night, to hear if the child's breathing properly. The worst attacks come at night. And so you're always kind of on edge. And you're always waiting for the worst— You *try* not to, but when the worst keeps happening, after a while you become conditioned to kind of—you know, waiting for the worst to happen. And whenever the child starts to wheeze, immediately you think: "Oh no! This is going to lead to another hospital visit!"

And you have to worry about the drugs that she has to be put on. We've been *told* the drugs are dangerous. They can cause bone deformities. And growth deformities. But if the child has to be put on the drugs to live, you have to put her on the drugs. Fortunately, she's only had to go on those steroids for short periods. If you have to go on them for a time, they can cause permanent damage. So there's the worry of *that,* too. So, you know, the whole family situation is very —is a very strained one. You don't get much sleep and therefore you're on edge. And then you have got the great worry, when the child is in the hospital, of whether she's going to make it or not. And I think that this—this kind of situation is very, you know, very strained and a very poor one to live under.

KATRINA: How often had she been to the hospital for this at the time you had the abortion?

LOUISE: Four times.

The last time wasn't quite as bad. I felt better. She was still on the critical list for—for two days. And then, of course, in Intensive Care for several days more before she could be brought out onto the floor. But, you know, it wasn't quite as serious as the others had been. Her—using medical, technical terms, her blood-gas tests—which are tests to show how much oxygen is in the blood; and oxygen of course is very important for being able to live, to survive—were better than they had been on previous visits to the hospital. Some of them have been *so* poor that—That is why they just couldn't tell us whether she would survive or not; because her blood gases were so bad.

And we prefer to wait for a couple of years just to see how she does. She's been doing quite well for about three weeks now. We're very pleased. And we're hoping that maybe even a climate change might help her. We're going to investigate all those possibilities. But we'd like to do that before considering having another child.

KATRINA: I'm thinking about parents of healthy children —particularly when they are critical—and wondering if perhaps they just don't *know*—

LOUISE: If you—if you have a healthy child, or children, you have *no idea* what it's like. I mean even if the child comes down with a childhood disease, and the mother's up a couple of nights with him—that's nothing. Because you know that the child is going to get over it. And, okay, the mother's *tired* after her experience with this. But how would she feel if she were going through years of this? Of not knowing. And under the *strain* of wondering if this child is going to—to live or not. I mean you—a person doesn't know what it's like unless she's been through it, really. They just have no idea of the strain and the mental anguish. I mean they have to think in terms of looking at their healthy child and thinking "What if this child had a—a disease or something, some really serious thing, and was going—and maybe he would be dead next week." You know, "How would I feel?" Then maybe—maybe they could get a *glimpse* of what it's like. But you really don't know until you've been through it.

KATRINA: When an asthmatic is not in the hospital, other than the worry every day of not knowing what's going to happen next month, are there any day-to-day things that are different?

LOUISE: Oh, certainly, certainly. Because she has to be given medication around the clock. Every four hours. And I have to be extremely careful with the house in terms of anything that she might be allergic to. Asthma is all related to allergies. You know, her room looks like a sterilized hospital room. No curtains or fancy frills or anything. Stuffed toys, I have to be extremely careful of what they've been stuffed with, and what the actual fabric is. And she cannot have certain foods. She has to have the hypoallergenic soybean milk, which has to be prepared especially for her. She can't have cheese or butter or bread or strawberries or anything like this. You really have got to go out of your way to find a proper diet for the child. And not be repetitious with the same old foods, day in and day out, which she would soon tire of.

KATRINA: She still had medication every four hours when she was twelve months old?

LOUISE: Oh yes, oh yes.

She's been off it for one week now. Completely off her medicine for one week now! She went to the pediatrician, had a check-up, and she was doing *very well*. And the pediatrician said, "Okay. Now I'm going to try her without medication."

And she's been off it. She had to have one dose, one morning. She woke up and she was wheezing. And I gave her a dose and it cleared it up, completely. She was fine the rest of the day. I didn't have to give her any more.

For the *first* time in over a year I have not had to get up at two o'clock and give her a dose of medication. [*laughs*] That means for the first time I am sleeping through the night. Mothers who know—you know, how in the beginning you have the two o'clock feedings, know how tiring it is when you have to get up and feed the baby and then go back to bed— Well, you can think if you have a whole year of this, it seems like a *vacation* when you're able to sleep through the entire night, finally.

KATRINA: Does your husband usually—

LOUISE: Sleeps through the two and six o'clock doses. He gets up about seven o'clock or so. But his profession is very demanding—he's a physician. And I was doing substitute teaching, but when my daughter became ill I didn't go in any more. I felt that it was more important that I be with her. So since I was home all day and could maybe take a nap in the afternoon if I got time or something, I didn't even ask my husband to get up to give her medication. He was *always* there when I needed him if she went into an attack or something. If he were home that night. You know, he would be there to help me. One night she was having an attack and we called the doctor. And it wasn't quite bad enough yet for us to take her into the hospital, so the doctor told us what to do at home. My husband had to give her an injection. We were doing everything possible at home. And my husband was up that night with me.

She did end up the next day going into the hospital, but, you know, we kept her going through the night, anyway.

KATRINA: When you know it's time to go to the hospital, how long do you have to get there? Do you have an hour? Half an hour? Do you hope to get there in five minutes? What is the—feeling?

LOUISE: Usually we hope to get there as quickly as possible. Of course once you get there the doctor has to examine her, and then they have to admit her and everything. You know, they take time once you get to the hospital. So you kind of want to get there quickly so that they'll get that time over with and give help to the child.

One time she did go in and of course they rushed her right up; they didn't even bother with anything because she was —she was blue. And they just rushed her right up, and put her on the respirator. As quickly as they could. That time going to the hospital, it was just— I was just praying for the —for the minutes. You know, I—She almost stopped breathing [*softly*] twice, going to the hospital.

The other times I didn't feel it was quite that big a rush. But we knew we had to get her there.

[*pause*]

KATRINA: Does asthma affect family life, things like where you can go for a vacation—?

LOUISE: Well, we were thinking about driving somewhere. But when it came right down to it we decided we really *couldn't,* because what if she had an attack on the way? You always have to worry, wherever you go, about her having an attack serious enough to put her immediately in the hospital. And what hospital she would be in, and, of course, who would be looking after her.

You have to think, too, about going into people's houses —about what their house might have as far as pets, cats and dogs, as far as wool rugs, as far as, you know, any type of thing like this that she could possibly be allergic to.

KATRINA: If you take her to play with another baby, do you have to think of that?

LOUISE: Yes, right. Right. And sometimes we just kind of experiment with her, because we— You know, when she's an older child and going to school and things, obviously she can't always be protected from everything. So we kind of experiment with her. We take her; and we see what the reaction is. If she has no reaction, then we sigh a breath of relief and think, "Well, we'll be able to go *there* again, anyway," you know, or "take her to play with *that* little child."

If we go there and she does have—we did go visit someone; and when we got back from visiting them, she went into an attack.

But we were able to stop it with an injection.

We go through all the possibilities: we have her on the medicine. And then if she starts wheezing and going into an attack on top of that, we have to try the injection. If the injections fail, then we've got no place to go but the hospital.

KATRINA: What about getting baby-sitters? Is that a different—?

LOUISE: Well, this is another thing. A lot of my friends have teenage sitters. I didn't really feel that I should have a teenage sitter, because of my child's condition. I felt that I needed someone who was aware of her condition, and would be able to drive, or know how to act in case of emergency. And I was afraid that if I had a teenage sitter and the baby went into an attack, the sitter would be frightened out of her mind and wouldn't know what to do; and, you know, it would be a bad experience for *her*. Maybe she'd never want to sit again, you know. And I didn't want to *scare* someone. I wanted someone older, who could face up to anything unexpected.

We've never had any difficulties when leaving her with a sitter that she's had. We—well, we didn't leave her that often, to tell you the truth.

KATRINA: Do you go to the movies at night?

LOUISE: We haven't been to the movies in years. My husband works—sometimes every other night. And the night he comes home he's in no shape to go to the movies. So we— you know, we lead a different kind of life than the average person. But I mean we've gone out when the occasion arose and we were invited out for some reason. As long as she wasn't wheezing, we felt it safe to put her to bed and go out. Of course we always left a number where we could be reached. And we made it clear to the sitter that if she woke up—she wakes up crying when she goes into attack at night. She starts crying and she just won't stop. I mean you *know* —and we just said that if she woke up crying, that the girl was to call us immediately. And this was a girl in her twenties. She has a profession, and she's a neighbor.

KATRINA: Would you go away for a weekend? You and your husband together?

LOUISE: Without her? Not now. Maybe—maybe in the future.

If she were a healthy child, of course we would.

But it would be—you know, it would be asking too much — I mean to go away and have an emergency come up, would just be a little bit too chancy right now. Not until she was doing better.

This is a limiting factor that we have to face. And we're just— And [*laughs*] we face it!

Of course, if she were pretty well out of the hospital phase, we would consider— You know, we would have considered having another child. Just because we'd planned to have two children; and my husband plans to have a vasectomy done afterward. And so if, you know, we had the other child, it would be out of the way, he'd have a vasectomy, and we'd have—we wouldn't have to worry! [*laughs*] For the rest of our lives!

So as soon as we found out I was pregnant, we went to the obstetrician and talked this over with him. You know, we explained to him the problem we were having with our asthmatic child and our worries about having another. And he knows us very well. And he said that, you know, he would understand; and he would think this was a perfectly legitimate reason for having an abortion.

I'm not a prude, and I do believe in abortions. And I'm very much in favor of New York State having the abortion program they do have. I think it would be unfortunate if they didn't, because— Okay, some people call it murder. But I think that there's a lot of murder going on in young girls who have nowhere else to turn; and who perhaps ruin their lives by going through with a pregnancy, or by having an illegal abortion in which they're butchered.

And I—I really couldn't think of it as being, you know, murder, to me. Because I had an abortion before I was quite six weeks pregnant. I had no feeling for the child. I could have never waited until the fourth month or so when the child was kicking. I would already have started to have feeling for the child, when the child started to act. And then I probably wouldn't be able to handle the situation of going through it! Or need counseling, anyway, to go through it. But having it as early as I did, I felt no responsibility to this child. And because of the fears that we did have, I thought it better not to bring it into the world. And my husband felt very strongly that we just couldn't have this child at this time.

So, you know, the doctor said he would set me up, and there was no trouble at all. He arranged for me to enter the hospital—I guess it was the very next week after I'd been to see him.

And—I went in. Of course I was scared! Because I'd never been through this kind of thing before. And I was scared.

I went in, and the nurses were very pleasant there. Everything was done very efficiently, very quickly. The nurses were talking to me and it was over before I even knew what happened. It was just—it's very simple. The doctor explained to me that it's a very easy process. Especially when they catch it within the first two months.

There was a special unit there in the hospital. Ironically, you walk through the maternity ward, where they had the babies, to get to it! And you walk to the very end of the corridor. Then it's all this one unit which is just for abortion patients.

KATRINA: Was it upsetting to walk through that ward?

LOUISE: Not to me, so much. Because I had justified in my mind why I was going through with it. I think for a woman who was perhaps unmarried and was facing a different kind of situation it might be very difficult to walk through and hear the babies crying and see mothers who had given birth. And then walk through to the end to have—to get rid of her child. For me it wasn't so difficult. You know, because I had settled it within myself. I had—I had "inner peace"—that I was doing the right thing. For a woman who didn't quite feel sure, I'm sure this would be an upsetting situation. However, I think they're cramped for space. And when the New York liberalized abortion laws went in, they just had to find the only space they had available. I think this is part of the problem. Maybe they could put another elevator in, that would deliver you closer to the unit.

But everybody in the unit was *very* pleasant, very *understanding*. And there was never anything said like, "How could you do this?" No derogatory remarks at all.

The process was very easy. My doctor told me that everything was fine and, as soon as I felt that I could get up and walk around, that I could leave. About an hour after I'd had the abortion, I was feeling fine; I was sitting up and I felt that I could walk. And the nurse came over and helped me. I went into the bathroom and cleaned myself up. We went down, I got dressed, and I left by noon! [*laughs*] So it was —it was a matter of just a couple of hours. And everything was—As I said *because* of the New York State law, I was allowed to have a very pleasant experience in which I didn't have to worry—and fear for my life.

I—I know right after I had the abortion, I shed a few tears. Because I think it was just kind of a feeling of: it's all over with now; I don't have to worry about it. You know, I had built up I think within myself just this worry of being pregnant. And—and these extenuating circumstances. And not knowing, at first, how to turn, and what to do. Then finally it was all over and I just felt *relief*.

And then I went *home* to my *own* child, and we *played* in the afternoon! And that was the extent of it. I don't feel any remorse. I'm glad that it's over with and behind me. And hopefully our child will do better eventually and we will be able to have another child.

I love children, and I would never— I could never really, I don't think, take even a, you know, a fetus's life, unless I really felt that there was—that I could justify it. And I also believe in keeping population under control. But I think it's best if you can do it other ways. I think abortion should be the last thing that you turn to. You know, there are other methods of contraception that hopefully will come about in the years to come that will, you know, kind of eliminate even having to have abortions.

The problem with the birth-control pill is just that it's got too many ill side-effects for too many of us. I took the pill for two years when we were first married, and toward the end of the second year I was having *so* many problems; I was having to see a doctor quite frequently. And finally he said, "You've just got to go off this pill. You *can't* stay on the pill." And at that time we thought, "Okay, that's fine." Because we were about—you know: we know who we are, we know where we're going, and we are ready to have a child. So I went off the pill and we just didn't bother with anything. And a few months later I conceived.

Now, of course, we have the same old problem! [*laughs*] I did *try* the pill again, after the abortion. I did go back on the pill and I tried again, without success. I was having a lot of effects again.

KATRINA: What about the diaphragm?

LOUISE: Oh, this—! I was examined, after I had the baby, for a diaphragm. And I'm not a fit. Apparently after having the baby it kind of stretched me out to a funny shape, and the diaphragm just—I wouldn't be a good fit for it. The gynecologist told me point blank; he says, "I'll *give* you a diaphragm, if you want it that badly. But," he said, "it's not going to work. So there's no sense in you *having* one." Also the coil wouldn't be good for me. He ruled out both of those on his examination. So we *had* to turn to a male contraceptive. Because there was nothing more *I* could do. And rhythm is just a joke! You can't depend on that.

So we turned—and my husband—of course my husband isn't thrilled [*laughs*] about having to use a prophylactic!

But, it's the only thing we have now. So we just have to rely on that and a little bit of common sense; a little bit of rhythm, you know, as far as common sense goes.

We kind of would like to have one more child. Just because I think our existing child would be better off if she had someone else! You know. A family of two is always nice, and there's always the chance that you—on the second try, you'll get what you didn't have the first time! Which would be nice. But our decision is going to have to rest on how our existing child does, with her condition.

And of course, you know, we could get lucky and have a child without— There's always hope. But there's every reason to believe that it would have *some* degree of difficulty. Now the doctor did say the next child would not necessarily be as severe as our child is now. But it would probably have some problems, to *some* degree. And, you know, once you've been through it— I mean, if our daughter pulls—does pretty well and pulls through this, then we won't feel that— After all, with the next child, we'll be more experienced. Already, as her attacks went on, I became a little more conditioned to the whole thing. I understood what was going on, and what to do, and I felt more sure of myself. And I think once this starts happening, then it's, you know, it's not quite as bad.

But even if we had a *healthy* child, somebody would have had to suffer; you see? If our daughter were still in and out of the hospital, either the second child, or she would have had to suffer. And that's not fair, either. Even if the second child were *healthy,* and able to be at home, it might not have my attention because of *her* being so ill and needing me.

KATRINA: I want to ask you about asthma being emotionally caused . . .

LOUISE: Not in that young a child.

Oftentimes with an older child, it can; or even with an

older person, it can be brought on emotionally. Actually some asthmatics, as they grow older, can bring on an attack. They can get angry and say, "Because you've done this I'm going to have an attack." And actually bring on all the symptoms and cause it. Now, you know obviously this is emotional asthma. In her case it's a medical situation. The origin, of course, is genetic. But this is completely medical. I mean her X-rays show— If you took X-rays of an emotional asthmatic, their tubings and stuff would not have the cuffings and swelling that a true asthmatic would have. And she does have that on her X-ray.

KATRINA: You mentioned, when we met, that you hadn't told your parents, or your husband's parents, about the abortion.

LOUISE: Well, we had thought about telling them. But then we weren't really sure how they would feel about it. And we decided rather than upset them or feel— I think basically my mother would have thought we were doing the right thing. But she would have been very worried about *my* condition. You know? And I *knew* I was going to be all right! [*laughs*]

Neither set of parents lives close by, and so they would be sitting there worrying about me, and how I was doing and everything; and I just didn't see any sense to have them worry. Also I didn't want to cause any family problems by telling the family, and then having one member of the family maybe think that it was a terrible thing to do and *say* so. And then it would cause a little bit of strain on the family relationship. We're—we're *close* with our families. And we prefer to keep everything as is. We just decided that it was our own personal decision. We're grown-up now and we can make — We can make these decisions and do these things without having to— We don't tell them *everything!* And I'm sure they don't expect us to tell them everything. You know.

We just thought that it was best not to say anything. Because you take the chance of causing any kind of friction. I mean even internal friction. As far as like my mother saying, "Well, you did the best thing." And my father thinking maybe we didn't! [*laughs*] You know! Whether it'd be—maybe cause a little argument there. It just wasn't worth it.

And they, of course, are very concerned about their grandchild. And her well-being. So that I—basically I don't think they would disapprove.

The only other person I really did talk to was a very good friend of mine. And she's a nurse, and we're very close. We both have children the same age, who play together. And she'd been over to my house. And I just felt that I had to talk to somebody.

And—I told her, and I talked to her about it. She said— she was really great. Because I was still in the—kind of the stage of debating, thinking, "Am I doing the right thing?" And she said, "How could you do anything else *but?* You really have no alternative." She said, "If I were in that situation I'd do exactly the same thing." She just made me feel better about the whole thing: that she would have made the same decision. And then I—I didn't feel that I was doing something, you know [*pause*] wrong.

But as far as telling a lot of people— Well, I think it's mostly *fear* of what—it was mostly fear of what other people would think of us—if they found out. Not that I— I'm not one of these people who gears my whole life to what other people think. I do, you know, pretty much what I please. And they go along with it, or else they don't. You know, they like me, or they don't like me.

But uhm—in this instance I was worried. Because I was afraid that people would think— I mean there *are* people, obviously, who think that you're some cruel, horrible *monster,* to even consider this. And I know—I have some close friends who are Catholics. Who, had I told them, would have just gone off the— They would have thought that we were just the *worst* people *possible.* Even though they *know* us!

They would think that for us to be able to do this we must just be the worst people possible, and have *no feelings*.

And it's just really the *opposite*. We feel very—you know, we have very *strong* feelings. We *do* care, we *are* concerned. We don't want to be considered *murderers* in any way. Because we're not. We're *pacifists*—by *every* standard. And, you know, my husband makes his life by saving lives. We just— You know, neither one of us would want people to think of us that way. My husband, I don't think was as much concerned, perhaps, as I was. Maybe I— [*laughs*] you know, maybe I'm a little insecure.

But a lot of people still look down on this as a means of —well, getting out of an unfortunate situation. And they're the ones that make you feel unsure, make you feel guilty somehow. When there's really nothing to feel— I really don't believe there's anything to feel guilty *about*. I know I did the right thing. But I think if somebody were to attack me, verbally, about this, over a period of time, I might *begin* to feel badly. Not because I didn't do the right thing, but because they can't *see* why I did it.

I actually kind of feel sorry for them! You know?

ELLIE

ELLIE: I was a war bride from Australia. In 1943, in Sydney, I married an American Marine. I came across the Pacific during the last six weeks of the pregnancy, and I got to Washington two days before the baby was born.

Now my own background was— I've had a lot of analysis, so I can pretty well piece together what happened. Two very sick parents; and I was an only child. My husband was no good. I couldn't even find him when I got to this country; finally the Red Cross found him for me. He did come to see me in the hospital once after I had the baby. He rejected both of us completely. I then followed it up by rejecting the baby myself. I can look back and see it now.

Uhm—

It's funny, I'd forgotten all this; flipped out of my mind. It came back to me last night. I was thinking what I'd tell you of it. And I *couldn't* sleep.

KATRINA: Did you know he was no good when you came over?

ELLIE: No, I didn't. I didn't know anything. I was twenty years old. I was so stupid at that age! I knew nothing about people—Americans, or anything else. I'd danced my way through my adolescence, you know, and refused to go to school, and just wanted to have a good time. So— I was certainly brought up short!

Uhm—I'm trying to think of the sequence of events. We left the hospital; and the baby got sick. It turned out she was allergic to milk-fat. And I was dragging her all over Washington to well-baby clinics, and this and that. I finally got up to Herndon Saint Andrew's, where she'd been born. And— I don't know—they changed the formula, or gave me something, whatever it was. We hadn't had any—either of us— barely had any sleep since she was born; and that was about six weeks. I'd found an apartment. It was a four-flight walk-up; and we had an icebox, a *real* icebox. The man used to come up and bring the ice about twice a week. So this was a long time ago. This was 1943.

And uhm— Then I think— Oh yes: I got sick. I came down with TB then. Post-partum. I don't know if you ever remember hearing of Grand Island Memorial Hospital over in Virginia. It was a big TB hospital for the District of Columbia. There was a lot of TB around in those days.

So anyway, I came down with TB. As soon as there was a place, the baby was sent out to board in the well-baby ward at Municipal Hospital. And I waited to go into Grand Island.

I had to wait until after Christmas, I remember. And I was all alone that Christmastime. I didn't know anybody in Washington except my mother-in-law, who was an illiterate Roumanian. So I couldn't communicate with her much. And she resented me, I don't know why. The people she worked for—she was housekeeper for a family called Grant. Anyway, a very nice family. And they were very kind to me.

My husband was still in the Marine Corps, in camp. During those months, while I was waiting to go to Grand Island, he came down a few times to see me, but not often. And obviously I—even *I* could see that I didn't have much in the way of a husband.

KATRINA: At what point did you realize that he wasn't—?

ELLIE: After I got into the hospital at Grand Island, I think. I didn't want to believe it before then. Because I was scared, I was alone in this town. Trying to live on eighty bucks a month even in those days wasn't so easy.

KATRINA: But you didn't realize it as soon as the baby was born?

ELLIE: I must have realized it. But I didn't want to face it. I must have known.

And I wasn't going to go back home. Because down in Australia everybody had said, "Oh, if you marry an American he'll leave you and go off with another woman." [laughs] So I wasn't going to go back!

And uhm—So— I don't know, I just— I think I—I must have had some kind of a nervous breakdown, but didn't know it. And nobody else did.

Uhm—anyway— Then finally— I found somebody out in Anacostia who would board the baby. There was another war bride who had come across on the ship with me, and she knew of somebody out there who would take the baby. So she went out to board in Anacostia, and I went off to Grand Island. Which at that time I think had about eighteen-hundred patients. And it was really a wild place.

I spent a year in Grand Island. And during that year, I told my husband—he came out to see me *once* at the hospital—I told him I thought that we might as well get divorced. And he said yes. He very happily wanted to get divorced.

I did get out of hospital. I was lucky there. I was one of five patients on that ward who was discharged that year. In fact, maybe it was less than that. I don't remember anybody else being discharged. They just died in those days. There was no cure, you know, except bed-rest; you couldn't get it there. And it was really a terrifying experience. I know four people died the first week I was there. Right on the ward. Hemorrhaging. And after a while you get sort of used to it. But it wasn't any joke.

Uhm— Then I came out of hospital, and I saw her. And she just wasn't my baby. I hadn't seen her in a year anyway. So she didn't look the same, she didn't know me. The woman who was looking after her, she regarded as her mother.

I managed to get a job. I began to know a few more people; and I felt better. I used to go out and see the—baby. On weekends. But I had no rapport with her whatsoever.

Well, one thing that did happen—

[*pause*]

Now I know why it all turned out the way it did. I *knew* it would have been all right if it had been a boy; and I didn't know why— But I would have been able to struggle through to keep the baby; you know, women can do *enormous* things when they *have* to— But because she was a girl, I rejected her completely. And I didn't know why I did. So, years later, I found out that either I identified her with *myself,* or with my mother.

So uh—

KATRINA: Had you been rejected by your mother?

ELLIE: No. Not— Well, that could be. She was a very possessive type; that can be a form of rejection. Very dominating. [*pause*] I had a pretty difficult childhood. I lived in four countries before I was five years old. And— Oh, well, a lot of things. Bad things. They had a very unhappy marriage.

So uh—

The big problem was that I nearly killed the baby. I've often said—I understood the battered-child syndrome.

She wouldn't stop crying and I couldn't get any sleep. This was before I went back to Herndon Saint Andrew's and they helped me. But I really must have been cracking up at that point.

KATRINA: This was before you went in the TB hospital?

ELLIE: That's right. I had TB and didn't know it, you see, so I was— I was really quite sick. And she cried day and night, because she couldn't keep her food down. Because of this allergy to milk-fat or what-have-you. And I went over to her one day—

You're the only—the second person I've ever told this to. But you might as well know it, since it's for this particular purpose.

I put my hands around her throat like that. And I was just within an ace—of strangling her. And uh— She was then, I guess, just about six weeks, because it was after that I managed to get some help. But even at that age she *knew,* and she just *froze.* Just like that. It was the most terrifying thing to see.

So I got up and I put on my coat, and I walked out of the house and walked around the block. And thought, "What in hell am I going to do?" I mean that, to me, was the ultimate disaster. To kill your own child. Now, it seems to be getting increasingly common. But I can understand how it happens.

Then, apparently, I just turned her off completely. So she stayed out in Anacostia until she was four years old. And she was very happy out there. It was a pretty bad section, I think, Avenue B. And it wasn't a very fancy home. They were Italian and ignorant. But at least she was happy there. They genuinely loved her. And that was good.

Meanwhile I went my merry way. I was introduced to a doctor here in D.C. I had made friends with the nurse in his office and she was determined to marry me off.

So she sort of talked us into it. I wasn't in love with him. But I thought, "Well, I was in love with the last one; and that didn't work out. And I'm not doing myself any good." You know, I wasn't very good at supporting myself. And I was *always* afraid of the TB coming back.

That's finally gone. Now they've got drugs for it. You can't imagine what a weight that was off the shoulders of people like me, you know, who'd had it. It had been almost like a death sentence.

Anyway, he decided he wanted to marry me, so I said I would. Uhm— But he didn't want another man's child around.

And so I—what happened around about this time, I'm still very cloudy about. I really don't remember. I must have blocked out a great deal. But I do know that I went to one of the big adoption agencies and I said that I wanted the baby adopted. And I think I must have explained to the people out in Anacostia, but I don't remember. I'm sure they were plenty upset. And I think also Jim did a lot of the arguing for me. So that probably helped. At any rate, the agency made the arrangements and they told me, you know, I could choose the income group, and the kind of people, and all that.

So this is '47. And I chose about ten to fifteen thousand a year. Which isn't much now. But then it would put you in the middle income, not *too* wealthy, but not too poor. So they said they'd let me know in a year if that adoption didn't work out and they had to re-place her. But I never heard. So I presume it did.

And then with my second husband I went off to Oregon. It wasn't— He was very good to me in his own way. It really wasn't a very good marriage. And I kept thinking that he was sort of neurotic, that there was something wrong. He got drafted into the Army—that was the time of the Korean War —and various things happened. Finally it turned out that he was a paranoid schizophrenic. By that time he had two guns, and he was practicing with them all the time. We were living in Arizona then, and he was stationed at Theodore Roosevelt Hospital. The Roosevelt psychiatrists broke it to me gently that he was very sick indeed. I said, "What's the diagnosis?" And they told me.

They wanted me to get a divorce from him, but not to leave— You know, he was due to get out of the Army, like in April, something like that—to give him a month or two in between the time he was going to be out of the Army, and the divorce.

They also told me not to tell anybody about it. I don't know what the Army was up to. I think they didn't want him stuck on their hands. Because then they'd have been liable for his hospitalization. They were just barely keeping him out of hospital, you see. So I think they wanted to sort of usher him out of the Army and let him go bye-bye all by himself. I don't know. Maybe it was just that the medical corps at the Army didn't want it known that they had a real live lunatic on their staff! He was running one of the wards there. And he had to be supervised constantly.

Anyway, I got divorced. He went back to Oregon, and re-married, and then killed himself about fifteen years ago. Which is what they had predicted he would do. And I came back to Washington. Where I have been since then.

But I've never heard another thing about Annie, or what happened.

KATRINA: But you do know she was adopted into a family when she was about four?

ELLIE: Yes. She was four years old, right.

I don't even remember which agency it was. Might have been Columbia Charities or something. Isn't that an agency? Some name like that. It's all so long ago. I could choose the type of people. That's all. And they will never tell you anything after that.

I never attempted to find out. I think I really didn't want to see her anymore. And I couldn't understand at the time. I felt—I thought I should have felt guilty; and I didn't. I felt quite clear in my mind that this was the right thing to do. *Now* I can understand why. But I didn't *know* then: I considered myself a terrible threat to her, you see.

KATRINA: Ah.

ELLIE: And I wouldn't have any more children. I'd be scared to death.

KATRINA: Because of—?

ELLIE: I nearly killed her.

KATRINA: And that's the one reason, is it? Or are there other reasons you're a threat?

ELLIE: I don't know.

KATRINA: As far as you know?

ELLIE: As far as I know, yes, that was the primary reason. [*pause*] Well, one psychologist explained it to me: that I could have identified her with, as it were, the bad part of me, the part that *I* rejected. This would have been, you know, very unconsciously; I mean I wasn't at all aware of it. That I was trying to destroy that part, you see.

But, you know, it's past history, and nobody will ever know for sure just how many factors were involved. The fact that the husband rejected her and rejected me has to play a big factor in it too. You become really animal, I think, over the whole process. The civilization drops away completely.

So I've never regretted it. I'm curious, I'd like to know sometimes, you know, where she is, or what happened to her. But since then I have had absolutely no desire to have children at all. I don't even want to go near children. And I've never gotten over that.

I did also have an abortion, as a matter of fact. It was a year after I got out of Grand Island. That would be 1945, I think. I managed to get pregnant and got an abortion. At some hospital right here in Washington. Oh, I know what it was; they signed me up for a legal abortion because of the TB. I still had one lung collapsed. There was no problem at all; it just took two doctors to give their permission—you know, their recommendation that I should terminate the pregnancy. So I had that done.

KATRINA: Was your motivation the TB, or the not wanting to have children?

ELLIE: Not wanting to have children. That was the only thing I was thinking of. Actually TBs do fairly well if they're pregnant. Because it splints the lung. So they do quite nicely. There *was* no real reason. Except that I wasn't married and didn't have any money and all the rest of it. But *my* main reason was that I just didn't want to have anymore children; no matter *what,* at any cost. And I never got pregnant after that.

And it's interesting—I'm nearly fifty now, so I'm in the menopause, and I'm starting to menstruate very irregularly. I haven't had a period for about two months. And I'm quite pleased at this point, you see. Because I don't have to worry about being pregnant anymore.

KATRINA: Did you feel any regret at taking the child away from the home in Anacostia?

ELLIE: Uhm—

KATRINA: Why did you not leave her there with the foster parents?

ELLIE: No. I wanted to have something better for her. You see, it was a home that she'd have never gotten anyplace with. She might have been happy, right? There were two boys of about fifteen and sixteen, but no father. There was an old grandmother and a mother. And they weren't going to go anyplace. She never would have been able to go to school, or at least to college, anyway. She was a very pretty and very bright little girl. And she wouldn't have had any opportunities at all, on Avenue B. That's a pretty deadly existence.

So I felt that if there was going to be a change made, then I should give her a chance to get into a better background. Where she might have a chance to do something with her life. I know that was my motive there. I think, inasmuch as I was able to, I was protective of her.

KATRINA: Along with the rejection of her, you had caring feelings as well?

ELLIE: Uh— [*pause*] I must have had, I presume. I didn't feel it, though. I had no normal maternal instincts. Except I remember when she was very tiny—before we both got so sick—I remember I started to feel slightly proud of her. And that was the first time. That was after we'd been out of the hospital maybe about three weeks. She was about a month old. And I was starting to get interested in her, as a baby; you know, when they start to smile and that kind of thing. So *probably* if I'd had a halfway break anywhere along the line, it might have been all right. If the husband had stood by or *some*thing. But there just wasn't a chance at all; and I cracked.

KATRINA: When you arrived in Washington, you had two days to go? She was born two days later?

ELLIE: That's right, yes.

KATRINA: Why did you take the journey so close to the—?

ELLIE: For some reason, I was desperate to get out of Australia and get over here. I think all this must have been boiling up. My mother was going crazy at that stage anyway. She didn't want me to leave. She didn't want me to get married; you know, came down and visited me on my honeymoon, and this kind of stuff; really nutty. So I wanted to get away from her. But also I figured it would be much better to have the baby here in Washington than to have her in Australia.

I'd been brought up with the idea that to have a baby was the most *painful* business on the face of the earth. And I was *constantly* regaled with stories from my mother about how she was "torn to pieces having babies"; you know, and I would listen to all this.

By the time she was actually born— I kept waiting for this terrible pain. I was all set, you know, for death by a thousand cuts! And I was extremely surprised. I don't remember any pain to speak of except a slight ache in my back. Of course, they knocked me cold. I don't know what they gave me, but I was out for about eight hours. And during that time, apparently, the baby was born. I didn't know anything about it. I was very surprised. But that was one motive I know that I had in coming over here; because I always heard that Americans were much more liberal with anesthetics, you know, in childbirth.

And they nearly caught me in San Francisco. They wanted to put me in a Catholic hospital to have the baby. And I said, "Oh no." No, the Catholic women always have to go through it the hard way, you see. So I was hellbent on getting to Washington to have the baby here.

I wonder what else happened? I remember— My husband left Australia a few weeks after I was married. By that time I was pregnant. He went up to the Solomon Islands. This was before Guadalcanal, and the war hadn't started moving north yet. Then from there, I guess he was going back— Yes, that's what happened; he was sent back to the States.

And I was very determined that when I had the baby I wanted him to be with me. That would seem to have been very important, for some reason. I think maybe that's normally important, I don't know.

And I couldn't—there were no ships going up. They put me on the first ship that they could get me on. And I don't know how I got them to do that, even. Because I wasn't supposed to travel at that stage. And, I mean, the American government didn't want me to. But I went down to see the consul, the American consul, and I don't remember what I said to him, but at the end of fifteen minutes he said, "All right, you can go."

And why it took so long— It should have been only about a two-week trip. But first of all, we zig-zagged the whole way across the Pacific. And we stopped off at New Caledonia; and they just dumped us in a little hospital place there; and we sat there waiting for another ship. It took two weeks before another ship came along. Then they wanted to keep me in New Caledonia. But I was determined to go on. I insisted on continuing across the Pacific.

KATRINA: Were you happy about being pregnant?

ELLIE: [*pause*] Uhm—I don't remember being either happy or unhappy. It didn't seem to *mean* anything to me. I certainly knew I was pregnant. I made all the preparations.

KATRINA: You had not planned it.

ELLIE: No! No. [*laughs*] In those days I planned nothing. If you can remember being twenty, I mean life is one grand sweet song—or should be.

I certainly don't think I was particularly happy about it. But I hadn't really rejected the baby before she was born. And of course at that time I kept thinking it was going to be a boy. I was determined I was going to have a boy. So when they came in to me in the hospital and said, "You have a beautiful little girl," that blew the whole thing, as far as I was concerned.

But I hadn't even heard of psychiatry in those days. So I didn't even question myself as to *why*. Which I think anybody would now. Why should I feel like this? I just knew I did, and I accepted that, you know.

If I'd thought about it, I'd probably have thought I was pretty nutty.

KATRINA: And do you think that if you'd questioned and thought about it, you might then have been able to overcome the feeling?

ELLIE: No. I don't think so. No, that wouldn't have been possible. Because, even with insight, you are still going to go through the same mechanism. I mean, it was a very powerful thing. I *had* to—I had to get rid of her somehow or other, you see.

I was so happy to go into Grand Island, believe it or not. To go into hospital. I was probably the only happy patient that ever walked in there. Because it let me out of this problem, you see.

I didn't have— I don't know what women normally think about when they're pregnant. They seem to— I guess they— they're looking forward to *having* the baby, because they're familiar with babies. I had never seen a newborn baby in my life. So when I saw this, I thought, "Good gosh, did I give birth for that?" You know, hands like this, spots all over its face. My idea of a baby was probably something about nine months old. All pink and plump; you know, with a hat on. So I was very shocked there.

KATRINA: Do you think you were uninvolved with your pregnancy?

ELLIE: Yes, I would say I could very well have been uninvolved. That's true; I don't remember feeling anything much. Except that I knew that I had to get to this country. And that was very important. And I didn't seem to have any plans for afterward, at all. I don't remember planning anything.

This was just one big push, to get here in time. I came across the country by train. They wouldn't take me on a plane. I was five days from San Francisco to Washington. And I was determined I was going to make it.

And then when I got to Washington, my husband's mother came down to meet me at the train. And I had cabled them, you know, "Please get a hospital ready, arrange everything." They had done nothing. It was early September; pretty hot. And so I had to start out right away to find a doctor and a hospital. Knowing the baby was due any minute.

I went to one doctor; he said he couldn't afford to take me, because I was being paid for by the Army plan, whatever it was. But he suggested another one, who managed to get me a bed in Herndon Saint Andrew's. Somehow or other. And then he told me to go home and rest.

So I went home. And the next morning I went into labor. Once the arrangements had been made! And I was so stupid and so ignorant, the first thing I had done was put my money in some bank right near where I was staying, which at that time was the Grants' apartment; you know, where my mother-in-law worked. It was very nice of them to let me stay there. Labor started at eight o'clock in the morning. I thought, "Oh God, I've got to get money back out of the bank so I can pay the hospital." So I trooped over to the bank. And I'm in the first stage of labor the whole time, you know. It never occurred to me the water could burst or something, me standing right there in the bank. It didn't. Apparently it didn't right 'til the end. Anyway I never knew about it. It wasn't until quite a while later that I found out there was water that was supposed to come out. I didn't even know what was happening to me! God, what an idiot I was!

So then I went up to the hospital. My mother-in-law took me. My husband didn't show up. Nothing; at all.

KATRINA: Did you suspect at that time?

ELLIE: No. I'll tell you, I think I took it for granted that's the way husbands were. Because of my own background, you see. My own father was a useless sort of person, who never did anything right, at least according to my mother. And I think there was some truth in it! So I guessed that's the way the world was. I was shaped to think that husbands were cold, and not in the least bit helpful; and I sort of didn't even expect him to come and see me. He showed up a few days later. Came just that once. But he didn't want to see the baby. The nurses were very angry with him; I remember that.

That's another reason I think: I wanted her to have a better break than she'd had with her own parents, emotionally. And I felt that, you know, a good adoption agency would make sure of that. And also, if you're adopting a baby, you're much more likely to want the baby. Because you wouldn't go to all that effort to adopt her, otherwise. So, I felt she'd be far more secure.

And thank God I didn't take her into that second marriage. That would have been unbelievably bad. You know, first with all the trouble she'd had in the early years, and then to have a stepfather who was psychotic. And dangerous.

KATRINA: So you really—you never planned life with her?

ELLIE: No. I don't ever remember, pregnant or not— Except, as I say, I think the thought was with me that if this was a boy, *then* I could do something. It would have been all right. But with a girl it was absolutely out.

Ellie · 349

KATRINA: So you knew practically from the moment they said, "You have a beautiful little girl," that you weren't going to be spending your life with her?

ELLIE: Well I didn't think of it consciously. But I'm sure that's what was going through my mind, "I'm in a trap and I've got to get out of it." But at the same time, "I must do my best," you see. In other words, I do take her home, and I do feed her; I take her around to hospitals. See what's wrong with her. I do my best.

KATRINA: You weren't consciously thinking: "I should find an adoption agency; I should find foster parents—?"

ELLIE: Oh, no. In fact, I put it off far longer than I should. See, I shouldn't have waited four years. If I had had a psychiatrist to talk to at that point, I might have come to a decision much earlier. But I just sort of put it off and put it off. I don't know now why I put it off. I think there must have been some conflict there. [pause] I think there would have to be.

KATRINA: You said you later went into therapy?

ELLIE: Yes, many, many years later.

KATRINA: Is it related to this, or not particularly? The reasons why you went in, and the going—

ELLIE: No. The reasons I went in had nothing to do with Annie at that point.

After my second divorce I thought, "I ought to get analyzed." By this time I must have read a book somewhere along the line about something. At least I was aware that there was such a thing as a psychiatrist. And uh— I wasn't stupid, but I was extremely childish. I grew up very, very late. I was thinking as a child would think. You know, with that directness, without thinking beyond.

So I came back to Washington. I still had some friends here from before. Got a job in a law firm. And went into analysis. Five days a week. He only charged me $7.50 an hour. So it was— I should have known better. I mean, you get what you pay for! So I just got worse. And at the end of two years he announced that he'd been very hostile to *all* of his patients. It wasn't just me.

So I was very upset with all the time and mental energy and goddam money that had gone into this. I was living on a hundred bucks a month in a cold-water flat to be able to finance this thing.

So, I got nothing out of that. But then I went to a therapist twice a week, and he more or less patched up my ego again.

But nothing came up about the baby during all that time.

And much later on I did talk to a psychologist over something that happened, a specific thing, and . . . I was working for a man whom I really adored. But I had always suspected him of being a bit faggy. And apparently he reached the age of forty-nine and cracked up. This is not too long ago. He fired me, and he hired a boy. And we'd been very good friends. I was really crushed by that. I haven't gotten over it yet.

So on that occasion I went to see a psychologist. She knows us both; she works in the same building. We have a social relationship, so I couldn't stay with her; but she's very good. And in the process of talking about this particular situation, she questioned me. She's the only one who ever did. She was very surprised to hear I had ever had a child. And she wanted to know more about it. And then this particular incident came up. So I told her about *that*. It obviously did have much more effect on me than I realized. I just buried it, you see.

KATRINA: So you've never really worked with a therapist on—?

ELLIE: On that area. No! No, I haven't. They were all obsessed with my bad marriages; they thought that was the main problem, or something. They never— I don't think any of them were very good!

KATRINA: Have you had more than the two you mentioned?

ELLIE: Yes; well, only briefly. The therapist whom I liked and I think had helped me— He certainly helped me get over the analysis. No doubt about that. Anyway, he retired from practice, and then I didn't see anybody for a long time. The next time I went was—oh, about five years ago. I went to a psychiatrist for a while. Because I knew my mother was going to die, and I was very apprehensive; you know, I thought, "Oh God, probably all the guilt will kick up now." I had been to see my mother, spent three months with her. She was even worse than she'd been when she was younger. So I came back here, and then I thought I'd better see this psychiatrist.

And so I just saw him for a few weeks. Then, right on schedule, as announced, my mother died. She practically planned it, I think. And I was—I didn't have any reaction at all. That went off beautifully. I woke up in the morning feeling fine.

And I've actually, until this last episode about my boss, I've felt much better than when my mother was alive. Because she was a constant drag on me. The kind that makes you feel guilty all the time.

KATRINA: What was her response to your solutions about the baby? To your problems and your solutions?

ELLIE: Well, she came over to this country when I was married to Jim. And she said, then, if she'd known I was going to have the baby adopted, that they would have taken the baby themselves, she and my father. But she didn't offer to at the time; when she knew that the baby was boarded out, and that I was working, and so on.

Well, we didn't speak for a long time. After I first got married, she was behaving very neurotically, storming around the house and saying, "You don't love me anymore," and all this kind of stuff. And finally she stormed out and said she was going to work in the outback, in the bush country. As far away as she could possibly go! So I just thanked— Thank God she's gone! You know, one less problem to worry about. So I came over to this country, and I didn't write her for a long time. Then I got a letter from a friend who said that she'd been very ill. She'd had a bleeding colon, and this and that. So I felt sort of sorry for her at this distance. I started writing her again. And this friend was not supposed to have told her anything about what was happening with me. But she apparently did.

KATRINA: Did she make you feel guilty about your choices with the baby?

ELLIE: I don't think she made me feel guilty about that. She made me feel guilty about herself. How lucky I was to be young. How lucky I was to be pretty. What a miserable life she'd had. Stuck with my father all these years. Always ailing, you know. So she made me feel guilty in that sense. I always felt I was over-privileged compared with her. And as somebody once pointed out, I managed to wreck my own life thoroughly enough so that no matter how hard she tried, she couldn't catch up with me! [*laughs*] You see.

KATRINA: In the years since the adoption and the fostering and the fear of being a battering mother—how much has it affected your life now? Do you think about it now?

ELLIE: No. I hadn't thought about Annie until my friend Phoebe said to me the other night that you were doing this book. And would I mind talking to you. And I said, "No," you know, "I don't mind."

And it wasn't until last night I thought, "Boy, it's really coming back. It's hitting me *now*. Uhm—and maybe I should have left well alone."

But it'll go away and it doesn't matter.

But I don't—It's not—it's not guilt I feel. Because I know I did the right thing, you see. So nobody could make me feel guilty for having had her adopted. But I feel *now* that it was much too important a thing in my life. It affected my whole life. But I didn't realize it. And the problem itself: in other words, I couldn't go into a normal marriage, because naturally you'd want to have children. Well, I didn't. So after I left Jim I was pretty sure then that I would never marry again. I never have. That's twenty years ago.

But I think that was the main reason for having Annie adopted: that I definitely considered myself a danger to her.

KATRINA: And that you could remain a danger if she remained in the foster home?

ELLIE: Uh—Probably. Uhm— I had to get her out of my life. Because I was duty-bound, you know, to go and see her and— I felt—I felt everybody must be thinking I'm a lousy mother. Which I certainly was, anyway you look at it! You know, it's an embarrassment to me, right? So uh—it simply never occurred to me that I had psychological problems. I didn't know. I mean I just assumed this is the way life is, you know. And I couldn't understand how other people could have little *girls* and *love* them. It was a big mystery to me. But I felt there was something deficient in myself. I lacked this maternal instinct. And that puzzled me, on that level. Because I had sort of thought that one was born with this kind of thing. If you're a female you're supposed to have a maternal instinct. Well, what happened to mine? [*laughs*] And everybody is supposed to love their children or something. Well, I didn't love mine, you know.

So—and I just—I don't like children to this day, I don't like them. And whether I consider myself a threat to *all* children, I don't know.

KATRINA: Do you feel you were wanted by your family?

ELLIE: Not by my father, no; I was totally rejected by my father. He was nearly fifty when I was born. And he didn't know anything about children. Couldn't *stand* me, you know. He just wanted to sit in a corner and read and smoke all the time. And at the age of three, I remember I'd always be pestering him, trying to get some affection out of him, you see. And he would usually cuff me—or throw me halfway across the room if he thought Mother wasn't looking. So—uhm—No, he definitely rejected me.

KATRINA: And your mother wanted you, do you think?

ELLIE: She, well, yes, she—she claims she did. She was very possessive of me. But she herself was so sick that she tried to turn me into like a girlfriend rather than her own child. So that I was her confidant. She was a very *brilliant* woman. She was well known and respected throughout Australia; an important figure on the intellectual scene. But *emotionally* a complete baby.

And uhm— When I started becoming a teenager, you know, and started rejecting her and had my own dates and what-have-you, she began to get very upset. So in *that* sense, she may have rejected me in a mother-child relationship. But she did substitute a very close *companionship*. As though I was a—almost like an *elder* sister. I was making all the decisions for the two of them by the time I was nine years old. You know, what houses to buy, and where I should go to school, and that kind of thing. I was the head of the family, at nine. So it was really a crazy background, you know?

KATRINA: Yes.

Did they—did they want a boy?

ELLIE: My *father* did, yes. Oh yes, we went through all that bit. They were both from very old families. My mother's family went back to somewhere around 600 A.D. Very old Welsh family. And my father's family had lived in the Hebrides, off the west coast of Scotland, for about eight hundred years. They were all seafaring people. They were late, late Vikings that came down about eight hundred years ago. It seems the eldest son in my father's family was, in alternate generations, either called Douglas or Antony, see. There was a boy born before I was. But apparently it was a transverse baby. And the baby was born dead.

I was born a year later. Uhm— So he was very disappointed that he never had a son to carry on the old family name.

And in my mother's family, they always had more women than men. It had once been a family that owned half of Wales. But there was nobody left, you see. So—there was just sort of *me*, and I'm a *girl*, right? Can't carry on the name, any way you look at it! There was a lot of talk about that. I think everybody would have preferred a boy.

However.

Maybe that's why *I* wanted a boy. Who knows?

But I don't think I ever wanted children. In any stage of my life. And also, I was a child myself until I was at least thirty. And I think as long as you're a child you don't really want to have children of your own. I think you have to be fairly mature to want children.

KATRINA: One thing that's particularly interesting to me about your story is that it's very, very similar to someone else who also gave up a child for adoption—

ELLIE: Oh yes? Then there has to be a—that's an interesting aspect of it: that in just sixteen or seventeen cases you would pick up two very similar stories. Because that means there are lots—a lot more who have gone through similar things.

KATRINA: Yes!

ELLIE: It could be very helpful. I think people are often criticized very much for giving— People have said to me, "*How* could you do it? *I* would never have let her go." You know. Which didn't help *me* very much.

KATRINA: Yes; how do you feel about that?

ELLIE: I wished I had been more of a person myself, so that I would have been able to marry normally and have children. I would like to be more of a . . . like the rest of the world. Because I know that I was born emotionally crippled. Not *born*. I *became* emotionally crippled, with all this background and all these problems. And I know that I missed a lot in life for that reason.

And I've had a difficult time in this country. I've had to work very hard. And I didn't have any real training of any kind. So the only jobs I've been able to get are pretty rough ones. And I will have to go on like that. Because I don't think I can do anything else. Uhm— So you're sort of faced with the prospect of just hard work . . . and very little . . . uhm—happiness—in a whole lifetime.

So I regret that aspect of it, you see.

KATRINA: And the fear of child-battering, she *also* . . .

ELLIE: Yes; well, I think this is pretty well rule-of-thumb, when the mother is up against too much emotional strain. As they say, the child is probably an extension of the ego. And the child gets clobbered. It's self-destructiveness, really. That's what it boils down to.

I expect many normal mothers may go through the same process, only they're not so alarmed by it. But *our* kind react very violently. We're very much afraid of what we might do. And we might. And some of us do. That's the big problem. You hold it down and then you let it out too much.

KATRINA: Apart from the incident you told me about, were there other, smaller incidents?

ELLIE: No! That was it.

KATRINA: It came to you out of the blue—?

ELLIE: Yes, absolutely, yes. I'd been holding on and holding on. Of course, right after that I was up at Herndon Saint Andrew's and they took an X-ray and found out that I had TB. So it was *urgent* to get her away from me, you see, in case she became infected. I was going around with a mask on my face, feeding her at arm's length, you know, so she wouldn't catch my TB. It took them at least two weeks until they managed to find board for her, at Municipal Hospital.

KATRINA: The one thing that I still don't quite understand is *when* you were rejected by your husband, or when you knew it—

ELLIE: I think that I had probably felt it the moment I landed at San Francisco and I couldn't find him. But that was sort of like part of an expected pattern. As though I knew what was going to happen. I probably married him for that reason. If he'd turned around and behaved properly, I probably would have rejected him immediately. I don't know.

But I think that's when I knew it. Because I remember sitting in a hotel room, calling all over the country trying to find him. I knew several of his friends, you know, by correspondence. The Red Cross finally helped me to track him down. He'd been sent to a camp in Pennsylvania.

KATRINA: Did he have to approve the adoption, too?

ELLIE: Oh yes. Sure; they wouldn't do it without his permission.

KATRINA: Was it hard? Or not?

ELLIE: No. My second husband went and found him. He was out in Salt Lake City. So Jim tracked him down. And they had some sort of discussion about it. And he was very happy to sign her up for adoption. His only stipulation was that she was not to go into a Catholic home. Which was interesting: he'd been Catholic! I said I didn't care what kind of a home she went into as far as religion was concerned. Just as long as it was a nice home.

KATRINA: Did you ever see the Anacostia family again?

ELLIE: No! Never! Oh, they were pretty mad at me, I'm sure. But I think they blamed the husband more than anything else—for having talked me into it. Which really wasn't justified. It was me, I know. I was just happy to have an ally. Somebody I could blame it on, so that I didn't look so bad socially, you see.

KATRINA: How is it now? You don't talk about it socially?

ELLIE: No, as a matter of fact, it's almost—it's so far back it's—it's forgotten, you know.
Sometimes people say, "Do you have any children?" and I—I'll just say, "No," or— It depends on the circumstances;

I might say, "No, I had a child in World War II but she was adopted." And nobody is going to ask too many questions after that unless they're really insensitive.

So as I say, it's just gone and out of my mind. I just don't think about it at all. Haven't for years.

[*pause*]

KATRINA: You said you were curious about Annie.

ELLIE: Yes, oh yes! I'd like to know how she turned out; you know. What happened. Did she get married? Did she become a . . . drug addict? Or, you know—After all, she'd be—How old would she be now? Over twenty-five, wouldn't she? Born in '43. She'd be twenty-nine. So I would like to see how her life's turned out; you know, what happened along the way. And extend my apologies for having loused up her early life.

But I don't feel as though it's my *daughter,* if you know what I mean. It's just another human being, that I have some interest in.

My good friend—I have a very good friend, and her nephew got married about two years ago. And we nearly flipped. Because we hadn't seen this girl. She was in the Midwest. We knew she was blonde and blue-eyed. She was born in 1943, and her name was Anne Eleanor. So we nearly died. We couldn't wait to see her. And it wasn't the same girl, of course. But it was a funny coincidence, you know. Born the same year with the same name. And they also call her Annie.

KATRINA: Did you give her your name as a middle name, or not?

ELLIE: Yes, well, apparently everybody in my mother's family has been called Eleanor. Back for God knows how long.

KATRINA: So you did. . . .

ELLIE: So—it's a name that I would have handed— It's a good name, anyway; it's a useful name; I'm Eleanor; my mother was, I think the Gaelic version of Eleanor—Ellen. And so on, as far back as we know. Anne was just after my husband's mother. But I liked the combination—of Anne Eleanor.

KATRINA: Do you worry about, or do you think about her reading this?

ELLIE: My God, never thought of it. She *might* at twenty-nine, she might—she *could* pick up a book like that. I mean, she would *know* that she was adopted.

I wonder if that would be bad? She wouldn't—Of course it would give the age of when she was adopted. . . .

KATRINA: Do you think there's something we can do? Something we can perhaps change—What do you think? Why don't you tell me which details, and then I. . . .

ELLIE: Listen, maybe it wouldn't matter.

Because, after all, if she did read it, and if she did think that could have been her, it would *explain why*. And I think an adopted child must always wonder *why* the mother left. And it might even—I think people very often—certainly as children—feel that if they're rejected, it's their fault. Who knows what that might have done to her?

Although I did—when I put her up for adoption, I said I wanted to be absolutely sure that if she needed psychiatric care she would get it. That she had to be in the kind of a home where it would be supplied. Because she'd had such a rough time over the previous four years. And I think that she probably would have needed some. I think it's very unlikely that she could have gotten away unscarred, going through all that.

So she might very well read it. But I think it might be good, if she was able to identify with it. She's had no way she could find out. And she may have *wondered*, all her life, you see.

KATRINA: You've mentioned that it was quite some time before you knew your motives, your true motives, in having Annie adopted. How long was it until—?

ELLIE: I didn't—I didn't know until uhm—I'm just trying to think when it was. Uhm—the end of July. Only about two months ago, that's when it was. This psychologist, that I just went to for a few sessions, she pointed this out to me: that the reason that I put Annie up for adoption was because I was afraid I would do her harm.

KATRINA: And you hadn't known that, all that time?

ELLIE: I had never told anybody *about* this episode. Naturally I'm not very *proud* of trying to kill my own child. Right? So it had never come *up* before, with *any*body.

You're the—outside of this psychologist and myself, you're the only other person who has this information. Which I feel is very vital for this kind of story. Otherwise there would have been a big missing link. So I *had* to tell you.

So, therefore, *besides* that there *is* no guilt about having her adopted. You see what I mean?

KATRINA: Yes; right.

ELLIE: Because that got her *out of harm's way*. The psychologist told me; and I said of *course* that was the reason. But I had never known it. I was very surprised. She said, "Absolutely." Well apparently it's a well-known syndrome. And of course she's seen it many times before. For some reason or another I just hadn't come across it. But then nobody had *known* that I ever had this episode happen to me, you see. Because I wasn't about to tell anybody about it.

KATRINA: Even *without* the episode it could—a trained person might have seen that this is what you were doing.

ELLIE: They should have seen it. But they never seemed to think that there was anything particularly unusual about that period in my life. I always said it was the worst part of my life I'd ever had.

But it's an interesting coincidence. That it's only recently that I found this out. And then you come along, and you're writing a book on the subject!

KATRINA: But then you must have *wondered,* all along, what your reason was!

ELLIE: I just thought I lacked maternal instincts. I simply didn't want to have children. That's all I knew.

But I didn't know that there was a positive reason there, you see.

KATRINA: So you had to live with a certain amount of self-hatred . . . for thirty-odd years?

ELLIE: Well, yes, you regard yourself—and I still do—as an abnormal human being. You learn to live with that. I mean, what can you do about it, right? You can't go back and start all over again. And— So I have sort of *adapted,* you know — But I—I *do* feel it. I mean I've had to give up marriage, and home, and *everything,* you know, that women normally want. Because of this *damn* thing. However, you know, I can look around and see how a lot of people are worse off than I am. I can't complain too much.

KATRINA: And this was just two months ago. Do you feel a load off now? Do you feel different as a result of it?

ELLIE: Well, no, because— If it hadn't been for this big fuss with my boss— And that's the only reason I went to see the psychologist. Because the last day I was at my job, I was feeling so terrible. I really adored my boss. I thought he was the most wonderful man. He was always so good and kind and everything. And he had a complete personality change, you see. He suddenly became sort of attacking everybody, and practically ruined his career. All sorts of things going on. So I'm heartbroken. Here I've got no job. I've been living on unemployment; and I've lost my beautiful boss. And all my associates. I'd been in that office long before he was there. It was like my own office, you know. I was very possessive about it. So I was terribly upset. And the last day I'm there this psychologist gets into the elevator, and we talk about it.

Then I called her up and I said that I'd like to see her for a few sessions and see if I could get myself straightened out. And she was just asking me about my background. She had assumed that I had no children. And I said, oh no; yes, I had a baby. She was very surprised. And that's how it came up, you see; she asked me the circumstances. So if it wasn't for *that*, two months ago, I would have never turned up this material for your book, see. Because I think this—this particular episode—is the clincher of the whole story.

And there may be many other people who have gone through similar things. I wouldn't be surprised. And a book would be of considerable help, I think. To get an insight like that would have helped *me* many, many years ago. I don't know how much more I may have punished myself for what I did, you see. After all, the next man I married was a psychotic. And a dangerous one at that. So, that could have been part of the picture. Now if somebody had gotten hold of me at that age, it would have been much, much better. Now it's too late. [*laughs*]

KATRINA: Well, no. No, no—

ELLIE: Oh yes, it is, really.

KATRINA: As long as you get the insight *some*time—

ELLIE: Before the end of your life. I think— I've always felt that I would like to know. . . . That's why I went to analysis—to *understand: What* motivated me to do all these various things? I had an odd life, you know. And I'd like to know why I did that—What life's all about.

And why I didn't use all my talents. I can paint, I can write; I do nothing with it, you see. So, even if I come to a sticky end—I'd still like to know *why*. I think that's important.

FRANCINE

Interviewed in May 1972

FRANCINE: I was attending Jefferson College in South Carolina. And I was doing student teaching in a city called Pinesville, about ninety miles from Jefferson. I was placed in a high school. Consequently I—uhm—For the first time, I actually had "an affair," I guess. With the coach there at the high school. Mostly because he was very athletic, had a beautiful build, and sort of reminded me of [*laughs*] I guess the kind of man I really wanted to have an affair with first. And it wasn't a matter of being passionately in love. But more of—because I was twenty-one and I'd never slept with anybody! [*laughs*]

It's really weird!

I felt it was time, and I just couldn't wait. I mean, I wanted to know what it was really all about. I felt that I was excluded from so many conversations! I would either ask a dumb question or would absolutely know nothing about what was going on. And as I said, I was attracted to Andrew, but not really that much physically. I wasn't really that turned on, you know, by the whole—by sex itself, you know.

Uhm—let's see. Well, that was in the spring of the year I was graduating. I was to graduate that July from college. And I did! I finished my student teaching, went home for a short vacation, came back to school; and I graduated July seventeeth. I went back to my hometown, and believe it or not, took a job, teaching.

And I realized around that October, that I was pregnant. Well, of course I had—I mean I sort of kept *thinking* I was. Because I wasn't having a period. But I had gone to a doctor in a small town near the college, and he had said I had an infection. I had an infection along with the pregnancy! But I just considered the fact that I had an infection as the reason why I wasn't having a regular menstrual period.

KATRINA: You conceived about—?

FRANCINE: Oh, it must have been, I'd say, about April.

KATRINA: And you didn't figure you were pregnant until October?

FRANCINE: Well, I finally went to a doctor in my hometown. I was *told* I was pregnant. [*laughter*] Only six months!

KATRINA: What—what were you thinking?

FRANCINE: I was thinking, "I *hope* I really do have some kind of ghastly infection!"

It really was something very simple, though. Doctors call it a yeast infection. You know, it's really nothing complicated. They gave me some suppositories and it goes away. That was it.

Well, at any rate, after that I resigned from my teaching job and came to New Jersey to stay with my brother. He had an apartment in Newark.

KATRINA: How did you take the fact that you were pregnant?

FRANCINE: Well, I was very—I was *distraught. Insane!* With disbelief. Couldn't believe it. I really could not believe that it actually happened.

KATRINA: Even though you must have looked—?

FRANCINE: Not very much. I'm very slim as you can see. And I've always had sort of a paunchy stomach. I was just a little bit more than this. About the way I'd be now after eating a very big meal and *full*.

But I finally calmed down. My family—I come from a very large family. You know, I've got five brothers and two sisters, and they're sort of scattered everywhere. Most of them are older than I was. And everybody was just sort of saying, "Okay," you know, "Well, you're pregnant." This sort of thing. I wasn't *driven* out of the house in *shame* or anything. I think they sort of felt sorry for me, too, because I—was kind of lost, you know. Frightened by the whole idea of *having* a child, period. You know, going through that whole business.

KATRINA: Had any of them said before—?

FRANCINE: "Could you be pregnant?" No, nobody really thought about it. I didn't act or feel pregnant; that was one thing, you see. I was still playing touch football with my brothers, and all sorts of weird, mad things.

KATRINA: But during that six months, it was crossing your mind from time to time?

FRANCINE: Right, right! I kept thinking how horrible it would be!

KATRINA: And *why* did you not go to a doctor?

FRANCINE: I just sort of put it off. I think subconsciously I kept thinking: "If I don't go and nobody ever tells me, then nothing's going to happen!"

KATRINA: You were a full college graduate, right?

FRANCINE: Right! [*roars with laughter*] Interesting? It's kind of funny now; it wasn't so funny then.

KATRINA: And so your family— You went right back and told them?

FRANCINE: Yes. Well, he was like the family doctor, and he had known all of us. So he asked me if I would tell them or should he. At first I said, "You'd better call up and tell her." And then I said, "No, I'll tell them." But when I came back to the car—my brother had driven me—he said he could tell from the look on my face what the doctor had said. So it was, you know, enough— Well, my mother sort of put two and two together. I—I still think to this day that she probably suspected it; waiting for that.

KATRINA: When you went to the doctor, was it to find out if you were pregnant? Or to see how your infection was doing?

FRANCINE: Just to see how I was doing, period. I think— my mother insisted I go, because she had gotten tired of playing a little game with me. Because I think she was really suspecting it.

KATRINA: And then everybody was pleasant and sympathetic? Or . . . ?

FRANCINE: *Oh* yes! No one was—you know, carried on. Except my older brother. He sort of cried. He said, "Poor little sister." Well, to him, you know, I was still a little girl.

But he's really quite sweet. They were all very nice, I must say. Oh, we're a very close-knit family. There's a lot of us. And we're very close to each other.

KATRINA: Do you feel that's unusual?

FRANCINE: Not for Southern families, I don't think. I feel it's something you sort of grow up with.

Maybe too, though, it was the influence of my parents. Because my father grew up sort of—he had two brothers, but he wasn't really close to them. Because in the old days in the South, see—well, first of all, there's alw—there's, there *was* at one time—that colored thing, you know. And my father's brothers were children from his mother's marriage to a white man. And he was the darkest of the family. So he was pretty much sort of ostracized. Not so much by his siblings, but by, you know, other people. I mean, to look at my uncles, you wouldn't assume that they were Negro. You'd assume they were Caucasians, or anything but. Not, you know, not—not—black. So he didn't have a really normal, warm childhood.

And my mother had one brother whom she wasn't really that close to. So she, in turn, sort of made the family "a real family." You know. In terms of really being *warm* and superloving. And she sort of passed it on to the rest of us. We're big on touching, and feeling, and, you know, just that real thing that you can feel. So I think it was mainly due to *them,* and the way they brought us up. And, in fact, I think we grew up kind of liking each other anyway. Being different, but yet having real affection for each other. I like to talk about my family.

KATRINA: Yes, they sound wonderful.

FRANCINE: They're really great people. There's not a single one that I don't like.

Most people are—strangely enough—are appalled at the fact that, you know, we're always in constant touch with each other. We're scattered everywhere. But, nonetheless, everyone knows where the other is, and what they're doing.

KATRINA: Are white people more surprised by this than black people?

FRANCINE: I see that *Eastern* whites seem more surprised by this kind of thing, yes. I talk about my brothers and sisters each chance I get, but it seems that, you know, it's just not a common thing. People don't go around constantly mentioning "my brother" and "my sister" or this, that, or the other. We were exceptionally close. And still are. Although both our parents are dead, you know, we're like— Well, my older brothers and sisters sort of—It was the kind of thing where the older ones look out for the younger ones too, you know.

KATRINA: So you came North—for what reason?

FRANCINE: Well, I was pregnant and I just didn't stay there.

KATRINA: Why would you not have stayed there?

FRANCINE: Uhmm. For a lot of reasons. I didn't want to. Because I had taken a teaching job in the same community where I lived. And at that time it was still sort of—uh—the small-town thing, you know, about being seen, and having to see people, and possibly explain or— You know, just not really wanting to see people staring or making comments. So I just got on a plane and came to Newark. My brother had suggested it might be better if I did. Because it's a large city and, you know, I can be alone when I want to. And just not really have to see people if I didn't care to.

KATRINA: And now that you knew you were pregnant, were you realistic about it?

FRANCINE: Yes. I started making plans. The only unrealistic plan I made was thinking I was really going to keep the baby with me.

It was really—it was kind of a *fun* pregnancy. Because everybody was really great. [*laughing*] I went and bought lots of clothes. And I went *out* with— My brother introduced me to a really *great* friend of his. This was a really nice young couple, who lived in the building; and he was a student minister. And uh—then there was Sam, who was—was really tall, and nice-looking, and just great, you know, a good, nice, kind, sweet guy. He was like a couple of years older than I was. And single. So he— I think about it many times now, and I wonder how he must have felt, you know, taking this pregnant girl around to all of his old friends. I think he had a steady girl friend; but he spent an awful lot of time taking me out, to movies and, you know, shopping—stuff like that. And after the baby was born he sort of did the whole bit, rushing over with flowers, and all that. You know, he ran out and bought millions of things.

KATRINA: To be kind? Or—?

FRANCINE: I don't know. I— Well, he died. [*pause*] Oh, about when the baby was around four months old. He was killed by accident. Two guys were fighting. He was stabbed accidentally, for someone else. It was—it was really— I couldn't believe it. It still seems incredible. It's been quite a while ago, now.

KATRINA: But his relationship was not romantic as much as sort of "older brother"? Or is it unimportant?

FRANCINE: I— Just before he died— Well, after the baby was born, I found a job. And we'd go out, after work— Well, anyway, I better tell you this part of the story:

I moved in with John's mother. He's the young student minister. She had a nice big house on Clifford Avenue, and I moved in there with her. And she took care of the baby. She's like a real grandmotherly type. She was constantly on the phone with my mother and my brother. And, you know, she got to know my family and sort of became another—a substitute grandmother-mother kind of thing. She took care of the baby, beautifully. I mean she's just a sweet, old, warm, loving lady. She just sort of throws her arms around you and, you know, makes everything all right. And I found a job. I made quite a few friends on the job, and I would have people over, and she was taking care of the baby.

KATRINA: So you were very comfortable, really?

FRANCINE: Oh yes! I never—I mean I never went through any *changes*. You know, in terms of the—just things I needed, like clothing or— The hospital bill was paid by my brother. All at one time, you know. I had a doctor, who was nice. He was really a sweet guy, too. Everything went beautifully. Delivery wasn't hard. I mean people were *there*. You know. All the time. My brother, his friends, Mrs. Walker.

KATRINA: So from the time you knew, you were really looked after and . . . ?

FRANCINE: Right!

KATRINA: And happy?

FRANCINE: Hm-hm!!

KATRINA: Were you "thrilled"?

FRANCINE: *After* it was over. Because as I say I had made friends, and everything looked better. The only thing I was hung up about was the whole *idea* of having a baby at this stage of the game. No husband. You know. "What am I going to do, now I've got a child?" You know, it's not the way to start a marriage. But that even worked out, too!

So I was a little worried about, you know, practical things. As I said, Mrs. Walker took care of the baby, and I worked.

And then my mother sort of got anxious! She sent my brother up here on a plane, one Friday. And he took this little tiny baby, and all of her stuff, and got the next plane back to Mississippi with the baby.

KATRINA: Your mother was "anxious"—?

FRANCINE: To take care of it. She sort of didn't think someone else should be doing that. And she should.

And they grew so attached to her. My father was really out of his mind. But uh—I think I left something out here. There's something I meant to tell you and I can't—

Oh, yes; about Sam: after the child was born, as I said, Sam started taking me out socially. And I think he was getting interested. And I knew I was interested in him. I wasn't madly in love with him, but I liked him quite a bit. And it was like a *normal* relationship. Not, you know, "You've had a baby." None of that really came into it. But he was sort of always there and playing with her and seeing her. This kind of thing. It was really good. And then, as I said, within a few months after she was born— She must have been—about four months old I think. And he died.

So I just sort of picked up. I started looking around for another job. Because the first job I took was in an office. It was clerical—really *dumb*—work. And I took the exam for my teacher's license. While I was waiting for that, I was offered a job with the Department of Welfare. I had no plan for social work. I was going to teach young children to talk in French! But in the meantime I got hired by the City. The pay was better, so I didn't even bother to leave when I got my teacher's license. And I met Eddie there. He was also working for the Welfare Department. But between that time I was dating a lot of really nice guys I had met.

KATRINA: How old was your daughter when she went . . . ?

FRANCINE: To stay with my parents? She must have been about— Born in January, February, March— It was sometime like April, when she went there. Then that next Christmas I went down, flew home and saw her. They would send me pictures every week, this kind of thing.

KATRINA: How did you feel about the separation?

FRANCINE: At first I didn't— I wasn't— See, I wasn't there with her all day anyway. So it was just a matter of her being taken care of and my not even having to worry about her at all. You know, getting up in the morning and doing anything for her. Or coming home at night. I mean I was more free to — And I think my mother realized this. I didn't think about it at the time. [*laughs*] I'm sort of slow to react, you know? But later I realized that must have been part of it. Because she felt I should have had *time,* completely to myself, to get my life together. Which is what I really started doing.

I started dating a lot. And I met a lot of really interesting guys. Almost got married to a guy from Rhodesia that I'd been seeing for about four months. And he always referred to Nancy as "the child." You know, "the child," and how we'd dispose of it while we went on to live in the bush. In Africa. And I wasn't too cool! Because it's like a thousand dollars one way from the States to Africa. And I wasn't about to give up, you know, my family, friends and everything, and go off and live that kind of life.

Another young man that I was working with was super-ambitious and was always planning all these great things we were going to do and all the money we'd have. But I was still going out with, you know, other people, too. And I met Eddie in the Welfare Center, where I was working. And within a month we were married!

Eddie is really a very nice man. A very *good* kind of person; you know, and he loves kids; and animals, and—You know, that kind of good. So he immediately started making plans for the baby to come and stay with us. We were married in March. And the baby came up in April. My mother brought her to us two weeks after we were married.

I sometimes tease Eddie now, about marrying me because I had a child already. You know, "You just married me for my baby." And that's the way it seemed. They were inseparable. Everywhere he went he was taking this kid and showing her off. And I got pregnant—when was it? In August, I think. We got married in March and I got pregnant in August. So it worked out that our second child was born in May, a year later.

KATRINA: Were there any formalities of having to adopt her? Had you *told* the first father—the biological father—?

FRANCINE: *Finally* I did. I called him from New Jersey. [*laughs*] Safely! five hundred miles away! Because I really didn't want him complicating things. Even as—uh—crazy as I was in those days, I didn't—I *knew* I didn't want to get married. Getting married, to me, was more frightening than having a baby. [*pause*] Can you believe it?

Because I knew that we just didn't have anything— From the marriages *I* had seen, Andrew and I didn't have that.

KATRINA: Did you tell him before you had the baby?

FRANCINE: Well, like a month before. I called him down in Pinesville and told him I was pregnant.

KATRINA: And how did he react?

FRANCINE: Mad. Wild. Insane. He thought I was the world's greatest idiot. He was angry. He acted like a real madman at first. And then I just sort of said . . . I think I said something really dumb like, "Well, you don't have to worry about it." You know. And I didn't realize how it had really affected him. I do regret though that I— But there was nothing I could do really. I couldn't handle having him around and making claims on me and that kind of thing.

KATRINA: Did he want to be a part of it?

FRANCINE: He was in love with me. Sadly. You know. And I really couldn't handle that. Because it just wasn't the way to— I didn't feel that wild about him. He was attractive and, you know, good for me at the *time;* but I couldn't have a continuation of that.

KATRINA: But he would have liked to?

FRANCINE: Mmm-hm! He would have. He just didn't know how to go about it. I just said I was in Newark and, you know, nobody told him where I was staying.

KATRINA: But if you had given him your address—

FRANCINE: He would have been on the next plane and come up.

KATRINA: And married you?

FRANCINE: *Wanted* to. Tried to.
He appealed to my parents and my brothers, and my sis-

ters; and everyone else he could get his hands on. But nobody put him— Fortunately my family didn't say. "Oh! you should get *married*. There's this *nice man* that wants to marry you." They didn't fall in that, you know, bag. So that was good.

And they knew that I was more frightened of getting married. "No, no, no!"

KATRINA: Well, but when you met the right man you weren't so frightened?

FRANCINE: Oh no! It was the most right thing in the whole world to do. It was just sort of knowing— My mother told me, a long time ago, that it's something you know; and that it happens one time. And it does!

KATRINA: Were there any problems about his wanting to have possession of the child? Or—

FRANCINE: Andrew? The child's natural father?

KATRINA: Yes.

FRANCINE: No, he didn't really— Well, he couldn't actually. Nobody had told him "She lives on Richmond Street, you should go up and see her." And by the time Nancy was fourteen months old, Eddie and I were married; and a friend of ours who was a lawyer did all the paperwork, in terms of getting the birth certificate changed. It was just a matter of getting a long white form and you fill it out and Eddie signs it, and we sent it in with the birth certificate. So his name is on the birth certificate, actually.

KATRINA: Did you see Andrew after you left college?

FRANCINE: I didn't see Andrew except in Pinesville, South Carolina, for my student-teaching. And not *ever* again.

So I didn't have to, you know, handle anything with him.

KATRINA: Did you think of giving the baby up?

FRANCINE: No.

KATRINA: Why not?

FRANCINE: I just never really thought about it. It—it's never even entered into *my* thoughts; or anyone else's.

I think it's probably part of my background too. You see, we don't—fewer blacks give up children—than when, you know, the average white girl would. And especially, too, because black babies are harder to place than white babies. And I wasn't going to take a chance on it. And I just never thought about it. I thought about it later, you know, in thinking what options I had had—foster care, or, you know, placement. But—I mean the child was part of a family.

And my father had said— I mentioned to him about, you know, the *name*. And he said, "She'll have her name." You know, "It's no sweat." He's really great like that—

KATRINA: Meaning that she'd have your maiden name? Or that, "She'll get a father one of these days."?

FRANCINE: *And* she'd have a name, his name; you know, *our* name! She was part of a family. And nobody ever really thought about it.

My family was *status* conscious. You know, there was— It wasn't as if it's something that happened, you know, every year or something. But it was just a matter of being something you had to deal with. Nobody was hung up about—uh —after the fact. I was *pregnant*. There was nothing to do but then plan for it, you see. My folks were not the kind to sit around—They taught us, "You don't sit around and cry about something. You just go on and do what you must do." I mean you don't sit around saying, "Who's to blame?" and, "Why did this have to happen?" It happened! You know, you *live* with these things. This is why now I can't stand to have something that needs to be done, or a situation comes up, and have to sit around and *talk* about it. Let's get busy and do something. I don't want to be hassled with the whys and hows. Just let's do what we have to do, from here. And this is sort of the way this was done.

I could see *me* sitting around crying through a whole pregnancy, probably. Under any other circumstances.

At that time I was—you know—I think immature for twenty-one. Not mature at all.

KATRINA: Considering you now—and this story!

FRANCINE: I think I grew up more after I married—Eddie. That's when I really started to grow. That's when I really started being a *woman*.

I think about it now; and I wonder how could I have been — You know, how was I like that? How *could* I? But I didn't really grow up. Until after I had a baby, and worked sort of—not really on my own, because I had a watchful older brother, who sort of looked out for me. And screened all my dates and—

Do you know the day—now the day I got married—well, he let us have the apartment. And he moved in with my brother who was living in Orange with his wife and son. Well, when he knew I was getting married, he had accepted a job in Gary, Indiana. A job that he had been after for years. The job finally came to him; but he didn't accept it until *after* he knew that I was getting married. You know. And he, within—like my mother came up about two weeks later and brought the baby to us. And *then* George sort of made his exit. But he did not leave New Jersey until I got—didn't even consider taking the job in Indiana until I got married.

And so my mother came and brought Nancy up. She was just young enough to not be hassled by who—you know, her surroundings more or less. She sort of just— Well, of course, she was more attached to Mother than she was to me, I was really a bit of a stranger. But after a while, you know, she sort of fell right into it. And I think it was probably Eddie's way *with* her that—within a month with us she started babbling, and the first thing she said was, "Daddy." You know, she—things started just fitting in. And it's been that way ever since. It's a funny thing: this child is more like Eddie than our other one. People are always saying, "Isn't she just like her old man!" I think maybe it could be because of his influence. Like when Diane was a baby— Well, Eddie does things just *naturally*. You know, here's this tiny newborn infant, and he's changing diapers and feeding her and— Eddie is the kind of man who runs out and does the diapers, comes home and folds them up, makes lunch, mops the floor, folds the clothes, hems their dresses, washes their hair; that kind of thing. And I think this is probably why they're so close to him. That, coupled with the fact that Eddie believes in being *with* them. You know, not have a certain time to play with them, but he just believes in taking them to places, and being with them, and showing them things, and—sort of just a real relationship from the time they were big enough to get out. And he spent an awful lot of time with Nancy, too, while Diane was in the infant—feeding, diapering, and sleeping stage. And Saturdays they would spend the whole day in the park or horseback riding or something. That kind of thing. And consequently they have grown very close to each other. Their relationship is like a really deep, quiet, abiding thing. Whereas with him and Diane they're just, you know, sort of loud and rambunctious. She's really *high* spirited. Diane has like *spirit* that just can't be corralled. Nancy is more subdued, very ladylike, very proper. Even at eight, she's— I can just see her now as a woman, as a young woman; when she gets older. Very sweet, very sensitive.

KATRINA: Who looks after the children now?

FRANCINE: He does! Well, he works in an office in the Bronx, and his hours are sort of flexible. He takes the big one to school in the morning and he picks her up at three, when school is out. And the little one goes to kindergarten from nine to two. He picks her up at two o'clock, and he keeps her in the office with him. And sometimes he's had to make visits—he's in social work—and he'll always. . . . All of his stuff is done around their schedule. It's not like here. I have to be here from nine to five—or in the field, if not here in the office—from nine to five. He doesn't necessarily have that.

Our work set-up, it's what people are starting to discover just recently. You know, that men can take care of the children. But Eddie and I have been doing it for a long time. Before it got so popular! My friends used to see him—come over and find him mending my pants [*laughs*] or doing the washing and the ironing, and it never made him uptight at all. Ever. It just never bothered him. *Now* it's okay. I mean more and more men are doing it, with their wives working. *Even* when I *wasn't* working you could come and find Eddie —he'd walk in and start washing the dishes or whatever needed to be done. He's never once said, "Why don't you make dinner?" or, "It's time for you to make dinner," or, "Is dinner ready?" I mean if—if it's six o'clock and I haven't started it—if I'm doing something else, he goes on and he starts cooking.

KATRINA: Was his family situation similar to yours?

FRANCINE: No, not at all. Totally different. I mean really his childhood was not very good at all. And he's—anything he achieved, he achieved more or less on his own; with no help from— His parents were separated, and he was sort of brought up around grandparents, and a lot of cousins. It was like the kind of thing where his mother's parents raised them along with some other of their children's children. That kind of thing.

He started college on a basketball scholarship and working two jobs, and really scrambling for everything. He left after two years and went into the Army, and then he came out and finished college on his GI Bill. He taught a few places, and then he started working for the Department of Welfare. And after, like, being in the Department for seven years, he decided to go and get a Masters in Social Work!

And now he's in the process of really looking for a position that is responsible. While he was doing his Masters, he started a job training program for parolees, and he's really kind of interested in working with ex-convicts. Rehabilitation, that kind of thing. He's really into that working with people. He likes it better than, you know, being in administration or whatever; you know, that aspect of it. He likes to be out *with* people, dealing with people.

Eddie, he's just a very simple kind of person. He's just not *showy* at all. I mean, he's the kind of person who would not be noticed at all. You know. And he really is outstanding. You could just walk right by. There's nothing spectacular about him, looks or anything. But he's got a lot going for him.

There's another thing, too, about Eddie and Nancy. *Physically* they are alike. She looks more like Eddie's daughter than Diane. Diane is petite, almost. Well, she's like average size; Nancy's big, like Eddie. Nancy's very tall and she's eight years old and wears a size ten. She's all legs and arms and just—and Eddie's tall and long-legged, too. And so it stands to reason that people say, "Oh, she's just like her old man," you know.

KATRINA: Have you discussed with her . . . ?

FRANCINE: No, not yet.

KATRINA: Have you planned about it?

FRANCINE: Right. I think when the time comes, she'll— It's reasonable that we were married in '65, and she was born in '64! I think that when she's really old enough to understand it, she certainly will be told. Eddie had said, "When it would make a difference." You know, when we felt it would matter to her, or when she'd be interested in knowing. But I think at this point, it's— She— First of all, I could say to her now, you know, "Eddie's not really your Daddy." And she would think I was *crazy!*

So there's no point in wasting a lot of time worrying.

GAIL

Interviewed in April 1972

GAIL: It's kind of strange, thinking how to start it. I guess I should start with: the guy that I became pregnant by was my boyfriend for over two years. We had been seeing each other, steadily, ever since high school. When I met him, we were both sophomores in high school. His name was David.

And when I got pregnant it was—let's see, I found out I was pregnant in September of 1969. He had just left for college. He goes to Schenectady U. And I was at a junior college near where I lived. And, you know, we had been dating steadily; we had been talking about marriage after college. And it was just kind of taken for granted that it was going to be "David and Gail" all along. My parents had accepted that and treated him like their son.

Then uh— It was kind of like we were taking a chance all along. I wasn't too careful as far as birth control was concerned. Sometimes we took the precautions, and then sometimes not. I don't know why, we never really got into me getting the pill or anything like that. And we knew we were taking this chance.

And this one time—we all of a sudden realized, "Hey, it wasn't too smart." We just kind of felt, right away, that I was going to be pregnant. It just occurred to us, "We shouldn't have done that." It was really strange.

KATRINA: But the other times it didn't occur to you?

GAIL: Right.

No, it never occurred to us really. It was just this strange premonition. And this was like about maybe two or three weeks before he left for college. And I was upset with him leaving, too, and I guess *he* was upset with it. It was a whole, you know—a lot of separation anxiety there.

So, he left for school, and it was just kind of on my mind that this possibly might be it; I could be pregnant this time.

And my period didn't come. It got to be like thirty-five days since my last period. And David called from college. The *first time* that he was away at college! And he called, "How are things going?" "Oh great! David, guess what?" And he kind of figured, "Well, don't worry about it, maybe you're just going to be late—" Something like that.

The following weekend I came to visit him at Schenectady. The entire weekend I was sick. I hadn't gotten my period. And we just said, "Well, this is it." I hadn't been to a doctor or anything like that. David said, "Don't worry about it, we'll get married. There's no problem. It's okay; I still care about you." And I was pretty happy about it because I did want—that's what I wanted.

I went home, and the first thing on my mind was telling my parents. I wanted to get that over with right away. And, you know, get married as soon as we could. Things like that.

KATRINA: When you said, that's what you wanted—?

GAIL: I wanted to be with David. I wanted to marry David. I wanted to have his baby. I'd thought about it. I had all sorts of fantasies about it. And that's what I wanted. At least that's what I thought I wanted at the time.

So I decided I'd better tell my parents. Decided to tell my father first. I don't know if I was closer to my father; it just seemed he would be able to understand more, because of things he had shared with me. My mother is very naïve; and I felt it would be much harder to tell her. Also David and I had figured my father wouldn't be too bad about it, because we figured he knew what was going on and it wouldn't be such a shock.

When I came home from visiting David that weekend I was still very sick, and they just took it for granted I had a virus. The following night, my father and I were alone. And I got very upset and nervous, knowing I was going to tell him. I started crying and everything; he was asking me what was wrong. And so I told him I thought I might be pregnant. And—he hit the *ceiling*. He had the *completely* opposite reaction of what I expected. He started *screaming* at me and telling me I was *stupid*. And why didn't I use some sort of birth control? Not only that, why did I *do* this?

It was really bad. He gave me the whole bit: "How am I going to tell your mother?" And he just *really* flipped out, and really upset me.

Well, he had to go back to work; he left. And I called David. David wasn't there. David didn't know I was going to be telling my parents.

My father came back before my mother did. So when she came in, she was very surprised to see my father home from work. She asked what was going on. My father told her. She started crying. It was a really bad scene: her and I were sitting there crying; my father was screaming.

Right away he said, "You're going away. And you're giving up the baby." I said, "No, wait a minute. This is *my* baby. This is *David's* baby. I think it's up to us to decide." He says, "Oh, well, what do you suggest?" And I said, "We decided we want to get married and keep it."

He says, "No. You're not going to. You're going away and you're giving up the baby. That's all there is to be done about it."

And I was—like I was just so amazed. I had never *considered* that. I had never *thought*, you know— I never thought of people doing that.

KATRINA: Was it very much out of character for him to suggest it?

GAIL: At the *time*. Knowing what I knew of him at the *time*, I would say *yes*. Now—I guess it's because of having gone through all this—I realize my father is full of surprises.

He was *extremely* disturbed about it. And *his* way was the only way. He wouldn't listen to me, no matter what I had to say about it. I realize now that it was a great shock for him. And he was extremely *hurt* by it. He felt it reflected on him. He was having guilt feelings; the whole thing.

I finally got in touch with David to tell him that I had told my parents. And he was just kind of . . . he was upset that my parents had reacted that way. Also my father says to me "You're *not* telling David's parents." He felt as soon as anyone else found out, the whole town would find out. Because we are from a small town.

Uh—that upset me. I felt that wasn't fair. I felt his parents had the right to know, and when I told David, he didn't seem to say one way or the other how he felt about telling his parents, and what my parents had said about that. He just said, "Don't worry, it's going to work out. We'll get married. Your father will cool down in time, don't worry."

So finally—you know, my mother was still hoping that I wasn't pregnant— I went to the doctor and it was positive: I was pregnant. And he told me I was due the end of May, 1970.

KATRINA: How was your mother that evening? Was she—agreeing with your father?

GAIL: Oh, constantly; that's the way my mother is. Like through this whole thing, anything my father said, she went along. She is completely submissive. That's a whole big thing that has to do with my relationship with my mother, too. Anything my father says is right. And so she went along with him. She was—she didn't say much of anything that night, now I think about it. She was crying most of the time.

For about a week or two, things were very tense. They would hardly talk to me. I was going to classes at the junior college. I didn't really know anybody there, so I wasn't too upset about people finding out. In a way I was kind of proud of it. Because I was having David's baby; and I was proud I was having David's baby, because I did *care* an awful lot about him.

It was also kind of an ego thing for me, because David was very popular in high school. Everybody knew David and liked David. And so people used to look up to me, you know, because David cared about me. And the fact that I would be having his baby was kind of impressive, I thought.

I was going to the doctor regularly. My father said I ought to start looking into places to go away. So I decided, okay, even if he does send me away, there's a chance I can still keep the baby. I figured, "I'll work on this with him in time."

I went to the library, got out some books, wrote to some places—mainly in Albany because I wanted to be near David, wanted him to be able to visit me as often as possible —and all of them wrote back saying I should contact agencies where I lived. One suggested that I get in contact with Family Services Institute. And I called them. And I was assigned to a social worker. Her name was Susan Provantz.

I was *very* nervous about going to see her for a first interview. I had never spoken to *any* sort of professional, you know, in the field of social work, psychology, anything like that. And I walked into her office and, right away, things just clicked. It was beautiful. I sat there and I poured out my entire life story to her. In about an hour and a half, two hours, she knew everything about me. It was just a very beautiful relationship that started up right then.

She got into things about what alternatives I had. Abortion wasn't legal at the time, so I really couldn't consider it. Although my father *had* mentioned asking the doctor about it. But I wouldn't do it. Then *he* was going to go to the doctor and ask him about it. But he decided he'd feel foolish.

KATRINA: Would you have had an abortion?

GAIL: Uh—I don't think so. Not at the time. Mainly because— I mean, times have *changed* now, with it being legal. At the time it was a very mysterious thing and, you know, I had no— I knew of a girl who did have an abortion, but she had to go through seeing different psychiatrists and getting signatures; and I didn't want to go through that, either. And it was just the idea that I *wanted* the baby, and I *wanted* to marry David.

So I started seeing the social worker, Mrs. Provantz. She was fantastic, she was really great. She talked to my parents. She talked to David the one time he was home, and talked about him telling his parents.

David kept saying he was going to tell them. Because he realized things were really tense at my house and it was going to take a lot to change my father. And if we *were* going to get married, we would definitely need his parents' support behind us. So he kept saying he was going to tell them. And he never did.

KATRINA: Why not?

GAIL: I don't know. I figure it was because he was extremely nervous; he was very afraid of telling them. David was his parents' favorite son. His older brother had had to get married because he'd gotten a girl pregnant. And there was a whole big deal about how his mother had packed Bill up and sent him away so he wouldn't have to marry the girl. [*laughs*] It was a big mess.

As I was seeing the social worker, she was telling me about the different places I could go; and that even if I did go away I could still keep the baby. She kept stressing that it was *my* decision. Not my father's. And I *could* keep the baby on my own without marrying David. I could have the baby, give it up for adoption . . . maybe we *could* get married without my parents' consent. And like just what that would *involve,* with having my parents, you know, disown me. Because my father had said he would disown me if I kept the baby.

KATRINA: Even if you married David?

GAIL: He wouldn't *allow* me to marry David! And if I married David it was like I was no longer his daughter. Which is really difficult to consider, because I am an only child. That adds, you know, all sorts of other problems into the whole thing.

My social worker gave me the name of this place in Springfield. It's a maternity home called Webber House Maternity Hospital. She made arrangements for my parents and me to go down there. To just see what it was like. This was over Thanksgiving vacation.

When we got there, I was very nervous about it. I didn't know what to expect. They showed us around; it was very much a dormitory sort of thing, except that they had a hospital built right in there. With the delivery room. At most of the maternity homes, you stayed there until it was time to deliver and then you went to a hospital. In this, it was all in the same building. It was very nice. I was just—it was just such a *shocking* thing to see maybe thirty girls, thirty *pregnant* girls walking around, living together in this place. It was exactly like a college dormitory, except everybody was pregnant. My father was very ill-at-ease at the place. And my mother was kind of taking in the whole thing, saying, "Yes, it's very nice." When I got back, I told Mrs. Provantz I liked the place, and if I *had* to go someplace I wouldn't mind going there.

So—time marches on. We get into December and it's time for Christmas vacation. Things are *still* very tense at home. My father was hardly speaking to me. Giving me very disgusted looks. I was beginning to show already.

KATRINA: How pregnant were you?

GAIL: I was about four months pregnant then. I began showing very fast, because I'm small.

The pregnancy itself was going along fine. I was very healthy. But I was having very, very strong emotional problems. I was *constantly* upset. *Cried*—most of the time. *Slept* a lot—as an escape. Just kept fantasizing what it would be like being married to David. Where we would be living. I pictured us living in his house; you know, with his parents. And him coming home from school on weekends to visit. [*laughs*]

Finally, over Christmas vacation David says he's going to come home, he's going to talk to my father. Now this was a big thing, because my father didn't want to speak to him. When David used to come home on weekends and come over to my house, nobody would speak to each other. The four of us would sit in the living room watching television—and not a word would be said.

So uhm—he came over. I had warned my father ahead of time that David wanted to speak to him. So we sat down. It was like—we sat there for like *four* hours waiting for somebody to say something. And nobody said anything. I was kind of upset with David, too; that he didn't make any move.

Finally my father walked into the kitchen, giving David the break. So *David* went into the kitchen, *I* went into the kitchen; my *mother* came into the kitchen. [*laughter*] And David says, "We don't agree with what you want for us. We want to get married, and we want to keep the baby."

My father *blew* off and says, "It's *not* possible; there's *no* way you can do it." So he asked how David intended to do it. He says, "Well, we'll both work. We'll have a baby-sitter for the baby. We'll get a little cheap apartment in Schenectady." Now that I think about it, having a cheap apartment in Schenectady is ridiculous! [*laughs*]

So my father completely blew up. That's all David said for the rest of the night, my father wouldn't let him get a word in. My father actually, literally, sat there with his back to David and directed everything he was saying to me. He said that he realized that it was my decision and—and if I decided to keep the baby he would not let me come back into the house.

He said he did not consider it a grandchild; he never would. My mother said she did not consider it a living thing. And this completely flipped me out. I mean, while she's saying this I can feel the baby moving inside of me. And I kept thinking "How can she say that? She's been pregnant; she knows what it's like to feel the life inside of her." I just couldn't understand how she—a woman—could say something like that.

My father went on with this whole big deal about: if David and I wanted to get married later on, after college, fine. But he just would not let us get married now and keep this baby. And also the whole bit, "What will the neighbors think?" And, "How will we tell your grandparents?"

KATRINA: Do you feel that if you had just come to him *not* pregnant and said, "David and I want to get married, now," that he would have—?

GAIL: That's funny. I never thought about that. [*pause*] I don't know. I really don't think so. He wanted me to go to college *so* badly. He didn't want anything to interfere with that.

KATRINA: The reason I'm asking the question is: Was it because the getting married was because you were pregnant? Or was it— How much was it also that you were too young to get married? What was the real thing that made him so insistent?

GAIL: I don't know. I think a very strong combination of both. I think even if I hadn't been pregnant, and David and I had wanted to get married, he wouldn't have agreed to it. But, you know, *maybe* he could have been swayed. This way, there was no swaying him at all.

That night was a total *disaster*. I really thought I was going to have some sort of breakdown, I was so upset. When David left, we walked out to the car together. He said this was it, he was going home to tell his parents. And not to worry; that probably within a couple of days I'd be moving into his house to live with his parents.

And this—I had been hoping for this. This was great. Because I wanted to get out of the house.

The next day, he didn't call all morning. I was so upset, I couldn't imagine what had happened. I finally called him. He said he didn't tell them. When I asked why, he said, you know, his little sister was there; and all sorts of feeble excuses he made up. And he left for school without having told them.

Around the end of January— I had already written a letter to Webber House, telling them I wanted to come and stay there. Arrangements were being made: this was what I was going to be doing. I had finished out my first semester. I couldn't go back to school because I was due the end of May. I was really showing. I was doing nothing. I was just sitting home. My parents would hardly let me out of the house, for fear somebody would see me. The only time I left the house was to go to the doctor.

When I went to the doctor one day, this one girl who had graduated the year before us was there. She was also expecting. There were like *five* couples, between our class and the class ahead of us, who had—the girls were pregnant at the same time I was. They all got married—except me.

KATRINA: Were they all pregnant before the marriage?

GAIL: Yes; yes. And it was kind of this big scandal. You know, everybody found out about me, because this girl had seen me at the doctor's office. It got back to the high school we had gone to. The entire faculty knew. Everybody knew. Word was getting back to David's parents. But they wouldn't believe it.

It was just kind of strange, you know. I knew everybody else was getting married. Everybody was having hassles about it, too. And I just kind of figured, "Well, we still will be married, too."

David didn't have to face any of this. He was away at school. And he didn't tell anybody at school. Not anybody. And so he didn't have any problems with it.

One afternoon, I got a phone call from David's brother. Saying that his father wanted me to come over for dinner that night. Meanwhile, *David* calls and says he's gotten a call from his father that morning; his parents knew. His father wouldn't tell him how he found out. But that he knew and they were very upset with David that he couldn't come to them and tell them.

So I went to dinner at David's house that night. David was still away at school. When I got there, the only person there to meet me was his younger brother. His brother was about thirteen. And I'm, you know, dressed up in my maternity dress! [*laughter*] The whole bit. And I go in. I'm sitting and talking to his brother. Even the ten-year-old daughter was out, sleeping over at somebody's house. His mother comes downstairs, *completely* ignores me, goes and starts fixing dinner. It was just *such* a mess.

Finally, his father got home. We had dinner. Meanwhile his mother hardly says anything to me. His father was very nice to me.

Afterward we go into the living room. It was like— Did you see the movie *Lovers and Other Strangers?*

KATRINA: No; I don't think so.

GAIL: Oh— Well, then you missed the one scene there. I go in the living room. And David's father just looks at me and says, "So what's the story?" And that was like the big thing throughout that movie; that's all the father kept saying.

So I said, "Well, gee, I'm pregnant," you know? [*laughs*] "And David and I would like to get married. My father doesn't want us to."

And he said it was a shame that David was in college; but he would back us up in anything we decided. If we wanted to get married, he'd help us out as best he could. If I decided to go away and give up the baby, well, that was my decision. He wouldn't hold it against us. *But* he was not in favor of giving the baby up for adoption. He felt it was *my* child, it was *David's* child. And it belonged to us. We should not give it up.

David's mother comes in. "You're not getting married! You're both underage, you have to have *my* permission for you to get married." She says, "I will *not* sign for David. He's in *college*. I want him to get through college."

You see, they're—they've never had anybody in their family go to college. And *David* was just so amazing; he was offered scholarships from so many different schools. Like this was *really* it. And she constantly bragged about *her son*

David. And she didn't want *anything* to interrupt his education.

So I said, "Well, okay. I'm also considering going away and giving the baby up for adoption. That's what my parents want." And she says, "No. I won't approve of that. I do not believe in giving up babies for adoption." And she points to her son Kenny who's sitting there. "I never wanted *him!*" she says, "but I would never consider giving him up." And I just — How could this woman *do* this? You know? And— Ohh!

I said, "Well, these are the alternatives I have." And she says, "I also don't think you should keep the baby and wait around for David to graduate from college."

So, like the only alternative she was giving me was keeping the baby and living in the street. Because my parents would kick me out otherwise.

Then she gives me this— See, the year before, I had taken a summer job in a hotel in Maine, and then I quit and I came back. [*laughs*] That's another whole story. Anyway, she says, "While you were away that time, I read every letter you wrote to David. And this is what you've wanted all along," she says, "And now you have him. You have your chance to get David. To have him all yours."

And it's like—this woman, what's she doing? You know? She's reading my letters to David and everything. And I just couldn't believe it. Like she knew what was going on all along. And it was just—oh, it was really strange!

So we didn't get too much accomplished that night. [*laughter*] Except Mr. C., David's father, said I could do whatever I pleased. And David's mother said I couldn't do anything.

Another strange thing was: she kept comparing me with her daughter-in-law who had had to get married because *she* was pregnant. And in one sentence she was saying the situations were completely different. And in the other sentence she was saying it was so similar. I left there so confused. Before I walked out the door she starts listing off places where David and I can get married without parental consent. Then she says, "If you do decide to get married you can come and live here." I'm thinking, "Ahh! What is this woman doing to me? She just gets done saying all this stuff; then she tells me she's prying into David's personal things. What's she going to do if I live there?"

KATRINA: But she'd also said earlier that you *couldn't* get married.

GAIL: Right, right. It was just very strange. I told her I would let them know what I decided to do.

I decided to go away. Whether I was going to keep the baby or not, I was going away. I just couldn't put up with what was going on at David's house, *or* at my house. I just couldn't wait to get to that place.

And when I got there, it was heaven. The people were so wonderful. The other girls—like my first day there I was really scared, because I didn't know what to expect. I didn't know whether the girls talked openly about their pregnancies, or not. I was put into a room with six other girls. There were about twenty-five or thirty girls in all. And it was just so *great*. Right away girls were asking, "Oh, when are *you* due?" and things like that. I didn't know too much about pregnancy or labor, and everybody's talking about it openly. Like, "So-and-so delivered this morning." And it was just: wow! My God! What's going on here? And it was really nice. Especially once I got to know the girls better. The whole experience was one of the best things I've ever experienced in my life—being at this hospital. I was there for three months.

And I learned so much about myself—that I had not known. Like before, I was always very much of a follower. I never initiated things. I was never—people never followed me for anything. And I felt very much inferior to most people.

When I got there, girls started looking up to me. I was a little bit older than some of them. I was eighteen at the time. There were some that were older than me, too, but most of them were very young. Their ages ranged from twelve to twenty-five. They had this magazine that they put out every month. And they elected me editor of the magazine. It was like after my first week there; and I was *really* excited. Because I felt this was a way of getting to know the girls, too.

And it was just really nice. My social worker from home used to come and visit me all the time, Susan Provantz. Meanwhile our relationship had gotten very close. You know, I looked forward to seeing her, *so* much. I still feel if it wasn't for her, I don't think I would have made it through. She was just so wonderful, I couldn't believe it, you know. She'd come and she'd keep saying, "Look what you are doing here! It's really great!"

I started realizing that, the way things were going, it was kind of late. I was already seven months pregnant; David and I wouldn't be getting married; and I wouldn't be keeping the baby. And I started thinking what kind of home could I give it, anyway? Obviously David wasn't all—you know, didn't want the baby that badly or he would have fought an awful lot harder than what he did. He didn't *do* much, you know, when you start thinking about it. Of course I wouldn't admit that, at the time. Because I was still very devoted to David. David was perfect, and all that. And he used to call once a week. I used to brag about "my boyfriend," who was standing beside me all the way. Whereas most of the girls didn't even know where the fathers of their children were. Most of them had broken up, and things like that. But, you know, David was still right there. And everybody was: "Oh, that's really nice! He calls every week, he writes to you occasionally."

But the whole experience was so wonderful. You *live* with your pregnancy. You *know* everything that's going on. Labor and delivery is nothing at all to be afraid of. My first night there, the girl that was in the bed next to me delivered in the middle of the night. You know? It was just—it's nothing! it happens *every* day to your best friends. You see them in the morning, walking around with nothing wrong.

KATRINA: Then afterward did she come back into the room?

GAIL: No, they stay on the hospital floor then, and they leave right from there. But there's like Visitors Passes allowed, and you get to see them.

I'd say it was divided half and half as to the number of girls who were giving up their babies. Every girl had such a *completely* different situation. And different reasons for keeping their baby; and different ways they were going to be able to keep it. And like I really got to consider *so* many alternatives. I was gaining an awful lot of confidence in myself, just from things that were going on there. And, you know, there was a possibility I could keep it on my own. I realized that it would be like about the worst thing I could do, though, for the baby. I couldn't give—give the baby anything. No. I wanted—I *definitely* wanted my baby to have a father. And I knew David wasn't ready.

KATRINA: So you *did* know that at the time?

GAIL: Yes. I realized that, yes. I still felt that he cared very much about the baby, though.

While I was there, I *really* got back into the idea of college. I had never really had my head into it. It was just kind of: "This is what my father *said* I was going to do." And then I really got into it. And that's when I decided I wanted to get into social work. Mainly because of my social worker; and because of the way I felt toward the other girls that came to me, and asked me for advice, and wanted to talk with me. I just felt a confidence that I could handle it. I got to talking about it with my social worker, about the profession and everything. And she thought that I—that it would work out. And I felt if *she* had the confidence in me, *I* certainly should.

Anyway, I made arrangements with her that I was going to be giving up the baby. She kept saying, "Well, don't forget, you *can* change your mind." You know, "Don't be *so* set on it." And I said okay.

David came to visit me over Easter vacation. And he was acting *very* strangely. Like very guilty. And I was very excited about the baby. You know, the baby was moving around; and "David, feel the baby moving." And he didn't want to be bothered. It was just very strange the way he was acting. I thought maybe it was because he hadn't seen me in so long. Obviously it was quite a shock when I turned the corner and he saw me, you know, with my stomach out three feet. But like the whole day he was kind of awkward. And he couldn't look at me. He had trouble talking to me. I didn't worry about it too much. I figured it was the pregnancy itself. It was the whole thing, you know, the whole idea: here I was in this hospital; he didn't like the idea of me being there. He didn't like the place. Even though I did like it.

Meanwhile my parents were visiting me every other Sunday. Things were *great*. They would come, and oh! it was *fabulous* when they came to visit me! We'd go out to dinner. And, you know, they didn't care; they'd take their pregnant daughter out to dinner! Because they knew we wouldn't bump into anybody that they knew.

We'd talk about what was going on, about things I was learning there, and the good things that were happening to me. They were really great about it.

I had told them I was learning about birth control, I was going to start taking the pill when I left. My father says good, you know, good. They *knew* that they couldn't stop

David and me from seeing each other. And they weren't going to try to. They just wanted us to take precautions from now on. So they said.

KATRINA: "So they said"?

GAIL: It was like they were accepting it outwardly, but they weren't *really* accepting it.

One day they came to visit me—one Sunday—and they said, "Guess what? Your cousin Linda got married." This cousin is like two years younger than me. I was *amazed,* you know. *"Wow! Really?"* And they were just kind of quiet for a while. They said, "She was pregnant." Ah—so! Really! Gee. And then they started saying, "Well, we can understand why getting married was a good alternative for her. She would never be able to get into a *college.* She really had no future other than marriage. And children."

Funny thing was, I later found out that her father was the one who told David's father that I was pregnant. Because he didn't like how my father was handling the whole thing. He felt David's father should know about it. And when his own daughter got pregnant he allowed her to get married.

And I was just *really* amazed, that *wow,* you know, here my parents are talking about "Gee, isn't it *great* Linda got married; and she's having a baby." And I'm sitting there thinking, "Yeah. Sure." I could understand their point, but, I mean—what are they saying to me? You know? Here I am in the exact same situation. And it would be a *crime* for *me* to get married.

But it's great that she did it. Just because *she* wouldn't be going to college.

Uh, *then* my father. . . .

KATRINA: But, how did you feel about it? Did you feel hurt? Or angry? Or—?

GAIL: When they first told me about it, I accepted it and said, "Yes, I can understand what you're saying." And I didn't really start thinking about it. It was so much of a shock in the first place. And I was happy for her, I really was. I couldn't see her going through what I had been going through at the hospital. I really couldn't see her coping with that. And I was very happy for her.

Then—my father just about gets that out of his mouth, when he starts talking about me and David getting married! Not right then, but, you know, in the future. And he got into *all sorts* of things! Like about churches, because David and I are at the opposite extremes of being Protestant. About maybe he would allow David and me to get *engaged* the summer after next. You know, David would be a junior then. And we could get married the summer after that, after he graduated. And he's talking about, you know, *where we would have the wedding*. Whether it would be his church or my church, or some other church. Where we could have the reception.

And I was just—! I was totally blown by the whole thing! I realize now that he was doing it because he felt he had to give me some kind of reassurance after he had just gotten done blowing this whole thing to me about my cousin. I guess he—he felt guilty. He *obviously* felt guilty. And he was trying to repay me in some way, by showing me, "There is a future. Things are going to be fine."

And I got really excited thinking about marrying David, getting engaged the following summer. I called David, and I was really excited about it. He says, "What are you doing? You're letting your father run your whole life." He says, "What if we're not ready to get engaged next summer? What if we don't want to? What if we want to get married now?" He says "We *did* want to get married, and he wouldn't let us. Why do we have to go according to his plans?"

And I got very upset. I realized that it was true; I

shouldn't let my father run the whole thing. But just the idea of, you know, getting engaged, getting married—that's what I wanted so badly. And I was very upset about that. I started thinking, "David's doubting the whole relationship." I *should* have started thinking that *long* ago.

Afterward I got thinking about the whole thing with my cousin and I got very upset about it. I started thinking, "Why her and not me?" I started getting jealous of her. Also my father had said that they had considered not telling me at all until I got home. Which would have been disastrous. Just disastrous. If I had gone home and seen her standing there pregnant, with a wedding ring on her finger, I would—I really would have fallen apart. So I'm glad they told me when they did.

KATRINA: Was there a chance you could have just gone off and married David right then and there?

GAIL: [*pause*] No. Because like David's alternative was getting married, both of us working, him going to school, and the baby in a day-care center or something. And I decided, "I don't want anybody else raising my baby. That's *my* baby. *I* want to raise it." You know, it would—it would be raised the way the baby-sitter wanted it to be raised. I didn't want that. And there was really no other alternative that I could see, because I *would* have to work. I, you know, I realized that keeping the baby was out of the question, then. And so marriage was kind of out of the question for then. I don't know. It was just—you know—

The rest of the time at Webber House went smoothly. I was just kind of anxious to get it over with by then. I was still very close to my social worker. And she started coming up with, had I thought of names? Because we get to name the baby. There has to be a name on the birth certificate. Otherwise they just fill in "Baby." And I didn't want that. I had strong feelings about it. And this was something I wanted

David to share in. He felt, "What's the big deal? Don't worry about it." That upset me. And all of a sudden all these little things were falling in place, about how David was just kind of [*pause*] kind of drifting out of the whole thing.

And uh—I decided to name the baby after David and my social worker. So I had chosen the names David Lawrence for a boy, and Susan Victoria for a girl. Because the social worker's name was Susan. And she was so excited about that. She was just— Oh! It was—it was really something. She was just so honored that I wanted to name the baby after her.

So, finally the day came. I went into labor. Finally. David had said, as soon as I go into labor I should call him. This was really amazing, this whole thing:

He said I should call him, and he would get a bus and try to be there as soon as possible. I found out I was in labor like maybe, oh, nine o'clock in the evening. I called him, there was no answer. I started calling like every fifteen minutes. I was pacing the halls. The girls were pacing with me. And I was calling David. There's no answer. I left some money with this one girl to keep trying to call him. Because at about eleven they wanted me up on the hospital floor.

I went through labor. Everything went *fine*. The labor—heavy labor—only lasted maybe two hours. So it wasn't bad. The whole experience was just the most beautiful thing you could *ever* experience. It was natural childbirth. I was awake, I helped with the delivery. The whole bit with the breathing exercises and everything. It was just *so amazing!* Like I was lying there on the delivery table saying, "This is it! I'm giving birth!"

And I was just—I was just so excited about the whole thing. And I wanted a girl desperately. Oh! I wanted to have a little girl. I kept telling the nurses it was going to be a girl. And they said no, it was going to be a boy because it was kicking so hard; it was a football player—

When she was born— Like I kept thinking she was already

born. Because I had felt relief already. And they said no, they couldn't tell if it was a girl yet.

And then there was this silence. It was absolutely quiet, and I like waited. It was so amazing. Just this long silence, and then suddenly there was a cry! Oh! It was *so* beautiful. All of a sudden she started *crying*.

They said, "You were right, it's a girl." And I was just *so happy* that it was a girl. I was just—there's no way of explaining it. Then I saw her. They had her over on the— See, we could see the baby if we wanted. If we definitely did not want to see the baby, they'd turn our head and get the baby out of the room as soon as possible. But I had told them that I definitely wanted to see her.

And she was laying there on the table and they were cleaning her off. And this *tiny little thing*—just screaming! And it was so amazing, thinking she just came out of me. That's what was inside, kicking, and causing me so much pain sometimes, and—it was—like I felt I *knew* her. I guess you just feel that way through a pregnancy, because you get to know all the little movements. And you think you know her already. And it was just so amazing.

Then they laid her on another table that was closer to me. They were putting the drops in her eyes. And her eyes were blinking *wide open*. And it was just—oh! it was just such a beautiful thing. Just looking at her and thinking— I just could not—it was so hard to identify her with my belly, you know? It was amazing. And they rushed her over to the nursery to weigh her. She was kind of chubby: she weighed eight pounds four ounces.

By then I was really exhausted, and they were messing around with stitches; and I didn't think it would ever be finished.

Then I was allowed one phone call; preferably to my parents. And I figured I'd better call my parents. This was like four-thirty in the morning. I called. My father says, "What do you want?" "Calling at four-thirty in the morning, what do you think?" I said, "I'm on the hospital floor now." He says "Well, are you just going in or is it over?" I said that it was over. [*pause*] He just kept saying, "How do you feel, how do you feel?" He didn't ask about the baby at all. But he put my mother on the phone and right away she asked what—what it was. I said it was a girl. She got really excited. And I kind of knew all along that my mother was excited about it, but was hiding it. Because even before I left, she was—when I told her I could feel the baby kicking, you could—you could see this sort of excitement. And I know she would have really liked it, if I'd kept the baby. But she wouldn't tell me. And it wasn't until way afterward that I realized—really realized how she felt about it.

But at that time on the phone, she was just really glad that it was all over, too. And she was asking me how I was feeling, and the whole thing. They were going to come visit me the next day.

So I *finally* got into bed. And I started thinking about David. I really wanted him to know right away. Because I wanted him to be there. I got up, I guess this was then Friday? Saturday? It's amazing, I can't even remember. It was —Friday. I got up out of bed. I called. There was no answer. I called like every half hour. All day long. Couldn't get him.

That whole day I was feeling "enh," you know; some pain from the stitches and all. Didn't know what to do with myself. Kept going to the nursery window to see the baby whenever I could. And just—so totally *amazed* every time I looked at her, thinking, "She's my baby, she's my child." You know?

But all the while I kept in my mind: I am giving her up; I'm giving her away. And I had integrated that into my thinking. And so it wasn't much of a problem any more. And I wasn't hurt by the thought of it.

KATRINA: Did she come to you for feeding?

GAIL: Only the day before she left the hospital was I allowed to feed her. The girls who were keeping their babies were allowed to feed them. Otherwise we could see them through the nursery window, during certain hours of the day.

So then, Saturday, I got up at six o'clock in the morning to call, and I woke up David's roommate. He said he hadn't seen David in a while. He didn't know where he was. Called all day Saturday. Couldn't get him. Started calling on Sunday. Finally, Sunday afternoon, I got him. "Where have you been?" He said, "Ah, just out goofing around." And I said, "Well, uhm, do you know you have a daughter?" He got excited: "Oh really? Wow! When did this happen?" So then he started saying that he had gone up to Canada for the weekend, with some friends of his. He asked when I had been in labor; I said Thursday night. And he said, wow, Thursday night he had had this really strange dream. He said it was kind of scary because it was so real. It was me, and I was screaming; and he didn't know if I was screaming at him or what. And like we kind of figured out that it was happening while I was in labor, you know. He was just amazed by it because he had heard stories about where things like that happened.

And he asked if I had been thinking of him. That maybe I hated him because I was in pain. And I said I hadn't thought of him at all through the whole thing. Which was *true*. And that surprised me, too.

So he got excited. He said he'd be there to visit me as soon as he could. And I couldn't understand why he couldn't come right away. Because the schools were on strike; he didn't have any classes. It was just kind of, *why* couldn't he get there to visit me, you know? I was upset about that.

I got a call from my social worker. She had heard I'd had the baby. She was so excited. I said the baby was named Susan. She was thrilled. She said she'd be there Wednesday. She'd be picking up the baby and taking it to a foster home.

It had to stay in a foster home until it could be placed into its permanent home.

David came up Monday, and he was still acting very strange. Just like the time I'd seen him before. He was—he was—you know, very nervous. He was like playing with my fingers; like he didn't know what to do.

I asked him if he wanted to see the baby. He said yes. But he wasn't really enthused. His first glance at her, "Wow! She looks just like your father!" [*laughter*]

And then we just kind of stood there looking at her. And like I was watching him for a reaction—and there was nothing. And— I don't know, I guess I was disappointed. Because I was *so proud* looking at her through the window. "This is *my baby*." And he just—indifferent; sort of. I think it was maybe he didn't know how to react. He couldn't *relate* to the baby. He hadn't been through the pregnancy. And he hadn't been in contact with me that much during it.

He didn't stay too long. He was only allowed in the hospital for certain hours anyway. So he left and said he'd try to get back if he could. Otherwise he'd see me at home. Because he would be going home from school, soon. I was kind of disturbed by how he was acting. He just wasn't himself.

Saturday my parents came up. I asked if they wanted to see the baby. And my mother, "Yes, yes, yes!" She was jumping at the chance. She stood there looking at it. She was just— I could *tell—she wanted*—that—that baby as her grandchild, you know? She was looking at it. And she kept saying, "Oh, she looks exactly like *you did*."

My father was just kind of cracking jokes like he normally does. His way of escaping. You know, looking around the nursery, saying, "So this is what a baby factory looks like." Some very cutting remarks. And no real—no real reaction to the baby at all.

They were just really excited I'd be coming home soon. That was about it.

The day before the baby left the hospital—she left on the fifth day; I couldn't leave until the eighth day—I was allowed to hold her and feed her. And this had been a big decision, whether I should or not. I was afraid how I might react. But I figured, it's the *only* chance I'm going to get. I may regret that I didn't take the chance while I had the opportunity. So I did. It was *great*. Like I *never* really knew how to react to babies, especially infants. I walked into the nursery and she was crying. The nurse just said, "There she is. Go pick her up." I was afraid, you know, what am I going to do? Maybe I'll drop her or something. And like right away I just picked her up; I knew *exactly* how to handle her. When they talk about motherly instinct, my *God,* it's *true!* I was so amazed that I knew how to handle her.

She ate very well. She was a very healthy baby. She—she sucked very well. And while I'm feeding her, I'm examining her, you know. She had droopy ear lobes, like mine. She had a cowlick on the same side of her hair as mine. And—trying to pick out where she looked like David, where she looked like me. It was just so amazing. I just—I was just really surprised that I knew how to handle her. It was really something. I stayed as long as I could while feeding her.

The next day my social worker came to pick her up. I had made an outfit for her to wear that was going to be given to the adoptive parents. It was a blanket and a sweater and cap and booties. And my social worker picked out the prettiest little dress she could find. She just kept saying, "This baby is special to me." She said she brought along her best friend to hold the baby in the car. Because she couldn't see just putting the baby on the seat or in a car bed or something.

They got her all dressed and they gave her to me to hold for a few minutes before she left. And her eyes were wide open. She just kept looking around, as if thinking, "Where am I? What am I doing?" You know? And my social worker was really excited seeing her. She was really taken by her. And I kept, you know— I wasn't thinking so much "This is the last time I'll see my baby." It was just, "Here she is." And I enjoyed holding her and everything. And uh— I was trying to unwrap her from the blankets to see how the outfit looked on her. It looked *really* cute. She had this *really* fat face that hung out of the bonnet. Looked so funny.

And so I handed her to my social worker. She said she'd be in contact with me as soon as I got home. Because there were papers to sign and everything. And she'd let me know how the baby was doing in the foster home.

The home they were placing her in, this was the first time the woman was going to be a foster mother. And she was really excited about having a newborn infant in her home again. She had had children of her own. But, you know, a newborn infant is something special.

So my social worker left then, and I just— I felt very empty. Very alone. Because it was kind of like I could always run to the nursery window and see the baby when I wanted to. And she wasn't there now.

And uh— [*voice shakes*]

It was. . . . there were maybe five other girls on the hospital floor then. And it was just sort of the natural thing. Everybody knew when the babies were leaving; and we kind of—took special attention to that girl. So everybody was being extra specially nice to me.

Uhm—David called— I think he called that night. Or I called him, to tell him the baby left. [*pause*] He didn't say much. Oh, my social worker had said I could see her if I wanted to when she was in the foster home; and David could too. I mentioned that to him. He said, "Well, if you want to, go ahead."

When I got home— I was—I was kind of excited to get home by then. Thinking of the whole, you know, a whole summer ahead of me with David. And getting over this whole thing. Getting back into a routine.

KATRINA: And you were really thinking in terms of getting back with your relationship with David?

GAIL: Yes. Very much so.

So I got home. Things at home— Like with my parents, I figured everything was going to be good. Everything had been so great when they came to visit me. But it went back to exactly the way it had been before! I couldn't understand it. They were still giving me these *looks*. And I felt I had been *away* so long. I didn't know what people were doing; where anybody was. It was very disturbing.

My first day home, David didn't even come over. He—he had called and said if he had a chance, he'd stop by. And he didn't. That upset me.

Finally, I got to see him. And while I was there a girl called him, long distance. And I found out he had been seeing this girl at school. He had been seeing her since February, which was before I even got to the hospital. Not only had he been seeing her, it came out that they had been having relations. And he hadn't told her that I would— She knew he had a girlfriend back home. She didn't know I was pregnant or anything. She just felt it was, you know, kind of odd.

And I was totally—that upset me more than anything. [*pause*] He said, "Don't worry. I still care about you."

KATRINA: How did you find out that they had been having relations?

GAIL: I was looking through one of David's notebooks. Looking at some of his philosophy notes, because I was going to take a course in philosophy. And there was a *note* in there, from her to David. It was just kind of the whole thing. Like, you know, what they'd been doing, that she was *afraid*, things like that. And I—I fell apart. I really did. I was very upset.

KATRINA: Did you have a confrontation?

GAIL: Oh yes. I confronted David with it. And he, "Well, what do you want me to say?" You know. He says, "You were away a long time; I needed somebody." I said, "I was away a long time, and *I* needed somebody. But I couldn't."

And then it came out that that weekend—when I delivered—he was up in Canada with her. That *really* threw me. Because like I was upset enough that he wasn't waiting around, because he knew that I could go into labor any day. I mean it was bad enough he was away. But he was away with this girl. And—I don't know; he just—he seemed very insensitive about the whole thing. I still wanted him very badly, so I said, "Okay. I accept the whole situation. You are still seeing her occasionally." You know, the whole bit.

Well, then I had to go sign the relinquishment papers. I asked David if he'd *please* be there with me. Because I was very scared about signing the papers. He said yes, he'd be there. My social worker explained that even after I signed the papers I could still change my mind until the time I went to court. Because I had to go to court, and be confronted by the judge; and that would make it final.

KATRINA: What is the period of time?

GAIL: It depended how soon they could get the case into court. I signed the papers the week after I got home, and that was the middle of June. I went to court the last week in July. So it ended up being about a month and a half. During that time I could visit the baby at the foster home if I wanted to. I could have a picture of her, too, if I wanted. And I said that I didn't want it. Mainly because if I had a picture, it would just be the thought of, where was I going to keep it so I wouldn't see it? So it wouldn't remind me of her? And when I came across it someday, how would I feel about it? I decided not to go see her, because I figured I was doing pretty well getting over the whole thing of *not* having seen her. And I'd just have to start all over again.

Meanwhile, my social worker went to visit her and was constantly telling me how she was doing. The foster mother had gotten so attached to her, she was having separation anxiety about giving up the baby to its—uh—adoptive parents.

So David went with me that day. But while he was there, I just couldn't talk to my social worker. I couldn't talk to Mrs. Provantz at all! It was the first time that had happened. There was just like this *barrier* there. It was very bad. *David* wouldn't talk to her. I couldn't talk to him. Things were very tense. And I signed the paper. She says, "How do you feel about it?" And I said, "How can I feel?" And I *knew* I was having a lot of feelings about it, but I couldn't bring them out.

Then uhm—the court case came up; it was time for me to go to court. I asked David if he would please go with me. He said yeah, he would, he would. You know, "Don't worry about it."

The night before, he told me he wasn't going to go with me. That he had to work. Like he works for his father! He can get out of work anytime he wants to. He said he wasn't going to go. So I said okay. And this was the *biggest* thing. Because it was final after this.

KATRINA: This was a routine thing, this going to court—right?

GAIL: Yes. Right.

My social worker was going to be there. And she said there would be another girl there who was also going through relinquishment.

I get there and find out: the same day that they do the relinquishments is the same day they have the adoptions. So that all these proud parents are standing there with their children, waiting to make their adoptions legal. And I just —"What are they *doing* this for?" You know, it's a hard enough thing for any girl that was going to sign—you know, to make a relinquishment final. Now all these little kids and babies all over the place?

So I'm standing there. I was alone in the hall for a while; and this little boy—he must have been about two years old —he comes running up the hall and he stands in front of me, he looks up at me; gives me the *biggest smile*. And then, you know, his father called him and said, "Come on." You know, "We have to go." And I just fell apart. I'm thinking "Oh my God! My daughter's going to be like that someday and I won't see her. And I'll never see her standing there smiling."

My social worker came—came over then, and I told her what had happened. I just kept saying, "Oh, thank God that wasn't a little girl. If it was a little girl I really would have collapsed." And—it was just really something. I got myself back together and— Like I was still sure that this is what I wanted. This is what is to be done. There is no other way around it.

And I went in to talk to the judge. It was really strange. It was a very formal thing. You go in; there's a lawyer there; they swear you in. And they ask you these questions like: "Do you realize that—? Do you understand what you're doing? Have you thought about it? Where was the child born? What date?" The whole thing.

So then the judge gives you this whole deal about, "Well, I'm confident you know what you're doing, and you've made this decision on your own." And he says, uh—"After this day, you are no longer the mother of that child." [*pause*] And I'm thinking, *how* can he *say* that? How can *any*body *say* that to me? I went through nine months of *carrying* this child. I gave birth to it! That was *my* child! Nobody is going to tell me I'm not the mother of that baby! I'm giving it up so it has other *parents*, but I'm *still* the mother of that child.

And I feel that way about it now!

I walked out of there. My social worker was very concerned about how I was feeling. So I said I was going to be okay.

And I walked out. And I was just kind of in a daze. It was that same empty feeling again.

That night David called and asked how it went. I said "How could it go?" And he didn't seem to want to try to comfort me at all. [*pause*] And he never spoke about the baby from then on, really. Unless I brought it up, and I was always bringing it up in conversation. But he just didn't want to be—bothered by talking about it.

I continued seeing my social worker for a while after that. She kept calling, seeing how I was doing. She made arrangements for me to speak with a college guidance counselor. I decided on Albany State because of their school of social work. I really got into the idea of being a social worker.

KATRINA: Is there anything special regarding your parents after you went through the final—?

GAIL: It's just—you never mention the word—the name Susan Victoria—again. You don't talk about the baby. The whole thing never happened.

Except *one* day— I had decided to write a letter to the adoptive parents. She was placed in a home about two weeks after I went to court. My social worker fought for three hours with the rest of the agency to have her placed in this one particular home, because she thought the parents matched her perfectly. Finally they said she could be placed there. Mrs. Provantz told me about what it was like when they came to pick her up. That they were so excited. And I just kept thinking how I would feel, having somebody give me a baby; you know, if I couldn't have one and wanted one so badly. And I was just thinking *wow!* you know. They were just so excited, and they wanted her so badly. They were given the outfit that I made her. In fact, I think she had it on when they gave—when she was given to them. And, you know, they—they said they were going to *keep* it; they were going to *show* it to her when they told her about being adopted. So they would—she would know that she was not just "given away," or that "nobody wanted her." But that I did care about her very much.

Then I decided to write a letter to them, just kind of thanking them. And asking them to please give her a good home. As I—I was sure they would, anyway. But just so they would know that I wasn't having hard feelings about it; and they wouldn't have to have nightmares about me searching for her or something. I gave it to my social worker to give them. And she said like—when—when—the woman —when the mother read it, she just burst out crying—And —the father was really touched by it. And they were just so [*voice momentarily trembling*] thankful.

And that really made me feel good. I felt *great* about it. Because whenever I think about the thing, I just don't think of the fact that I gave her up. I think about how they felt getting her. [*sniffs, tears*] I always get misty at this point!

[*again fully composed*] The way I look at the experience now, I see the whole thing as very much of a learning—a learning experience. And very much of a *growing* experience for me. In my entire eighteen years before that time, I hadn't grown as much as I had in those three months at the hospital.

And I decided I really wanted to get into the field of working with unmarried pregnant girls; with unwanted pregnancies—whatever you want to call it. When I had the opportunity to get the job in the abortion clinic, I *jumped* at the chance. I mean I'm *very* much in favor of abortion.

Oh, there's another part of this story. About the bit with David and the girl he was seeing:

He continued to see her, occasionally, during that summer. When September came and he was leaving for school, I said, "What am I to expect? I know you are going to be at school with her, and it's going to upset me." He said, "I'm not going to see her anymore."

Meanwhile I started looking at the relationship, seeing there was nothing left. Like what else was there? You know? It had all gone downhill. I decided I ought to make the break, but I was too insecure just to say, "David, this is it, let's call it quits."

So—in fact it was the weekend I came for my interview here at Albany State—I was spending the weekend over at Schenectady U., with him. And we just kind of brought it out in the open that this is it. We realized that there was nothing much left. "We'll still be friends." You know, the typical line.

He told me he had a girlfriend. Meanwhile, I didn't know whether he was still seeing the same girl or somebody else, or what. He had *said* he had stopped seeing her. I had met her. She came to visit David in Fairview one day during the summer.

Well, over Christmas vacation, she contacted me. She wrote me a letter. She said she wasn't seeing David anymore, she heard that I wasn't, and she'd like to get to *know* me. She said she thinks maybe we could be friends.

I contacted her, and we got to talking about how David had lied to both of us. And I told her about the baby. Really flipped her out. Really upset her. And she goes and tells me that David had just taken her for an abortion the week before she had written me.

They hadn't been seeing each other. They were seeing each other steadily at the beginning of the semester, she said. But come November they just stopped seeing each other. He had started seeing somebody else. Then she found out she was pregnant. So he took her for an abortion.

That really flipped me out. I felt by doing that, it just kind of proved . . . the baby meant nothing to him. That it was just the *first* in a long *chain* of events that was going to be happening. And which would have no meaning. It really upset me.

This girl and I got to be very close friends. We're still friends. She's at Schenectady U., same as David. Their campus is only twenty minutes from here. And I see her like every week. She despises David; won't speak to him anymore.

David and I have gotten to— I went through many different changes with him. Through hatred. Through feeling guilty. To indifference. And now it's just kind of—sort of a friendship sort of thing. Even though I realize it's kind of forced. We still see each other, you know, every so often. He calls occasionally; we say hello. And uhm—I, you know— every so often, I bring up the subject of the baby. And it's nothing to him.

One day—one day he asked me if I was still having hard feelings about it. And I was amazed that he even brought up the whole subject. And I said no, that I had put it in its proper place. And I was using it for good purposes; not to hurt myself anymore. And he said well, that was good; he would have felt bad if he knew I was still feeling bad about it.

KATRINA: So you *did* feel bad about it?

GAIL: Yes, for a while. Every so often, like I got into these spells where I felt upset about it. But I didn't—I *never* felt that I wanted the baby back. Because I saw girls on campus with little babies, and I thought, "How would it be like for me?" And I felt I couldn't handle it. I'm very much into school now. I really enjoy it. I don't think I could handle both of them properly.

And I *want* to have children *so* badly now, I just *really* do. And, you know, I'm seeing Lee now. We've talked about what it would be like to have children. He knows I'm very much into this mother bit. [*laughs*] But we know that *now* isn't the proper time.

I'm very much in favor of abortion. But if I were to become pregnant now, I do not know if I could go through an abortion. I mean I *work* in a clinic, I *see* what abortion is about; there's absolutely *nothing* to be afraid of. But I don't know if *I* could go through it. I just know that as soon as I got on that table I would picture the entire delivery room, picture childbirth; the whole thing. And know I wasn't having a child. I think it would upset me immensely. Because I know what it's like to be pregnant now, I know what a wonderful experience pregnancy and childbirth is. I'm very anxious to experience it again.

KATRINA: And are you using contraception?

GAIL: Yes. I'm very *afraid* now. What's going to happen if it doesn't work, you know? *Now* I am taking the precaution. What if it doesn't work? Because that happens to people.

KATRINA: Did David take precautions with the other girlfriend—who had the abortion?

GAIL: Occasionally he would use a condom. That was it. Just occasionally, she said. *He* said he had used it *all* the time with her, because she *wouldn't allow* it otherwise, because she was afraid of getting pregnant. Speaking to *her*, she said occasionally he would.

So he was—he was—he had not learned anything. Not anything. At all. Through the whole thing.

KATRINA: You were saying, in the field of social work, that you specifically wanted to work with unwanted pregnancies.

GAIL: Yes. Definitely.

KATRINA: I was wondering in what area? Exactly how?

GAIL: In any area. Like—I guess my—my biggest fantasy is to work at Webber House Maternity Hospital as a social worker. They need them badly. The two they have there don't know what they're talking about.

The hospital has changed. I've been back there to visit since then. In fact, I took Deedee with me, the girl that David had been seeing. *Now* they don't have as many girls coming in who are giving up babies; because of abortion now. So they've opened it up as a general maternity hospital. And they're dealing with a very different type situation, where it's a *wanted* pregnancy. But it's kind of mixed up, because there are still unwanted pregnancies there too. And my big dream is to work there as a social worker. To work with those girls. I feel that I can give them so much—through my experience, and what I did with my experience.

Uhm— I like working at the abortion clinic. Because as I said, I am very much in favor of abortion. I can sympathize with these girls, the way they feel when suddenly they find out they're pregnant, and what do they do about it. And I just—I feel I can be of help in this area more than any other. And so I want to stay in that area.

KATRINA: You don't feel you'd direct people toward giving the baby up?

GAIL: Oh, never! Never. No; I don't think I could do that. In fact, I have never yet counseled anybody to have the baby. I'm also doing women's counseling on campus at Albany State; and there I am expected to present alternatives. Whereas at the abortion clinic you aren't really expected to. You figure they've already been counseled. If they're at the clinic, that's what they want. Although, you know, you keep an open mind for people who are doubtful. And also you have to, uh, be prepared in cases where there are girls who are over twenty-four weeks; who cannot have an abortion. So far I had one case like that at the clinic. She was someone who *definitely* should have had an abortion, because she was so *extremely* upset. Most girls, if they're too late, kind of accept it and say, "Okay, I realize that." But she had just denied the pregnancy all along. So it was a heavy thing for me to work with. And I—when I presented the possibility to her, she said, "No, no, I couldn't do that. Nobody can do that." I said, "*I* did that." And all of a sudden she stopped. Because she'd been hysterical before that, crying. At least it got her attention, if nothing else.

KATRINA: If there had been legal abortions at the time—?

GAIL: Yes, I'm usually asked that question! Would I have had one?

KATRINA: Yes.

GAIL: It's very, very hard for me to—consider it now. Having seen the baby and held her. And known her to be alive. It's very hard to think of her not having ever existed.
  Now, depending on the situation, I would probably consider abortion very seriously. The chances are I would have an abortion. I would *never* give up another child for adoption. Because I couldn't go through that again. And knowing I want a child so badly, if there was absolutely no way I could keep the baby, I would have an abortion, definitely.

KATRINA: If you "could never go through it again," how could you have gone through it once?

GAIL: Because I had a very good social worker. I was lucky. But going through it again I think would be too much. Because I *do* want children badly. And I would think,

"What am I doing? Giving away all my children? Will I ever have the chance to have my own?" I don't think I could handle it twice. It's—it's a very heavy thing.

KATRINA: What were the other girls like at the hospital?

GAIL: Oh, so many different kinds— There were girls from black ghettos. There were girls from upper-class America. Just *so* many different girls. They were sad, too, some of them. There was a twelve-year-old girl there who was having — Wait, no; she was fourteen. She was having her second baby and keeping it. She was twelve when she had her first one. Her parents were raising it. And they were kind of raising it as her—as her baby brother. I couldn't go through that myself. I just couldn't accept that. There was a girl ten. Ten years old. Who had been raped. And she was pregnant. I saw her when she came back for her six-week check-up afterward. I mean, this girl has been destroyed psychologically. Just destroyed. I mean she was sitting in a room with like six other girls, and she went berserk because there were people in the room. And it was just—it's the saddest thing.

Oh, the day I got there, a girl was in labor who was mentally retarded. She was twenty-six, but had the mentality of, oh, maybe an eight-year-old. Her entire family has been proclaimed "slow." Not necessarily retarded, but slow. When she was eighteen, she became pregnant by her brother. She had the baby and kept it. The baby died at home, when it was about two months old.

A social worker finally talked the family into placing the girl in an institution. She went to this institution; she was raped by an electrician. She became pregnant, and so they put her in Webber House. She didn't understand what was going on. I was there when they asked her if she wanted to see her baby, and she sort of said, "Yeah." They showed it to her through the window. And like it was a little doll to her.

And it was just—you know, she didn't know how to handle it. It was very strange.

There were a few girls who had been planning on giving the child up for adoption, and after they saw it they changed their mind. There were some who were in college and going back; some who were not going back to college. An awful lot of the girls were in high school. They had tutoring programs there at the hospital.

Oh, as a matter of fact, they just developed that into something really good. Because that still is a big problem. High-school girls are kicked out of school once they get to a certain stage. Some of the girls I knew were quitting high school. And a lot of girls had been kicked out of their homes by their parents.

One girl that I got to be very close with, she was about twenty-five. She was handicapped and had to walk with a brace. I found her story very sad. She's not a very attractive girl and so she's never really had that many boyfriends. She was teaching special education somewhere near New Haven. She met a guy who was going to Yale. He was from Iran. She desperately wanted a boyfriend, so she would do *anything* for him. She became pregnant; and, you know, she just kind of figured they'd get married. But when she told him she was pregnant, he told her he could not marry her. He had a wife and two sons back in Iran. She more or less had a nervous breakdown. She went home, to her parents. Her father beat her up and kicked her out of the house. And her mother wouldn't speak to her. Her brothers wouldn't speak to her. She's from a very religious background; she went to the church. The nuns took her in and made arrangements for her to go to Webber House. She was there almost the entire pregnancy. Most girls are only there during the last month or two.

KATRINA: How are things with your parents now?

GAIL: Well, we're going through a lot of different things now; involving my trying to separate from them, becoming more independent.

Every so often we refer to the— My mother really surprised me last time I was home. One of my aunts had a baby, and my mother went to see it. And she said, "You know, the baby looked just like Susan." And that was the first time she'd ever called the baby by *her name,* by the name I gave her.

Oh, another thing I forgot to mention was: like I told you I did write this letter to the parents. A couple weeks afterward I just mentioned to my mother that I had written a letter to them. And she asked what I said. I read it to her. And she burst out crying. Crying hysterically. I asked what was wrong. What she was crying about. She said, "Because—my grandchild."

And I just— Where *were* you? You know! During those nine months! You know—what—what were you doing? What were you thinking? She couldn't say anything then, because she wouldn't go against my father. But now that it was all over, then she could say it.

It's uh—I don't know. I think I have more hard feelings against her for doing that, than I do against my father for what he did. Because all along she was feeling something for it and she wouldn't admit it. At least my father was being honest about the way he felt. And she wasn't.

Uhm—it's kind of strange that—after my cousin Linda did have her baby, all of a sudden my aunt and uncle were grandparents. And they were talking about how great it was to be grandparents. And my parents just kind of sat there. Didn't say anything. I don't know; it was weird. Like my mother talks about being a grandmother. What it will be like. How she's going to treat her grandchildren. And once in a while I kind of say, "Well, you are," or, "You had the chance to be." Something like that.

KATRINA: Do you think about little children of the age that your child would be?

GAIL: Oh, definitely. She'll be two years old in May. May 29. And—uh—whenever I see a child about that age I—I try to picture— Mainly, I would just love to be able to *see* her. Just to see what she looks like. I'm just very curious as to how she looks.

My social worker saw a picture of her when she was about nine months or so. And she said she was really adorable. She had curly hair and a big smile. And she could see where she looked very much like me, and very much like David. And like, you know, it's hard to picture her. And I would like to be able to have a picture of her in my mind, for whenever I thought of her. Because I, when I think of her, there's kind of a blank. Or sometimes I can see the way she looked when I was feeding her. Or the last time I saw her. Or how she looked in the nursery.

KATRINA: How much does this affect your life now? How hard is it?

GAIL: Oh, it's not hard; at all. The only thing is like when I meet people. People that I want to be close to. I feel the only way people can understand me is by knowing this. And I'm not afraid to share it with anyone. Most of the people that I care most about, and that care most about me, know about it. Lee, the fellow I'm seeing now, knows all about it. And he's been more sensitive about the whole thing than anybody I've ever met. Which kind of makes me feel, you know, a lot better about *him*.

But, funny thing is, I found out that my father's favorite cousin—his very favorite cousin that he really grew up with —had had a baby and given it up for adoption. And she never told her husband about it. This was before she got married. She was in high school then. And her husband still doesn't know about it. And I cannot see living a lie like that. I would be *terrified,* everytime the phone rang, that somebody was calling to tell him. And the thing is, her husband is like the most *open-minded*—I think he'd be able to accept it so easily. But she would never tell him. And that's, you know, her prerogative. But I could never do that. I could never live with—live with someone not knowing that. She knows that I know about it now. My father told me. Because he kind of felt, "Well, *she* did it, why can't you?"

KATRINA: Do you think that influenced him all along?

GAIL: I suppose if she had never done that, he would not have been aware—as aware of the possibility.

KATRINA: How did that affect his reaction to you, when you first came with the problem?

GAIL: Well, I know he was very disgusted with *her* when he found out about *her.* And he probably identified me very much with her.

KATRINA: I mean, do you think it's *important?* Or really *not* important?

GAIL: [*pause*] In a way I think it would be, now I think about it. Because *probably,* if that had not happened to her, he would not have been as ready to consider the possibility of sending me away. He wouldn't have been so aware of these maternity homes being available.

So when this came up with me, his cousin started thinking about—she told my mother that all of a sudden she started thinking about her son. He would have been twenty-one then. And just, you know, thinking, gee, maybe he's even dating one of her nieces, or something. You know?

KATRINA: You spoke right at the very beginning about "separation anxiety." And I was wondering if there were anything from your childhood that puts more light on this than I—than I know?

GAIL: It's kind of funny. Because like I'm—I go for therapy once a week, too. And we've been looking at that. Uhm —I don't know. I have been an only child. And as far as I can see I've always had all of my parents' attention. So really I don't see where there was any separation anxiety before. Except maybe like I was—I became very dependent on my parents. And when they started going out and leaving me home alone, things like that probably upset me. But there's nothing— Like I never went away from home and things.

KATRINA: Did you feel you were a wanted child?

GAIL: I was *definitely* a wanted child. I was planned out to the day. I was born like four years after my parents were married. I kind of resent *that* fact, too, though. I resent the idea of being so *planned* out. Because by planning my birth, they decided on planning *every*thing, you know? And my mother almost died when I was born. She had complications and they didn't think she was going to live. Then when she found out she couldn't have any more children— They had wanted a boy. And so I said, "Well, how did this make you feel, that you had a daughter?" My mother gives me this thing, "We were happy we had a girl when we found out we could only have one. We figured she'd be closer to home; she'd remain closer to the family." Which means they had *that* planned. My father had *college* planned for me. He has a big wedding planned for me. [*laughs*] And a pregnancy just didn't fit in to the picture!

KATRINA: How much did your father insist on abortion?

GAIL: You mean because he had mentioned about asking the doctor about an abortion?

KATRINA: Yes; right.

GAIL: He was afraid to make any mention, because he knew it was illegal. I had mentioned that I knew of someone who had had one. I'm sure there was a lot of it going around. I had the feeling my doctor would have done an abortion if—if I really asked. Especially if my parents had contacted him.

My father told me that when I went to the doctor I should ask him about it. And I said I didn't know if I wanted to. He said, well, then he would come with me and *he* would talk to the doctor about it. But then he decided no, because he'd probably—the doctor would probably tell him he was a *fool*. Because it was illegal and, "How could he consider such a thing?" Also I guess he was very scared. He didn't know what an abortion was about. The only thing you ever heard about abortion, before it was legal, was about all the butcher jobs that were done.

And for myself, I was afraid that if I had an abortion, any chance of David and me getting married was completely out.

KATRINA: Do you think you got pregnant "in order to" marry David?

GAIL: Uhm, not really. I don't think I had really thought of it that much. I'd thought of what it would be like to be pregnant. You know, have David's child. I never thought of planning it out that I would become pregnant, or anything like that. Of course, it may have been there without me realizing it. But not consciously.

KATRINA: At one point I wanted to ask you— I guess you were talking about how you tell people, now, about it. And for a moment there I was wondering whether you think of it as a tragedy in your life? [*pause*] Or not? Or—and I don't know what I was thinking of, as *opposed* to tragedy—

GAIL: Hum— I kind of look at it as both a tragedy and— I'm very—I'm actually very thankful I got to experience pregnancy and childbirth. I mean, I think it's—for *any* woman it's like the ultimate of experience. And—uhm—I guess I—I feel fortunate I was able to experience it. And hopefully I'll be able to again. Uhm, definitely—of *course* it was a tragedy. But I *learned* more from that experience than I *lost* from it. I *definitely* didn't lose anything, any of myself. Except if you want to look at—I lost the child, and the child was me, a part of me.

KATRINA: And now you—how much do you—? suffer—? I guess I feel you *do*. I mean. . . .

GAIL: Yes, you do, to an extent. But I'm still very proud of it. I'm still very proud of having had that child. I guess I'm proud of myself for having been able to give it up, too. Having had the strength. I had never thought of myself as having any strength for anything. And this kind of showed me otherwise.

I'm thankful for all I learned from it. I mean even just simple things about how to take care of yourself during a pregnancy. I learned to be—not to be afraid of pregnancy. The next time I become pregnant I can devote—devote myself entirely to enjoying it.

Uhm—I regret the fact that David wasn't there with me, all the time, to share it. Or that there wasn't a man there to share it with me. The only people I had to share it with were like my social worker. She was more helpful than anyone at all.

KATRINA: You never mention any girl friends.

GAIL: I was never really that close to anyone except David. I never really had any girl friends. Because David was always there. Which was definitely a mistake. You definitely need to have girl friends. I mean that's a whole problem of mine, of being able to relate to women.

Of course, I got over some of that when I met my social worker. She was the first woman I could really relate to. Because I couldn't relate to my mother. Also I think I always patterned myself after my mother. Because *she* never had any woman friends. She devoted her entire life to my father. And, you know, my whole relationship with David, I realized, was patterned after the relationship between my parents. I was totally dependent and submissive to David. And I *definitely* do not want that in a relationship now. I've been fighting it very hard. Even in my relationship with Lee now, every so-often I see patterns arising. And I fight it, immediately.

And I'm learning to relate to women now. I mean, I'm doing women's counseling, I'm working in an abortion clinic, I've organized a women's group at school. I'm in contact with women more than I am with men now, as far as that goes.

KATRINA: I was wondering if you had any comments about the present sexual climate—

GAIL: There's a lot of talk about how times have changed and everything's so different. The thing is that's how it *appears*. But when you really get down and really talk to people, everything's the same. People feel just as confused about sex. It's still the exact same problems. And it's even *harder* now, because everybody *thinks* it's the opposite. Everybody thinks everyone's free and open. But people are really afraid to be.

I think the biggest problem—especially with the guys I've spoken to—they're very afraid of what it means to have relations with a girl: What kind of a commitment is it? I was *amazed* to find out that some of these guys, you know, twenty to twenty-five years old, have never had relations with women. Guys who I thought were like the biggest playboys in the world. And it's just—it just *amazes* me. Because I had thought it was completely the opposite, myself. Until I really started getting into talking with these people, and finding out what's going on in their relationships. I had thought, you know, every guy "has his first lay when he's sixteen" or something like that.

And the girls, too, they feel this tremendous pressure now. They feel that, without *considering* any alternatives, that's how the guy's thinking about it. And I'm learning, well, that's not always true. Because the guys are just as scared as the girls are. They figure they are responsible for anything that happens to the girl, and they're afraid of the responsibility. I have found that there are less *girls* that are virgins than guys. Of the people I know.

In fact I only know of one girl who is. And she's very hung-up about it. She doesn't know what to do about it. And with the guys—I was really surprised. Because it seems like most of the girls I know are having relations with guys. But *few* of the guys I know are.

KATRINA: Do you think this could be an improvement? More responsible than, say, David's—?

GAIL: Oh, yes! Definitely.

When I first met David—like I can see a change in David. Such an immense change between the time I met him when he was in high school, and the way he is now. The way he's been after he started going to college. I mean *now* I would say he's on very much of an ego trip. You know. Like he tells me about the seven girls he's sleeping with. Plus he has one girlfriend that he sees steadily. It's a very serious relationship. The two of them bought a car together, the whole thing. And it's—uhm—it's strange. I mean the change is incredible. Even people I know at home, who knew him before, they're amazed at how different he is; and they don't like the way he is now.

KATRINA: I wonder: if it hadn't been so *easy* for him—to have all the girls he wanted—

GAIL: It's funny: as you said about it being easy for him, it reminded me of something. In this relationship, my father didn't want to make it hard on David. Like the hospital—my father is still paying for the bill at the hospital. It came to over two thousand dollars. And he would not ask David to pay for any of it, because he didn't want to make it rough on David in college. My father was thinking in terms of the possibility of David and me getting married in the future. He wanted him to have a college education.

Afterward, when the child was—when the baby was in the foster home, I told my fath—my dad that I was now responsible for the baby; I would pay for the bill in the foster home. David took care of that. It came to like a hundred dollars or so. But other than that, David had no responsibility at all. Maybe if he had been forced to *pay* something for it, it would have been different. Maybe he would have been more concerned with what was going on at the hospital, if he was putting out the money for it.

And I never pushed him into a decision. It was kind of like, "Well, you know, make up your mind, and let me know."

KATRINA: *Why* didn't you, in November or whenever, just take off and get married?

GAIL: Hmm! Neither of us—I guess— We both felt too insecure to do that. I couldn't see myself taking a step like that; just leaving my parents' house. I was too dependent on my parents.

I guess David really wasn't sure enough. Even though I thought he was. I guess he really wasn't sure enough to do that.

Also, there was the hassle: we didn't know where we could go. We had no money. His parents didn't have any money. Any money we could get would have to be from my parents. And they probably wouldn't give us any, anyway.

KATRINA: Do you feel that you made the best decision under the circumstances?

GAIL: Oh, definitely. Any marriage that—between David and I—*definitely* would have been down the drain by now. David still is not ready for marriage. And I know even if he was, I'm just not the wife for him. He's not the husband for me, that's for sure. I need someone much more sensitive. Even now I see him as very insensitive, very immature. And he's just—it just wouldn't have worked. And it would have been torture for the—for Susan. For the baby.

Oh, another strange thing: David has this new girlfriend I was telling you about. Her name is Susan! I have the feeling that things are going to work out with them. I kind—I just kind of hope that every time he thinks of her name, he'll think of the baby. But I doubt it.

KATRINA: You *want* him to still think of the baby?

GAIL: Oh, definitely.

KATRINA: Why?

GAIL: Because I hope he'll learn from it. He'll remember it. And remember— Or— I hope like someday he'll *realize* the impact of it. What it . . . what a big thing it was. It wasn't just, you know, signing papers and saying yes and no. It was much bigger than that.

KATRINA: Is it a malicious thought?

GAIL: Probably. He hurt me. I guess I feel I want him to be at least a little hurt by it. I don't feel he suffered any pain at all through it. The only pain maybe he did suffer was when it came to us breaking up, he was afraid of hurting my feelings. That's why it—it drug out for so long.

KATRINA: And you were *very* hurt then? And you're— How much hurt would you say you are now? I keep—

GAIL: About the baby? [*long pause*] I don't think I'm too hurt. Lee insists I'm still hurting from it. My therapist insists I'm still hurting from it. They— I guess they both feel that I'm rationalizing the whole thing, about: "It was a *good* experience, I *learned* through it," you know. Uhm—

I feel that it's the only way to cope with it, though. You know? If I don't put it to good use, what can I do except sit around and cry about it? And there's still nothing that can be done. So I feel what I'm doing is right. At least I don't feel the hurt as much. If I felt it, there would be nothing I could do about it anyway. Every so often, when my defenses are down, I hurt about it.

I think anybody who did it would—would say that they did the right thing. Nobody— I don't—I can't see anyone who did it, sit—sitting down saying, "I did what was wrong. I did the wrong thing. I shouldn't have done that."

Because if they do that, they're just going to . . . totally fall apart.

INDEX

Abortion,
    as preferable to adoption, 31, 108, 182–83, 198, 263–64,
        292–93
    procedures, 39, 60, 133–34, 210–12, 224–25, 266

Abortionists,
    illegal, 59–60, 72–73, 77–78, 224–27, 240–42, 265–66,
        298
    legal, 38–41, 279
    See also Hospitals

Adoption, 270, 340, 359
    as only alternative, 244, 255–56, 259–60
    in one's own background, xii–xiv, 82–92
    institutionalization and, 292–93
    previous pregnancy and, 153, 168–79
    relinquishment proceedings for, 413–14

Adoption reform movement, xii, xiii, xv

American Civil Liberties Union, 236

American Society of Journalists and Authors, xix

An Adopted Woman, xiii–xiv

Burtchaell, James T., xvi–xxi